Handbook of Retinal Diseases

Handbook of Retinal Diseases

Editor: Judi Graham

AMERICAN
MEDICAL PUBLISHERS
www.americanmedicalpublishers.com

AMERICAN
MEDICAL PUBLISHERS
www.americanmedicalpublishers.com

Cataloging-in-Publication Data

Handbook of retinal diseases / edited by Judi Graham.
p. cm.
Includes bibliographical references and index.
ISBN 978-1-63927-687-5
1. Retina--Diseases. 2. Eye--Diseases. 3. Retina--Diseases--Diagnosis.
4. Retina--Diseases--Treatment. 5. Ophthalmology. I. Graham, Judi.
RE551 .H36 2023
617.735--dc23

American Medical Publishers,
41 Flatbush Avenue,
1st Floor, New York,
NY 11217, USA

ISBN 978-1-63927-687-5 (Hardback)

Contents

Preface

Retinal diseases are those diseases that affect the light-sensitive tissue found in the back side of the eye. There are various common retinal diseases and conditions, such as macular hole, retinal tear, epiretinal membrane, retinitis pigmentosa, retinal detachment, macular degeneration and diabetic retinopathy. Several retinal diseases have some symptoms in common, which include distorted or blurred vision, lost vision, seeing floating specks or cobwebs, and defects in side vision. There are various risk factors of retinal diseases, which include having diabetes, or other diseases, aging, having a family history of retinal diseases, smoking, eye trauma, and obesity. Optical coherence tomography, wide-field retinal imaging and dilated retinal examination are a few of the tests used to diagnose retinal disease. The treatment of retinal disease can be complicated at times and can include various treatment options, such as implanting a retinal prosthesis, shrinking abnormal blood vessels, injecting gas or air into the eye, evacuating and replacing the fluid in the eye, using a laser surgery, or freezing. This book unravels the recent studies on retinal diseases. Those in search of information to further their knowledge will be greatly assisted by this book.

This book is a comprehensive compilation of works of different researchers from varied parts of the world. It includes valuable experiences of the researchers with the sole objective of providing the readers (learners) with a proper knowledge of the concerned field. This book will be beneficial in evoking inspiration and enhancing the knowledge of the interested readers.

In the end, I would like to extend my heartiest thanks to the authors who worked with great determination on their chapters. I also appreciate the publisher's support in the course of the book. I would also like to deeply acknowledge my family who stood by me as a source of inspiration during the project.

Editor

1

The Role of Adrenoceptors in the Retina

Yue Ruan [1,*], Tobias Böhmer [1,2], Subao Jiang [1] and Adrian Gericke [1,*]

1 Department of Ophthalmology, University Medical Center, Johannes Gutenberg University Mainz, Langenbeckstr. 1, 55131 Mainz, Germany; tboehmer@joho-rheingau.de (T.B.); sjiang@uni-mainz.de (S.J.)
2 St. Josef's Hospital Rheingau, Eibinger Str. 9, 65385 Rüdesheim am Rhein, Germany
* Correspondence: yruan@uni-mainz.de (Y.R.); adrian.gericke@unimedizin-mainz.de (A.G.);

Abstract: The retina is a part of the central nervous system, a thin multilayer with neuronal lamination, responsible for detecting, preprocessing, and sending visual information to the brain. Many retinal diseases are characterized by hemodynamic perturbations and neurodegeneration leading to vision loss and reduced quality of life. Since catecholamines and respective bindings sites have been characterized in the retina, we systematically reviewed the literature with regard to retinal expression, distribution and function of alpha$_1$ (α_1)-, alpha$_2$ (α_2)-, and beta (β)-adrenoceptors (ARs). Moreover, we discuss the role of the individual adrenoceptors as targets for the treatment of retinal diseases.

Keywords: α_1-AR; α_2-AR; β-AR; retina; distribution; function

---

1. Introduction

Many ocular diseases, such as age-related macular degeneration (AMD), diabetic retinopathy, retinal vascular occlusion and glaucoma frequently cause severe visual impairment substantially diminishing the quality of life [1–5]. Permanent ischemia or ischemia-reperfusion injury of the retina and/or optic nerve have been implicated in the pathophysiology of these diseases [6–9]. Retinal ischemic conditions may lead to a direct loss of cellular function. However, they can also induce various secondary sequelae, such as retinal edema, hemorrhage, neovascularization, detachment and secondary glaucoma [10].

Since the retina is the tissue with the highest metabolic demand in the body, it is not surprising that retinal hemodynamic perturbations play a critical role in the pathogenesis of numerous ocular diseases [11–18]. The retinal vascular structure provides metabolic support for neural and glial cells while minimizing interference with light-sensing [19]. In this context, modulation of vascular diameter by local mechanical and chemical stimuli can be considered the main basic regulatory mechanism in the retinal circulation [20,21].

Receptor families comprising multiple subtypes with organ-specific patterns of neurovascular expression and function appear to be attractive candidates for the development of targeted therapies against diseases associated with abnormal tissue perfusion. One such intriguing receptor family is the adrenoceptor (AR) family.

The discovery of ARs by Ahlquist more than six decades ago has uncovered the adrenergic signaling pathways as pivotal regulators of systemic arterial blood pressure and other metabolic and central nervous system functions [22]. ARs belong to the superfamily of guanosine triphosphate-binding protein (G protein)-coupled receptors (GPCRs) and are targets of catecholamines, especially epinephrine and noradrenaline [22–25]. According to its pharmacological properties, amino acid sequence, and signaling mechanisms, the AR family is subdivided into three subfamilies, the alpha$_1$ (α_1)-, alpha$_2$

(α_2)-, and the beta (β)-AR subfamily [26]. Each class is composed of three subtypes (α_{1A}, α_{1B}, α_{1D}, α_{2A}, α_{2B}, α_{2C}, β_1, β_2, and β_3) (Figure 1) [27]. Members of the α_1-AR subfamily are widely expressed throughout the cardiovascular system [28]. They critically participate in the regulation of vascular tone and blood flow primarily by mediating the vasoconstrictive effects of catecholamines [28–35]. Remarkably, the expression pattern of individual α_1-AR subtypes and their involvement in mediating vascular responses to catecholamines differ considerably between individual vascular beds [34,36–39]. Members of the α_2-AR subfamily are expressed in both the central and the peripheral nervous system throughout the body. They are localized either pre- or postsynaptically and mediate inhibition of neurotransmitter release [40,41]. β-ARs are widely distributed at both the central and peripheral nervous system and are involved in important functions activated by circulating catecholamines, such as heart rate regulation, vasorelaxation, bronchodilation, and neurotransmitter release [42].

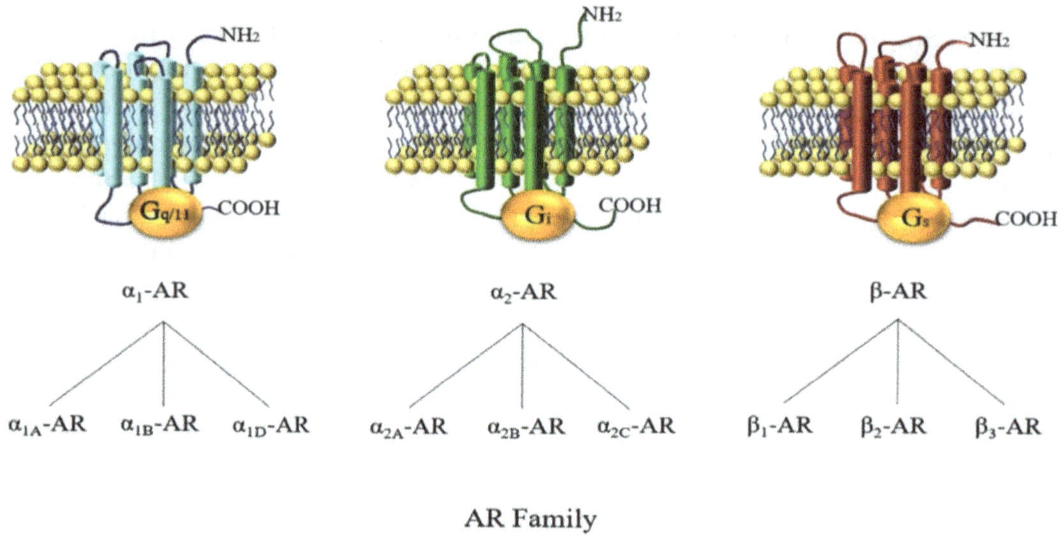

Figure 1. The three adrenoceptor (AR) subfamilies and their subtypes. α_1-, α_2-, and β-ARs mainly couple to $G_{q/11}$, G_i, and G_s proteins, respectively. To be more exact, the α_{2A}-AR subtype has an unusual dual pharmacological effect by coupling to G_i proteins when concentrations of agonists are low and mainly coupling to G_s proteins when concentrations are high [43]. β-ARs are mainly coupled to G_s proteins and both β_1- and β_2-AR are able to switch their G protein-coupling specificity from G_s to G_i proteins [44].

The purpose of the present review is to summarize the current state of research on the role of α_1-, α_2- and β-ARs in the retina. We provide an overview of the expression, structural distribution, and regulation of the individual AR subfamilies and their subtypes in the retina and discuss their therapeutic implications.

2. The Retina

The retina is a thin multilayer with neuronal lamination responsible for detecting, preprocessing, and sending visual information to the brain [45]. The neuronal lamination in the retina includes neural circuits containing six major types of neuronal cells: retinal ganglion cells (RGCs), amacrine cells, bipolar cells, horizontal cells, and the cone and rod photoreceptors [46]. Despite the retina's peripheral location, retinal neurons utilize the same types of neurotransmitters (noradrenaline, dopamine, and acetylcholine) as those of the central nervous system [47]. Since visual formation highly depends on the complex neuronal structure of the retina, a variety of detrimental factors, such as ischemia and oxidative stress, may result in the deterioration of retinal cell function and consequently lead to retinal diseases [48].

Two different circulatory systems are originating from the ophthalmic artery, the retinal circulation and the choroidal circulation, which both supply oxygen and nutrients to the retina [19]. While choroidal blood vessels are innervated and modulated by the autonomic nervous system, no sympathetic nerve fiber terminals have been found in or on the wall of human retinal blood vessels, suggesting that the retinal circulation lacks autonomic innervation [49]. Notably, retinal arterioles were shown to respond to local chemical factors, such as oxygen (O_2), carbon dioxide (CO_2), nitric oxide (NO), and hydrogen sulfide (H_2S) [50–52]. Although no evidence for sympathetic nerve fibers has been provided in the retina, catecholamines, including noradrenaline, adrenaline and dopamine, have been detected [53]. One possible source of noradrenaline in the mammalian retina are sympathetic nerve terminals located in the choroid [54]. In support of this concept, a decrease in noradrenaline concentration has been observed in the retina after removal of the superior cervical ganglion, which provides sympathetic input to the choroid [53]. This finding indicates that noradrenaline may originate from sympathetic nerve terminals in the choroidal circulation and reach the ARs in the retina by paracrine diffusion [55].

Dopaminergic amacrine (DA) cells, a class of retinal neurons, synthetize and release dopamine, which is the prevailing catecholamine in the retina [56,57]. In the bovine retina, noradrenaline was detected in the inner nuclear and plexiform layers, and Osborne suggested that retinal tissue can metabolize dopamine to form noradrenaline [58]. Also, amacrine cells have been detected in the retina, which differs morphologically from DA cells and can be detected only after a preload with exogenous noradrenaline [54,59]. It has been proposed that these cells contain only small amounts of endogenous catecholamines, but are equipped with high-affinity uptake properties for exogenous catecholamines [54]. There is also compelling evidence indicating that in addition to noradrenaline, dopamine can also activate α_1-, α_2-, and β-ARs, but may be less potent [60]. Importantly, members of all three AR subfamilies, α_1-, α_2-, and β-ARs, have been detected in retinal tissue, including blood vessels [61].

3. Expression and Function of ARs in the Retina

3.1. *α_1-ARs*

3.1.1. Expression of α_1-ARs in the Retina

In contrast to choroidal blood vessels, the retinal vasculature seems to lack autonomic, i.e., adrenergic, cholinergic or peptidergic innervation [49,50,62–64]. However, α_1-ARs have been found in retinal tissue of various mammalian species [65,66]. Particularly with regard to the intra-retinal vasculature, Forster et al. have demonstrated the presence of α_1-adrenergic binding sites in homogenates of isolated bovine retinal arteries and veins, which were few in number, but of high agonist affinity [61]. In homogenates of isolated murine retinal arterioles, our laboratory has found mRNA for all three α_1-AR subtypes, which were expressed at similar levels [67].

Several studies provided evidence that the cellular components of the three main layers of a vascular wall, i.e., endothelial cells of the intima, smooth muscle cells of the media, and fibroblasts of the adventitia, have the potential to express α_1-ARs [29–33]. Furthermore, evidence has been provided that individual α_1-ARs may exert distinct functions within one vessel [32,68,69]. For example, it has been suggested that in coronary arteries, endothelial α_{1B}-ARs mediate vasodilation by stimulating endothelial nitric oxide synthase, while α_{1D}-ARs localized on smooth muscle cells mediate vasoconstriction [68].

The cellular location of α_1-ARs within the architecture of retinal blood vessels is still elusive but may have relevant pharmacological and pathophysiological implications. For example, with regard to α_1-ARs located on retinal vascular smooth muscle cells, one would expect that the intact blood-retinal barrier prevents circulating hydrophilic molecules, such as catecholamines, from reaching these binding sites [70]. Conversely, they might become well-accessible in pathological states associated with an impaired endothelial barrier function [61,71]. Since a series of enzymes involved in catecholamine synthesis has been localized in retinal cells of different species, retinal vascular α_1-ARs may also be a target of agonists released from surrounding retinal cells [72–75]. From a therapeutic point of view, the blood-retinal barrier may be circumvented by administering α_1-adrenergic ligands into the vitreous body [76].

In addition to retinal vessels, Zarbin et al. localized α_1-ARs in the outer plexiform layer of the rat retina in vitro by semiquantitative autoradiography using [^{3}H]prazosin. The authors reported that α_1-adrenergic binding sites were only enriched in the outer plexiform layer [77]. Other research groups demonstrated that α_1-ARs are expressed on retinal pigment epithelium (RPE) of the rabbit and bovine retina, where they modulate K^+ and Cl^- transport and electrical currents [78,79]. Unfortunately, at present, antibody-based methods to localize α_1-AR subtypes within the tissue structure appear to lack validity, since a growing body of evidence indicates that many commercially available antibodies directed against individual α_1-AR subtypes do not specifically detect their alleged target antigen [80–83]. A combined approach of ligand-receptor binding techniques and immunostainings and/or functional studies in tissues from knockout (KO) animal models lacking the respective receptor subtype may represent a more suitable methodological alternative to determine the location and function of α_1-ARs within the retina, which remains a subject of further research [28].

3.1.2. α_1-ARs in Retinal Vascular Reactivity

In vivo studies performed in experimental animals and healthy humans have investigated the impact of systemically administered α_1-adrenergic agonists on retinal vessel reactivity. The results, however, are partly contradictory, which makes it difficult to draw unequivocal conclusions regarding the functional role of α_1-ARs in the regulation of retinal vascular resistance and perfusion. While Mori et al. observed a dose-dependent constriction of rat retinal arterioles in response to intravenous administration of noradrenaline, Alm et al. did not observe any effect of exogenously administered noradrenaline on retinal blood flow in cats [84,85]. Dollery et al. reported that intravenously administered noradrenaline decreased retinal vascular diameter in healthy humans, whereas other studies detected only a negligible impact of circulating noradrenaline and the α_1-adrenergic agonist, phenylephrine, on human retinal vessel diameter and blood flow [86–88].

In general, in vivo studies investigating the effects of systemically applied adrenergic agonists or antagonists on retinal vascular responses are hampered by considerable changes in systemic blood pressure induced by these ligands. Due to the pronounced autoregulatory capability of the retinal vascular bed, the resulting changes in ocular perfusion pressure may also induce compensatory responses of the retinal vasculature, which makes it difficult to discern between direct pharmacological effects on retinal vessels and their reactive responses to systemic blood pressure changes [70,71,88,89]. This methodological dilemma may, at least in part, explain the contradictory results of the in vivo studies outlined above.

Ichikawa et al. and Hara et al. reduced systemic influences by intravitreal drug injection and observed constriction of rabbit retinal arteries in response to phenylephrine, which was attenuated after application of the α_1-AR antagonist, bunazosin [76,90]. Additionally, in vitro studies using isolated eyes, retinal tissue grafts, and preparations of retinal arterioles also demonstrated a constrictive effect of α_1-adrenergic agonists on retinal blood vessels [71,91–94].

In this context, Hoste et al. reported that on the one hand, the contractile response of bovine retinal arteries to α_1-adrenergic stimulation was greatly masked under resting conditions [94]. On the other hand, retinal arteries became sensitive to α_1-adrenergic agonists when activated by circumferential stretch and displayed an enhanced myogenic vasoconstrictor response to elevated perfusion pressure during α_1-adrenergic stimulation [94]. In the study of Yu et al., the extent of vasoconstriction in isolated porcine retinal arterioles with intact endothelium in response to α_1-adrenergic agonists differed between intra- and extra-luminal drug application. Adrenaline and noradrenaline caused concentration-dependent vasoconstriction, which was larger when applied intraluminally [70,92].

Although the aforementioned in vitro studies found a constrictive effect of α_1-adrenergic agonists on retinal vessels with an intact endothelium, the reported vascular responses were mostly weak and had a relatively high threshold [91–94]. In a study conducted on murine retinal explants, our group has demonstrated that retinal arteriole constriction to α_1-adrenergic stimulation is largely masked by endothelial mechanisms and becomes more relevant when the endothelium is damaged [67].

findings, expression studies employing commercially available AR antibodies need to be interpreted with caution [82].

3.2.2. α_2-AR in Retinal Neuroprotection

The family of α_2-ARs is one of the pharmacological targets of the natural stress hormone, norepinephrine, and is involved in modulating cellular resistance and adaptation to stress stimuli [150]. α_2-ARs were first described as presynaptic receptors inhibiting the release of various transmitters from neurons in the central and peripheral nervous systems [151]. In vivo studies revealed that α_2-AR stimulation reduces ischemic injury in the brain [152]. This effect has been largely attributed to its classic presynaptic inhibition of signaling molecules released by blocking Ca^{2+} channels, activating K^+ channels, or reducing active release sites [153,154]. Neuroprotective treatment strategies for retinal diseases whose course includes neuronal degeneration have arisen a great deal of interest. Some studies have assessed the functional role of α_2-ARs in the retina in a variety of animal models through the mechanism of α_2-mediated neuroprotection. For example, Donello et al. suggested that activation of α_2-ARs might reduce ischemic retinal injury and preserve retinal function following transient ischemia by preventing extracellular glutamate and aspartate accumulation [155]. An in vivo study by Manuel et al. revealed neuroprotective effects of α_2-ARs in preventing RGC death after transient retinal ischemia [156]. In the study, pre-treatment with two α_2-AR-selective agonists, AGN 191,103 and brimonidine tartrate, has proven very effective not only in preventing rapid RGCs loss, but also long-term RGCs loss in a rat model [156].

Glaucoma with elevated intraocular pressure (IOP) often continues to progress even after the reduction of IOP to normal levels [5]. The progressive loss of vision in eyes with glaucoma is a result of RGCs degeneration, emphasizing the need for a neuroprotective therapy [157]. The α_2-AR agonist, brimonidine, and other α_2-AR agonists were shown to lower IOP mainly by reducing aqueous humor production and by increasing uveoscleral outflow [158–160]. In a rat model of chronically elevated IOP, pharmacological activation of α_2-ARs exerted neuroprotective effects in RGCs, irrespective of the IOP level [157]. In addition, the α_2-AR agonist, brimonidine, preserved visual function in glaucoma patients with low/normal IOP and high IOP, suggesting that pharmacological α_2-AR activation may exert neuroprotective effects IOP independently [161–163]. Various mechanisms underlying the neuroprotective activity of α_2-AR agonists have been proposed. For example, activation of α_2-ARs was shown to decrease the IOP-induced overexpression of intermediate filament glial fibrillary acidic protein (GFAP) in Müller cells, suggesting that activation of α_2-ARs may reduce stress responses in glial cells. [157]. Furthermore, the α_2-AR agonist, brimonidine, was reported to protect RGCs from the effects of chronic ocular hypertension through mechanisms involving α_2-AR-mediated survival signal activation and up-regulation of endogenous neurotrophic factors in the rat retina [164]. Another study demonstrated that α_2-adrenergic modulation of *N*-methyl-d-aspartate (NMDA) receptor function was an important mechanism for neuroprotection in experimental glaucoma models [154]. Brimonidine may protect RGCs by preventing abnormal elevation of cytosolic free Ca^{2+} evoked by NMDA receptors in RGCs under stress conditions [165,166]. Other studies suggested that brimonidine-mediated inhibition of the cyclic adenosine 3′,5′-monophosphate/protein kinase A (cAMP/PKA) pathway could be an important mechanism to protect RGCs from glaucomatous neurodegeneration [162]. Based on a recent study in a rat glaucoma model, Zhou et al. suggested that α_2-AR activation hyperpolarizes RGCs by improving the γ-aminobutyric acid (GABA) receptor response to spontaneous and elicited GABA release, thus reducing the risk for excitotoxicity and RGC injury [167].

Activation of α_2-ARs has also been shown to exert neuroprotective effects in other retinal diseases, such as light-induced photoreceptor damage, retinal detachment, and optic nerve injury [168–170]. For example, α_2-adrenergic agonists were shown to induce the expression of basic fibroblast growth factor (bFGF) in photoreceptors in vivo and to alleviate light-induced damage in the retina [168]. In retinal detachment, stimulation of α_2-AR signaling protected photoreceptors by inhibiting oxidative stress and inflammation [170]. Furthermore, in a mouse optic neuritis model, topical administration of the α_2-AR agonist, brimonidine, exerted neuroprotective effects against RGCs death by increasing retinal bFGF expression in the retina, particularly in Müller cells and RGCs [171]. In contrast, in mechanic optic nerve injury, activation of α_2-AR signaling promoted optic nerve regeneration via activation of extracellular-signal-regulated kinase (ERK) phosphorylation [169].

Activation of α_2-ARs was suggested to induce vasoconstriction in the vasculature distal to the ophthalmic artery, such as ciliary and retinal blood vessels [172–174]. While the α_{2A}-AR subtype was proposed to mediate adrenergic vasoconstriction in porcine ciliary arteries, no suggestion regarding the contribution of individual α_2-AR subtypes has been made for retinal blood vessels [172].

Only little is known about the functional role of individual α_2-AR subtypes in the retina. A study by Harun-Or-Rashid et al. showed that α_{2A}-ARs are expressed by chicken Müller cells and that pharmacological activation of the α_{2A}-AR subtype triggers a mitogen-activated protein kinase (MAPK)-dependent response with phosphorylation of ERK1/2 both in vivo and in vitro. Taken together, most studies indicate that activation of α_2-ARs raises neuronal resistance to retinal injury suggesting that the receptors may become potent treatment targets in various retinal diseases. However, the role of individual α_2-AR subtypes remains to be better characterized in the retina.

3.3. *β-ARs*

3.3.1. Expression of β-ARs in the Retina

In 1986, Zarbin et al. localized β-AR binding sites by [^{3}H]dihydroalprenolol in nearly all rat retinal layers (the outer nuclear layer, outer plexiform layer, inner nuclear layer, and inner plexiform layer), but with the lowest concentration in the outer nuclear layer [77]. In the human retina, β-AR binding sites were visualized by [125I] (-) iodocyanopindolol in vitro autoradiography [175].

Three distinct β-AR subtypes, β_1-AR, β_2-AR and β_3-AR, have been identified [176]. In 2001, the β_4-AR was hypothesized by Granneman as a novel state of the β_1-AR [176]. Six years later, the β_4-AR was considered by Madamanchi as a low-affinity state of the β_1-AR, which still needs pharmacological and genetic characterization [177]. Among β-AR subtypes, β_1-AR and β_2-AR binding sites were found in bovine retinal vessels and in the neural retina [178]. The presence of functional β_3-ARs has also been verified in rat retinal blood vessels [179]. By immunohistochemistry, β_3-ARs were localized in the inner capillary plexus of the mouse mid-peripheral retina, whereas β_1-ARs and β_2-ARs were localized in rat cultured Müller cells [180]. However, since many commercially available antibodies lack sufficient specificity for β-ARs, data based on antibodies need to be interpreted with caution [83]. Expression of β_3-ARs has been shown for the first time on cultured human retinal endothelial cells in 2003 [181]. In that study, pharmacological activation of β_3-ARs promoted migration and proliferation of endothelial cells [181]. Based on the wide distribution of β-ARs in retinal blood vessels and the neural retina, β-ARs are believed to play an important role in retinal vascular and neuronal function. The localization of individual AR subfamilies in individual retinal layers and structures is shown in Figure 2.

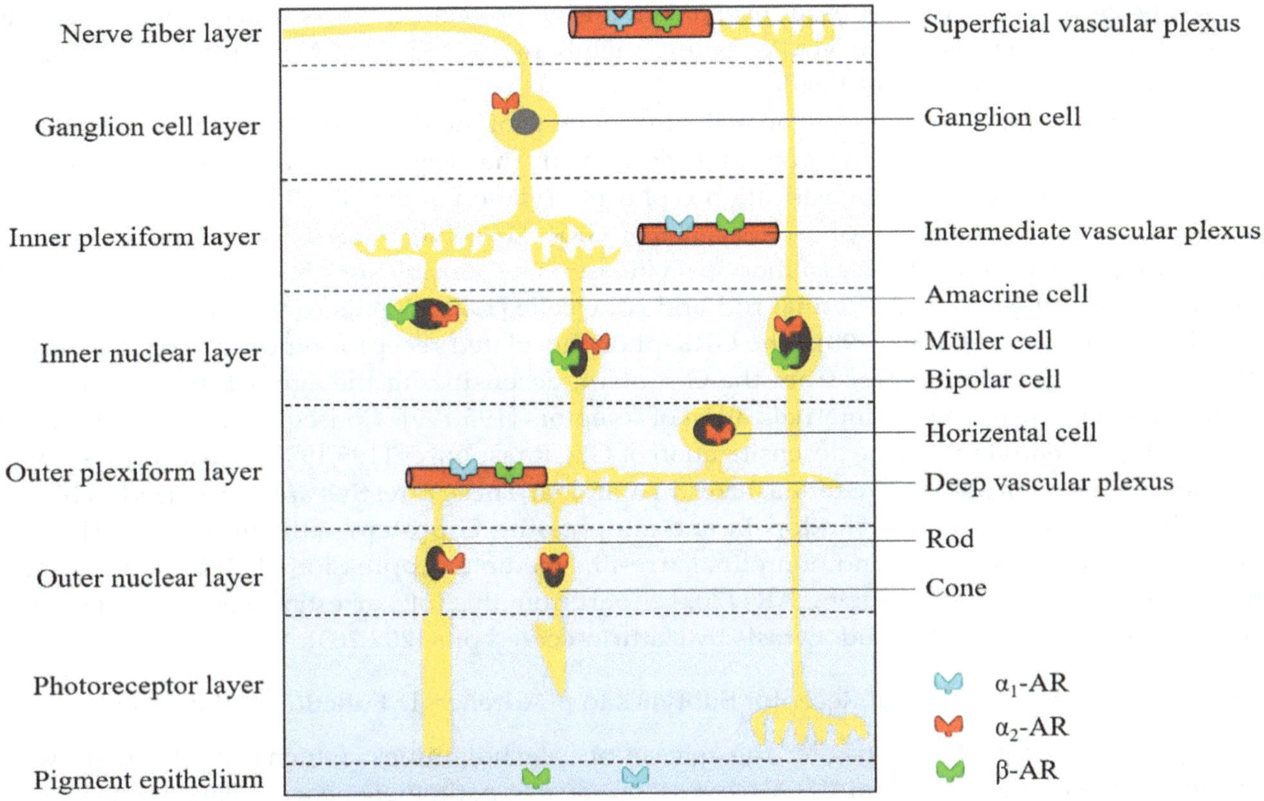

Figure 2. The distribution of ARs in individual retinal layers and structures.

3.3.2. Role of β-ARs in the Retina

Stress conditions, such as hypoxia, can cause catecholaminergic overstimulation in the cardiovascular system, which in turn may activate β-ARs [182]. A study in mice reported that the noradrenaline level increased by approximately 90% in the hypoxic retina compared to normoxic conditions [183]. Activation of β-ARs is considered to upregulate the hypoxia-inducible factor-1α (HIF-1α) and vascular endothelial growth factor (VEGF), which plays a key role in the formation of pathogenic blood vessels in various retinal diseases, such as retinopathy of prematurity and diabetic retinopathy [183–185]. The β-AR blocker, propranolol, effectively inhibited the increase of VEGF expression caused by hypoxia and the consecutive neovascular response in the retina [55]. Likewise, propranolol administered subcutaneously reduced VEGF and HIF-1α levels in an oxygen-induced retinopathy (OIR) mouse model, suggesting that β-AR blockade was protective against retinal angiogenesis and ameliorated blood-retinal barrier dysfunction [186].

Intriguingly, a novel β-AR agonist, compound 49b, was reported to decrease VEGF levels in the diabetic rat retina [187]. The effect of compound 49b was attributed to an increase in insulin-like growth factor binding protein 3 (IGFBP-3), which reduced VEGF levels via modulation of eNOS and PKC pathways [187]. These seemingly contradictory findings regarding the impact of β-AR agonists and antagonists on VEGF levels suggest that the effects may be mediated through diverse regulation mechanisms depending on the retinal disease and the experimental setting.

β-AR activation was also shown to increase human and mouse pericyte survival under diabetic conditions [188]. Conversely, a significant decrease in the number of pericytes has been reported in the rat retina after surgical removal of the superior cervical ganglion, which supplies the eye with sympathetic nerve fibers [189]. These findings suggest that proper β-AR signaling is essential for pericyte survival. An in vitro study proposed that β-ARs are involved in the regulation of inducible nitric oxide synthase (iNOS) expression [190]. Activation of β-ARs reduced levels of iNOS and other inflammatory molecules, such as interleukin (IL)-1β, tumor necrosis factor-α (TNF-α), and prostaglandin E2 (PGE2) in human retinal endothelial cells and rat Müller cells in an in vitro model of hyperglycemia [191]. The proposed mechanism for the protective effects was that the stimulating β-ARs decrease the levels of the MAPK family members, PKA, p38 MAPK, and p42/p44 MAPK, in human retinal endothelial cells [190].

Stimulation of β-AR by agonists can activate members of the G protein-coupled receptor (GPCR) kinase (GRK) family, which is the potential mechanism that leads to β-AR desensitization [192]. A first mechanism underlying desensitization is phosphorylation of the GPCR [193]. After coupling to activated receptors, G proteins are phosphorylated by GRKs [194,195]. Seven GRKs (GRK1–7) have been identified, at present [196]. GRK1, as a rhodopsin kinase, is responsible for phosphorylating rhodopsin, which is richly expressed in the retinal rod and cone cells [197]. β-ARs can be phosphorylated by a protein kinase termed GRK2 [198]. The GRK-phosphorylated receptor binds to arrestins, leading to the uncoupling of the receptor from the G protein, desensitizing the agonist-induced response, and subsequently mediating the internalization of receptors [195,199]. Consequently, the GRK-arrestin pathway plays a central role in the desensitization of GPCR responses [195,199]. Two arrestin subtypes were found to be expressed in the retina, arrestin-1 and -4. These arrestins are specialized in binding light-activated phosphorylated rhodopsin and suppressing G protein activation [200,201]. It has been demonstrated that retinal and nonretinal arrestins mediate suppression of GPCRs, suggesting a common mechanism for desensitizing ARs [202]. Apart from this role, arrestins were also shown to be involved in receptor-mediated endocytosis by clathrin-coated pits [202,203].

3.3.3. Contribution of Individual Receptor Subtypes to β-Adrenergic Function in the Retina

Hypoxia was reported to trigger the release of catecholamines, which have been shown to contribute to the increase in retinal VEGF expression, causing pathologic neovascularization [183–185]. In a mouse model of OIR, deletion of β_1- and β_2-ARs reduced retinal VEGF receptor-2 expression and abolished the development of vascular abnormalities in the superficial plexus of the retina [204]. In another study employing a mouse model of OIR, β_1- and β_2-AR blockade by propranolol was shown to reduce the expression of VEGF and to ameliorate retinal dysfunction [186]. Other studies demonstrated that ICI 118,551, a selective β_2-AR blocker, decreased retinal levels of proangiogenic factors and reduced pathogenic neovascularization in a mouse OIR model, suggesting that β_2-AR blockade may be effective in the blockade of retinal angiogenesis [205].

As we mentioned before, there are inconsistent results regarding the role of β-AR activation or blockade on VEGF expression and pathogenic vessel formation. While most studies reported on inhibitory effects of pharmacological β-AR blockade on VEGF formation some other studies observed blockade of VEGF formation by β-AR agonist exposure [55,182–186]. An explanation to these seemingly contradictory results provides a study by Dal Monte et al., which suggested that the nonselective β-ARs agonist, isoproterenol, can cause agonist-induced β_2-AR desensitization that downregulates the expression of β_2-ARs in the retina, which in turn exerts a downregulation effect on VEGF expression in OIR [183]. Jiang et al. proposed that β_2-AR KO mice exhibited certain features similar to diabetic retinopathy, resulting in retinal cell death [206]. A study in β_2-AR KO mice has shown a functional link between β-ARs and insulin receptor signaling pathways in the retina [200]. Furthermore, β_2-ARs can maintain insulin receptor signaling in retinal Müller cells, which potentially supports neuroprotective effects promoted by β-AR stimulation in diabetic retinopathy models [200]. Xamoterol, a β_1-AR agonist, attenuated iNOS expression in human retinal endothelial cells grown in high glucose medium [191]. Studies by Mori et al. have demonstrated that stimulation of β_1-, β_2-, and β_3-ARs can cause dilation of retinal arterioles in rats, thus, increasing retinal blood flow [207,208]. Moreover, the latest study by Mori et al. reported that retinal vasodilation by β_2-AR stimulation is mediated via a G_i protein by activation of large-conductance Ca^{2+}-activated K^+ channels [209].

β_3-ARs were shown to be involved in the neovascularization processes of various retinal vascular diseases [186]. For example, β_3-ARs were upregulated in response to hypoxia in an OIR mouse model with dense β_3-ARs immunoreactivity in engorged retinal tufts, suggesting that activation of β_3-ARs is likely to constitute an important part in pathologic angiogenesis [186]. It has also been demonstrated that the β_3-AR antagonists, L-748,337 and SR59230A, downregulated retinal VEGF release in hypoxia via modulation of the nitric NO signaling pathway [210]. Moreover, the β_3-AR agonist, CL316243, was shown to reduce retinal damage following intravitreal injection of N-methyl-D-aspartate (NMDA) in rats [211]. Furthermore, β_3-ARs, which differ from β_2-ARs with regard to a lack of GRK, are resistant to agonist-induced desensitization [192,212]. Taken together, based on the studies performed so far, the β_3-AR appears to be an attractive therapeutic target for the treatment of ischemic retinal diseases.

Notably, β-AR genes have genetic polymorphisms caused by mutations in the gene promoter, leading to changes in the expression of receptors and the regulation of signal transduction [195,213,214]. The mutations of ARs mainly affect receptor responses and are associated with some diseases [214]. An in vivo study tested the effects of two polymorphisms (codon 16 and codon 27) of the β_2-AR on agonist-mediated vascular desensitization, suggesting that the arginine at position 16 (Arg16) polymorphism (the substitution of glycine for arginine) of the β_2-AR is associated with enhanced agonist-mediated desensitization in the vasculature [215]. However, to the best of our knowledge, no association between genetic polymorphisms of β-AR genes and retinal diseases has been described, so far.

4. Future Directions and Clinical Implications

Although α_1-ARs play a potential physiological and/or pathophysiological role in the regulation of retinal vascular tone, retinal α_1-adrenergic vasoconstriction is largely masked by endothelial mechanisms under physiological conditions and becomes more relevant when the endothelium is damaged. Therefore, α_1-AR signaling pathways may represent therapeutic targets primarily in the context of retinal pathologies associated with impaired endothelial function. However, there are inconsistent findings regarding the subtype mediating adrenergic vasoconstriction in retinal blood vessels. While Mori et al. found that α_{1A}- and α_{1D}-ARs mediated vasoconstriction in vivo in the rat retina, Gericke et al. reported that the α_{1B}-AR-mediated adrenergic vasoconstriction in the isolated mouse retina [67,84]. It remains to be determined which α_1-AR subtype mediates vascular responses in the human retina. However, the lack of highly specific pharmacological ligands and antibodies for individual α_1-AR subtypes hampered the progress in this research area so far. From a clinical point of view, subtype-selective agonists and antagonists would constitute a therapeutic approach to specifically influence retinal perfusion.

It should be emphasized, however, that many issues remain poorly understood and need further investigation. The location of α_1-ARs in general and of the three α_1-AR subtypes in particular within the architecture of retinal vessels is still elusive but may be indicative of their vascular function(s) and relevant for their pharmacological accessibility. The endothelial mechanisms involved in masking retinal α_1-adrenergic vasoconstriction have not yet been identified. In retinal diseases associated with endothelial dysfunction, the actual pathogenic contribution of α_1-AR-mediated vasoconstriction remains an open question.

Various animal experiments and cell culture studies revealed neuroprotective effects of the selective α_2-AR agonist, brimonidine, in the retina [148,150,216]. In 2011, a randomized clinical trial reported on the neuroprotective effects of topically applied brimonidine tartrate 0.2% in preventing visual field loss progression in patients with low-pressure glaucoma, which supports the concept of direct activation of retinal α_2-ARs [163]. In contrast, another trial failed to show neuroprotective effects of 0.2% brimonidine tartrate in patients with non-arteritic anterior ischemic optic neuropathy [217]. In a pilot study on patients with retinal dystrophies, topical treatment with brimonidine suggested a trend towards reduced disease progression [218]. However, the number of patients (n = 26) was relatively small and the mean follow-up period (mean 29 months) relatively short, which does not allow to draw unequivocal conclusions. Taken together, the retinal neuroprotective effects of brimonidine obtained in various experimental disease models remain to be confirmed in large human trials.

Propranolol, which has a high affinity to β_1- and β_2-AR subtypes, is the only β-AR antagonist that has been tested in clinical trials, so far [55]. Propranolol 0.1% eye micro-drops have been developed and administered in a multicenter pilot clinical trial to analyze the safety and efficacy in treating preterm newborns with stage 2 ROP [219]. However, the second stage of this study was discontinued, since the fourth of the 19 newborns showed a progression to stage 2 or 3 with additional disease [219]. Based on animal studies, β_3-ARs appear to be involved in pathogenic vessel formation in the ischemic retina. Hence, future studies are needed to explore β_3-AR ligands in human ischemic retinal diseases.

5. Conclusions

In conclusion, the studies reviewed in this article provide evidence for the presence of α_1-, α_2- and β-ARs in the retina of various species, including humans. α_1-ARs function as stimulatory receptors involved mainly in the contraction of vascular smooth muscle, resulting in vasoconstriction. In contrast, α_2-ARs are primarily expressed in neurons and glia. Its pharmacological activation was shown to lower IOP and to induce neuroprotective effects in the retina. β-ARs are expressed in blood vessels, neurons and glial cells, where they were shown to contribute to the regulation of vascular diameter and to responses to hypoxia. The results of numerous in vitro and in vivo studies suggest that these retinal receptors are functionally active and, hence, may constitute potential targets for the treatment of several retinal diseases.

Author Contributions: Conceptualization, T.B., Y.R. and A.G.; writing—original draft preparation, T.B. and Y.R.; writing—review and editing, A.G., S.J., and T.B.; visualization, Y.R.; supervision, A.G. All authors have read and agreed to the published version of the manuscript.

References

1. Brown, M.M.; Brown, G.C. Utility values associated with blindness in an adult population. *Br. J. Ophthalmol.* **2001**, *85*, 327–331. [CrossRef]
2. Brown, M.M.; Brown, G.C. Quality of life associated with visual loss: A time tradeoff utility analysis comparison with medical health states. *Ophthalmology* **2003**, *110*, 1076–1081. [CrossRef]
3. Krishna, U.; Ajanaku, D. Uveitis: A sight-threatening disease which can impact all systems. *Postgrad. Med. J.* **2017**, *93*, 766–773. [CrossRef] [PubMed]
4. Biousse, V.; Nahab, F. Management of acute retinal ischemia: Follow the guidelines! *Ophthalmology* **2018**, *125*, 1597–1607. [CrossRef] [PubMed]
5. Quigley, H.A.; Broman, A.T. The number of people with glaucoma worldwide in 2010 and 2020. *Br. J. Ophthalmol.* **2006**, *90*, 262–267. [CrossRef]
6. Paulus, Y.M.; Gariano, R.F. Diabetic retinopathy: A growing concern in an aging population. *Geriatrics* **2009**, *64*, 16–20.
7. Rahmani, B.; Tielsch, J.M. The cause-specific prevalence of visual impairment in an urban population. The baltimore eye survey. *Ophthalmology* **1996**, *103*, 1721–1726. [CrossRef]
8. Kocur, I.; Resnikoff, S. Visual impairment and blindness in europe and their prevention. *Br. J. Ophthalmol.* **2002**, *86*, 716–722. [CrossRef]
9. Congdon, N.G.; Friedman, D.S. Important causes of visual impairment in the world today. *JAMA* **2003**, *290*, 2057–2060. [CrossRef]
10. Osborne, N.N.; Casson, R.J. Retinal ischemia: Mechanisms of damage and potential therapeutic strategies. *Prog. Retin. Eye Res.* **2004**, *23*, 91–147. [CrossRef]
11. Grieshaber, M.C.; Flammer, J. Blood flow in glaucoma. *Curr. Opin. Ophthalmol.* **2005**, *16*, 79–83. [CrossRef] [PubMed]
12. Toda, N.; Nakanishi-Toda, M. Nitric oxide: Ocular blood flow, glaucoma, and diabetic retinopathy. *Prog. Retin. Eye Res.* **2007**, *26*, 205–238. [CrossRef] [PubMed]
13. Flammer, J.; Orgul, S. The impact of ocular blood flow in glaucoma. *Prog. Retin. Eye Res.* **2002**, *21*, 359–393. [CrossRef]

14. Schmetterer, L.; Wolzt, M. Ocular blood flow and associated functional deviations in diabetic retinopathy. *Diabetologia* **1999**, *42*, 387–405. [CrossRef]
15. Dimitrova, G.; Kato, S. Relation between retrobulbar circulation and progression of diabetic retinopathy. *Br. J. Ophthalmol.* **2003**, *87*, 622–625. [CrossRef]
16. Mori, A.; Suzuki, S. Vasodilation of retinal arterioles induced by activation of bkca channels is attenuated in diabetic rats. *Eur. J. Pharmacol.* **2011**, *669*, 94–99. [CrossRef]
17. De La Cruz, J.P.; Gonzalez-Correa, J.A. Pharmacological approach to diabetic retinopathy. *Diabetes Metab. Res. Rev.* **2004**, *20*, 91–113. [CrossRef]
18. Wong-Riley, M.T.T. Energy metabolism of the visual system. *Eye Brain* **2010**, *2*, 99–116. [CrossRef]
19. Kur, J.; Newman, E.A. Cellular and physiological mechanisms underlying blood flow regulation in the retina and choroid in health and disease. *Prog. Retin. Eye Res.* **2012**, *31*, 377–406. [CrossRef]
20. Delaey, C.; Van De Voorde, J. Regulatory mechanisms in the retinal and choroidal circulation. *Ophthalmic Res.* **2000**, *32*, 249–256. [CrossRef]
21. Patton, N.; Aslam, T. Retinal vascular image analysis as a potential screening tool for cerebrovascular disease: A rationale based on homology between cerebral and retinal microvasculatures. *J. Anat.* **2005**, *206*, 319–348. [CrossRef] [PubMed]
22. Ahlquist, R.P. A study of the adrenotropic receptors. *Am. J. Physiol.* **1948**, *153*, 586–600. [CrossRef] [PubMed]
23. Alexander, S.P.; Benson, H.E. The concise guide to pharmacology 2013/14: G protein-coupled receptors. *Br. J. Pharmacol.* **2013**, *170*, 1459–1581. [CrossRef] [PubMed]
24. Piascik, M.T.; Perez, D.M. Alpha1-adrenergic receptors: New insights and directions. *J. Pharmacol. Exp. Ther.* **2001**, *298*, 403–410. [PubMed]
25. Civantos Calzada, B.; Aleixandre de Artinano, A. Alpha-adrenoceptor subtypes. *Pharmacol. Res.* **2001**, *44*, 195–208. [CrossRef]
26. Wikberg-Matsson, A. A1- and α2-Adrenoceptors in the Eye: Pharmacological and Functional Characterization. Ph.D. Thesis, Acta Universitatis Upsaliensis, Upsaliensis, 2001.
27. Bylund, D.B.; Eikenberg, D.C. International union of pharmacology nomenclature of adrenoceptors. *Pharmacol. Rev.* **1994**, *46*, 121–136.
28. McGrath, J.C. Localization of α-adrenoceptors: Jr vane medal lecture. *Br. J. Pharmacol.* **2015**, *172*, 1179–1194. [CrossRef]
29. Tuttle, J.L.; Falcone, J.C. Nitric oxide release during alpha1-adrenoceptor-mediated constriction of arterioles. *Am. J. Physiol. Heart Circ. Physiol.* **2001**, *281*, H873–H881. [CrossRef]
30. Gericke, A.; Martinka, P. Impact of alpha1-adrenoceptor expression on contractile properties of vascular smooth muscle cells. *Am. J. Physiol. Regul. Integr. Comp. Physiol.* **2007**, *293*, R1215–R1221. [CrossRef]
31. Hrometz, S.L.; Edelmann, S.E. Expression of multiple alpha1-adrenoceptors on vascular smooth muscle: Correlation with the regulation of contraction. *J. Pharmacol. Exp. Ther.* **1999**, *290*, 452–463.
32. Faber, J.E.; Yang, N. Expression of alpha-adrenoceptor subtypes by smooth muscle cells and adventitial fibroblasts in rat aorta and in cell culture. *J. Pharmacol. Exp. Ther.* **2001**, *298*, 441–452. [PubMed]
33. Ciccarelli, M.; Santulli, G. Endothelial alpha1-adrenoceptors regulate neo-angiogenesis. *Br. J. Pharmacol.* **2008**, *153*, 936–946. [CrossRef] [PubMed]
34. Guimaraes, S.; Moura, D. Vascular adrenoceptors: An update. *Pharmacol. Rev.* **2001**, *53*, 319–356. [PubMed]
35. Cotecchia, S. The alpha1-adrenergic receptors: Diversity of signaling networks and regulation. *J. Recept. Signal Transduct. Res.* **2010**, *30*, 410–419. [CrossRef]
36. Graham, R.M.; Perez, D.M. Alpha 1-adrenergic receptor subtypes. Molecular structure, function, and signaling. *Circ. Res.* **1996**, *78*, 737–749. [CrossRef]
37. Hosoda, C.; Tanoue, A. Correlation between vasoconstrictor roles and mrna expression of alpha1-adrenoceptor subtypes in blood vessels of genetically engineered mice. *Br. J. Pharmacol.* **2005**, *146*, 456–466. [CrossRef]
38. Marti, D.; Miquel, R. Correlation between mrna levels and functional role of alpha1-adrenoceptor subtypes in arteries: Evidence of alpha1l as a functional isoform of the alpha1a-adrenoceptor. *Am. J. Physiol. Heart Circ. Physiol.* **2005**, *289*, H1923–H1932. [CrossRef]
39. Rudner, X.L.; Berkowitz, D.E. Subtype specific regulation of human vascular alpha(1)-adrenergic receptors by vessel bed and age. *Circulation* **1999**, *100*, 2336–2343. [CrossRef]
40. Drouin, C.; Bobadilla, A.-C. Norepinephrine☆. In *Reference Module in Neuroscience and Biobehavioral Psychology*; Elsevier: Amsterdam, The Netherlands, 2017.

41. Hieble, J.P. Adrenergic receptors. In *Encyclopedia of Neuroscience*; Squire, L.R., Ed.; Academic Press: Oxford, UK, 2009; pp. 135–139.
42. Djurup, R. Adrenoceptors: Molecular nature and role in atopic diseases. *Allergy* **1981**, *36*, 289–307. [CrossRef]
43. Qu, L.; Zhou, Q. Structural basis of the diversity of adrenergic receptors. *Cell Rep.* **2019**, *29*, 2929–2935.e4. [CrossRef]
44. Magocsi, M.; Vizi, E.S. Multiple g-protein-coupling specificity of beta-adrenoceptor in macrophages. *Immunology* **2007**, *122*, 503–513. [CrossRef] [PubMed]
45. Amini, R.; Rocha-Martins, M. Neuronal migration and lamination in the vertebrate retina. *Front. Neurosci.* **2018**, *11*, 742. [CrossRef] [PubMed]
46. Masland, R.H. The neuronal organization of the retina. *Neuron* **2012**, *76*, 266–280.
47. Haider, N.B.; Cruz, N.M. Pathobiology of the outer retina: Genetic and nongenetic causes of disease. In *Pathobiology of Human Disease*; McManus, L.M., Mitchell, R.N., Eds.; Academic Press: San Diego, CA, USA, 2014; pp. 2084–2114.
48. Herzlich, A.A.; Patel, M. Chapter 2—Retinal anatomy and pathology. In *Retinal Pharmacotherapy*; Nguyen, Q.D., Rodrigues, E.B., Eds.; W.B. Saunders: Edinburgh, UK, 2010; pp. 5–14.
49. Hogan, M.J.; Feeney, L. The ultrastructure of the retinal blood vessels: I. The large vessels. *J. Ultrastruct. Res.* **1963**, *9*, 10–28. [CrossRef]
50. Ferrari-Dileo, G.; Davis, E.B. Biochemical evidence for cholinergic activity in retinal blood vessels. *Investig. Ophthalmol. Vis. Sci.* **1989**, *30*, 473–477.
51. Gericke, A.; Goloborodko, E. Contribution of nitric oxide synthase isoforms to cholinergic vasodilation in murine retinal arterioles. *Exp. Eye Res.* **2013**, *109*, 60–66. [CrossRef]
52. Liu, H.; Mercieca, K. Hydrogen sulfide and β-synuclein are involved and interlinked in the aging glaucomatous retina. *J. Ophthalmol.* **2020**, *2020*, 8642135. [CrossRef]
53. Hadjiconstantinou, M.; Cohen, J. Epinephrine: A potential neurotransmitter in retina. *J. Neurochem.* **1983**, *41*, 1440–1444. [CrossRef]
54. Nguyen-Legros, J. Chapter 5 morphology and distribution of catecholamine-neurons in mammalian retina. *Prog. Retin. Res.* **1988**, *7*, 113–147. [CrossRef]
55. Casini, G.; Dal Monte, M. The β-adrenergic system as a possible new target for pharmacologic treatment of neovascular retinal diseases. *Prog. Retin. Eye Res.* **2014**, *42*, 103–129. [CrossRef]
56. Hirasawa, H.; Contini, M. Extrasynaptic release of gaba and dopamine by retinal dopaminergic neurons. *Philos. Trans. R. Soc. Lond. Ser. B Biol. Sci.* **2015**, *370*, 20140186. [CrossRef] [PubMed]
57. HÄGgendal, J.A.N.; Malmfors, T. Identification and cellular localization of the catecholamines in the retina and the choroid of the rabbit. *Acta Physiol. Scand.* **1965**, *64*, 58–66. [CrossRef] [PubMed]
58. Osborne, N.N. Noradrenaline, a transmitter candidate in the retina. *J. Neurochem.* **1981**, *36*, 17–27. [CrossRef] [PubMed]
59. Frederick, J.M.; Rayborn, M.E. Dopaminergic neurons in the human retina. *J. Comp. Neurol.* **1982**, *210*, 65–79. [CrossRef]
60. Lei, S. Cross interaction of dopaminergic and adrenergic systems in neural modulation. *Int. J. Physiol. Pathophysiol. Pharmacol.* **2014**, *6*, 137–142.
61. Forster, B.A.; Ferrari-Dileo, G. Adrenergic alpha 1 and alpha 2 binding sites are present in bovine retinal blood vessels. *Investig. Ophthalmol. Vis. Sci.* **1987**, *28*, 1741–1746.
62. Ehinger, B. Distribution of adrenergic nerves in the eye and some related structures in the cat. *Acta Physiol. Scand.* **1966**, *66*, 123–128. [CrossRef]
63. Laties, A.M. Central retinal artery innervation. Absence of adrenergic innervation to the intraocular branches. *Arch. Ophthalmol.* **1967**, *77*, 405–409. [CrossRef]
64. Ye, X.D.; Laties, A.M. Peptidergic innervation of the retinal vasculature and optic nerve head. *Investig. Ophthalmol. Vis. Sci.* **1990**, *31*, 1731–1737.
65. Suzuki, F.; Taniguchi, T. Distribution of alpha-1 adrenoceptor subtypes in rna and protein in rabbit eyes. *Br. J. Pharmacol.* **2002**, *135*, 600–608. [CrossRef]
66. Wikberg-Matsson, A.; Uhlen, S. Characterization of alpha(1)-adrenoceptor subtypes in the eye. *Exp. Eye Res.* **2000**, *70*, 51–60. [CrossRef] [PubMed]
67. Bohmer, T.; Manicam, C. The alpha1b-adrenoceptor subtype mediates adrenergic vasoconstriction in mouse retinal arterioles with damaged endothelium. *Br. J. Pharmacol.* **2014**, *171*, 3858–3867. [CrossRef] [PubMed]

68. Jensen, B.C.; Swigart, P.M. Functional alpha-1b adrenergic receptors on human epicardial coronary artery endothelial cells. *Naunyn Schmiedebergs Arch. Pharmacol.* **2010**, *382*, 475–482. [CrossRef] [PubMed]
69. Jensen, B.C.; Swigart, P.M. The alpha-1d is the predominant alpha-1-adrenergic receptor subtype in human epicardial coronary arteries. *J. Am. Coll. Cardiol.* **2009**, *54*, 1137–1145. [CrossRef]
70. Yu, D.Y.; Su, E.N. Isolated preparations of ocular vasculature and their applications in ophthalmic research. *Prog. Retin. Eye Res.* **2003**, *22*, 135–169. [CrossRef]
71. Ferrari-Dileo, G.; Davis, E.B. Response of retinal vasculature to phenylephrine. *Investig. Ophthalmol. Vis. Sci.* **1990**, *31*, 1181–1182.
72. Hadjiconstantinou, M.; Mariani, A.P. Immunohistochemical evidence for epinephrine-containing retinal amacrine cells. *Neuroscience* **1984**, *13*, 547–551. [CrossRef]
73. Kolb, H.; Cuenca, N. The synaptic organization of the dopaminergic amacrine cell in the cat retina. *J. Neurocytol.* **1990**, *19*, 343–366. [CrossRef]
74. Nguyen-Legros, J.; Krieger, M. Immunohistochemical localization of l-dopa and aromatic l-amino acid-decarboxylase in the rat retina. *Investig. Ophthalmol. Vis. Sci.* **1994**, *35*, 2906–2915.
75. Chen, Z.; Jia, W. Immunohistochemical localization of dopamine-beta-hydroxylase in human and monkey eyes. *Curr. Eye Res.* **1999**, *18*, 39–48. [CrossRef]
76. Ichikawa, M.; Okada, Y. Effects of topically instilled bunazosin, an alpha1-adrenoceptor antagonist, on constrictions induced by phenylephrine and et-1 in rabbit retinal arteries. *Investig. Ophthalmol. Vis. Sci.* **2004**, *45*, 4041–4048. [CrossRef] [PubMed]
77. Zarbin, M.A.; Wamsley, J.K. Autoradiographic localization of high affinity gaba, benzodiazepine, dopaminergic, adrenergic and muscarinic cholinergic receptors in the rat, monkey and human retina. *Brain Res.* **1986**, *374*, 75–92. [CrossRef]
78. Joseph, D.P.; Miller, S.S. Alpha-1-adrenergic modulation of k and cl transport in bovine retinal pigment epithelium. *J. Gen. Physiol.* **1992**, *99*, 263–290. [CrossRef] [PubMed]
79. Frambach, D.A.; Valentine, J.L. Alpha-1 adrenergic receptors on rabbit retinal pigment epithelium. *Investig. Ophthalmol. Vis. Sci.* **1988**, *29*, 737–741.
80. Jensen, B.C.; Swigart, P.M. Ten commercial antibodies for alpha-1-adrenergic receptor subtypes are nonspecific. *Naunyn Schmiedebergs Arch. Pharmacol.* **2009**, *379*, 409–412. [CrossRef]
81. Michel, M.C.; Seifert, R. Selectivity of pharmacologic tools: Implications for use in cell physiology. A review in the theme: Cell signaling: Proteins, pathways and mechanisms. *Am. J. Physiol. Cell Physiol.* **2015**, *308*, C505–C520. [CrossRef]
82. Pradidarcheep, W.; Stallen, J. Lack of specificity of commercially available antisera against muscarinergic and adrenergic receptors. *Naunyn Schmiedebergs Arch. Pharmacol.* **2009**, *379*, 397–402. [CrossRef]
83. Bohmer, T.; Pfeiffer, N. Three commercial antibodies against alpha1-adrenergic receptor subtypes lack specificity in paraffin-embedded sections of murine tissues. *Naunyn Schmiedebergs Arch. Pharmacol.* **2014**, *387*, 703–706. [CrossRef]
84. Mori, A.; Hanada, M. Noradrenaline contracts rat retinal arterioles via stimulation of alpha(1a)- and alpha(1d)-adrenoceptors. *Eur. J. Pharmacol.* **2011**, *673*, 65–69. [CrossRef]
85. Alm, A. Effects of norepinephrine, angiotensin, dihydroergotamine, papaverine, isoproterenol, histamine, nicotinic acid, and xanthinol nicotinate on retinal oxygen tension in cats. *Acta Ophthalmol. (Copenh)* **1972**, *50*, 707–719. [CrossRef]
86. Dollery, C.T.; Hill, D.W. The response of normal retinal blood vessels to angiotensin and noradrenaline. *J. Physiol.* **1963**, *165*, 500–507. [CrossRef] [PubMed]
87. Polak, K.; Dorner, G. Evaluation of the zeiss retinal vessel analyser. *Br. J. Ophthalmol.* **2000**, *84*, 1285–1290. [CrossRef] [PubMed]
88. Jandrasits, K.; Luksch, A. Effect of noradrenaline on retinal blood flow in healthy subjects. *Ophthalmology* **2002**, *109*, 291–295. [CrossRef]
89. Garhöfer, G.; Schmetterer, L. Endothelial and adrenergic control. In *Ocular Blood Flow*; Schmetterer, L., Kiel, J., Eds.; Springer: Berlin/Heidelberg, Germany, 2012; pp. 311–346.
90. Hara, H.; Ichikawa, M. Bunazosin, a selective alpha1-adrenoceptor antagonist, as an anti-glaucoma drug: Effects on ocular circulation and retinal neuronal damage. *Cardiovasc. Drug Rev.* **2005**, *23*, 43–56. [CrossRef] [PubMed]

91. Nielsen, P.J.; Nyborg, N.C. Adrenergic responses in isolated bovine retinal resistance arteries. *Int. Ophthalmol.* **1989**, *13*, 103–107. [CrossRef] [PubMed]
92. Yu, D.Y.; Alder, V.A. Vasoactivity of intraluminal and extraluminal agonists in perfused retinal arteries. *Investig. Ophthalmol. Vis. Sci.* **1994**, *35*, 4087–4099. [PubMed]
93. Spada, C.S.; Nieves, A.L. Differential effects of alpha-adrenoceptor agonists on human retinal microvessel diameter. *J. Ocul. Pharmacol. Ther.* **2001**, *17*, 255–277. [CrossRef]
94. Hoste, A.M.; Boels, P.J. Effect of alpha-1 and beta agonists on contraction of bovine retinal resistance arteries in vitro. *Investig. Ophthalmol. Vis. Sci.* **1989**, *30*, 44–50.
95. Hoste, A.M.; Boels, P.J. Effects of beta-antagonists on contraction of bovine retinal microarteries in vitro. *Investig. Ophthalmol. Vis. Sci.* **1990**, *31*, 1231–1237.
96. Sercombe, R.; Verrecchia, C. Pial artery responses to norepinephrine potentiated by endothelium removal. *J. Cereb. Blood Flow Metab.* **1985**, *5*, 312–317. [CrossRef]
97. Bauknight, G.C., Jr.; Faraci, F.M. Endothelium-derived relaxing factor modulates noradrenergic constriction of cerebral arterioles in rabbits. *Stroke* **1992**, *23*, 1522–1525. [CrossRef] [PubMed]
98. Carrier, G.O.; White, R.E. Enhancement of alpha-1 and alpha-2 adrenergic agonist-induced vasoconstriction by removal of endothelium in rat aorta. *J. Pharmacol. Exp. Ther.* **1985**, *232*, 682–687. [PubMed]
99. Lues, I.; Schumann, H.J. Effect of removing the endothelial cells on the reactivity of rat aortic segments to different alpha-adrenoceptor agonists. *Naunyn Schmiedebergs Arch. Pharmacol.* **1984**, *328*, 160–163. [CrossRef] [PubMed]
100. Godfraind, T.; Egleme, C. Role of endothelium in the contractile response of rat aorta to alpha-adrenoceptor agonists. *Clin. Sci. (Lond.)* **1985**, *68* (Suppl. 10), 65s–71s. [CrossRef]
101. Egleme, C.; Godfraind, T. Enhanced responsiveness of rat isolated aorta to clonidine after removal of the endothelial cells. *Br. J. Pharmacol.* **1984**, *81*, 16–18. [CrossRef]
102. Alosachie, I.; Godfraind, T. The modulatory role of vascular endothelium in the interaction of agonists and antagonists with alpha-adrenoceptors in the rat aorta. *Br. J. Pharmacol.* **1988**, *95*, 619–629. [CrossRef]
103. Furchgott, R.F. The role of endothelium in the responses of vascular smooth muscle to drugs. *Annu. Rev. Pharmacol. Toxicol.* **1984**, *24*, 175–197. [CrossRef]
104. Miller, V.M.; Vanhoutte, P.M. Role of the endothelium in modulating vascular adrenergic receptor actions. *Prog. Clin. Biol. Res.* **1989**, *286*, 33–39.
105. White, R.E.; Carrier, G.O. Alpha 1- and alpha 2-adrenoceptor agonist-induced contraction in rat mesenteric artery upon removal of endothelium. *Eur. J. Pharmacol.* **1986**, *122*, 349–352. [CrossRef]
106. Verrecchia, C.; Sercombe, R. Influence of endothelium on noradrenaline-induced vasoconstriction in rabbit central ear artery. *Clin. Exp. Pharmacol. Physiol.* **1985**, *12*, 169–179. [CrossRef]
107. Jones, C.J.; DeFily, D.V. Endothelium-dependent relaxation competes with alpha 1- and alpha 2-adrenergic constriction in the canine epicardial coronary microcirculation. *Circulation* **1993**, *87*, 1264–1274. [CrossRef] [PubMed]
108. Berkenboom, G.; Unger, P. Endothelium-derived relaxing factor and protection against contraction to norepinephrine in isolated canine and human coronary arteries. *J. Cardiovasc. Pharmacol.* **1991**, *17* (Suppl. 3), S127–S132. [CrossRef]
109. Cocks, T.M.; Angus, J.A. Endothelium-dependent relaxation of coronary arteries by noradrenaline and serotonin. *Nature* **1983**, *305*, 627–630. [CrossRef] [PubMed]
110. Baumgart, D.; Haude, M. Augmented alpha-adrenergic constriction of atherosclerotic human coronary arteries. *Circulation* **1999**, *99*, 2090–2097. [CrossRef]
111. Vita, J.A.; Treasure, C.B. Patients with evidence of coronary endothelial dysfunction as assessed by acetylcholine infusion demonstrate marked increase in sensitivity to constrictor effects of catecholamines. *Circulation* **1992**, *85*, 1390–1397. [CrossRef]
112. Heusch, G.; Baumgart, D. Alpha-adrenergic coronary vasoconstriction and myocardial ischemia in humans. *Circulation* **2000**, *101*, 689–694. [CrossRef]
113. Schmetterer, L.; Polak, K. Role of nitric oxide in the control of ocular blood flow. *Prog. Retin. Eye. Res.* **2001**, *20*, 823–847. [CrossRef]
114. Zembowicz, A.; Hecker, M. Nitric oxide and another potent vasodilator are formed from ng-hydroxy-l-arginine by cultured endothelial cells. *Proc. Natl. Acad. Sci. USA* **1991**, *88*, 11172–11176. [CrossRef]
115. Moncada, S.; Higgs, E.A. Nitric oxide and the vascular endothelium. *Handb. Exp. Pharmacol.* **2006**, 213–254.

116. Palmer, R.M.; Ashton, D.S. Vascular endothelial cells synthesize nitric oxide from l-arginine. *Nature* **1988**, *333*, 664–666. [CrossRef]
117. Palmer, R.M.; Ferrige, A.G. Nitric oxide release accounts for the biological activity of endothelium-derived relaxing factor. *Nature* **1987**, *327*, 524–526. [CrossRef] [PubMed]
118. Ignarro, L.J.; Byrns, R.E. Pharmacological evidence that endothelium-derived relaxing factor is nitric oxide: Use of pyrogallol and superoxide dismutase to study endothelium-dependent and nitric oxide-elicited vascular smooth muscle relaxation. *J. Pharmacol. Exp. Ther.* **1988**, *244*, 181–189. [PubMed]
119. Koss, M.C. Functional role of nitric oxide in regulation of ocular blood flow. *Eur. J. Pharmacol.* **1999**, *374*, 161–174. [CrossRef]
120. Sun, D.; Huang, A. Nitric oxide-mediated arteriolar dilation after endothelial deformation. *Am. J. Physiol. Heart Circ. Physiol.* **2001**, *280*, H714–H721. [CrossRef]
121. Tesfamariam, B.; Cohen, R.A. Inhibition of adrenergic vasoconstriction by endothelial cell shear stress. *Circ. Res.* **1988**, *63*, 720–725. [CrossRef]
122. Kaneko, K.; Sunano, S. Involvement of alpha-adrenoceptors in the endothelium-dependent depression of noradrenaline-induced contraction in rat aorta. *Eur. J. Pharmacol.* **1993**, *240*, 195–200. [CrossRef]
123. Filippi, S.; Parenti, A. Alpha(1d)-adrenoceptors cause endothelium-dependent vasodilatation in the rat mesenteric vascular bed. *J. Pharmacol. Exp. Ther.* **2001**, *296*, 869–875.
124. Angus, J.A.; Cocks, T.M. The alpha adrenoceptors on endothelial cells. *Fed. Proc.* **1986**, *45*, 2355–2359.
125. de Andrade, C.R.; Fukada, S.Y. Alpha1d-adrenoceptor-induced relaxation on rat carotid artery is impaired during the endothelial dysfunction evoked in the early stages of hyperhomocysteinemia. *Eur. J. Pharmacol.* **2006**, *543*, 83–91. [CrossRef]
126. Cipolla, M.J.; Harker, C.T. Endothelial function and adrenergic reactivity in human type-ii diabetic resistance arteries. *J. Vasc. Surg.* **1996**, *23*, 940–949. [CrossRef]
127. Nakazawa, T.; Kaneko, Y. Attenuation of nitric oxide- and prostaglandin-independent vasodilation of retinal arterioles induced by acetylcholine in streptozotocin-treated rats. *Vascul. Pharmacol.* **2007**, *46*, 153–159. [CrossRef] [PubMed]
128. Resch, H.; Garhofer, G. Endothelial dysfunction in glaucoma. *Acta Ophthalmol.* **2009**, *87*, 4–12. [CrossRef] [PubMed]
129. Goto, W.; Oku, H. Amelioration by topical bunazosin hydrochloride of the impairment in ocular blood flow caused by nitric oxide synthase inhibition in rabbits. *J. Ocul. Pharmacol. Ther.* **2003**, *19*, 63–73. [CrossRef] [PubMed]
130. Chen, Z.J.; Minneman, K.P. Recent progress in alpha1-adrenergic receptor research. *Acta Pharmacol. Sin.* **2005**, *26*, 1281–1287. [CrossRef] [PubMed]
131. Zhong, H.; Minneman, K.P. Alpha1-adrenoceptor subtypes. *Eur. J. Pharmacol.* **1999**, *375*, 261–276. [CrossRef]
132. Gericke, A.; Kordasz, M.L. Functional role of alpha1-adrenoceptor subtypes in murine ophthalmic arteries. *Investig. Ophthalmol. Vis. Sci.* **2011**, *52*, 4795–4799. [CrossRef]
133. Docherty, J.R. Subtypes of functional alpha1-adrenoceptor. *Cell. Mol. Life Sci.* **2010**, *67*, 405–417. [CrossRef]
134. Han, C.; Li, J. Subtypes of alpha 1-adrenoceptors in rat blood vessels. *Eur. J. Pharmacol.* **1990**, *190*, 97–104.
135. Shen, H.; Peri, K.G. Distribution of alpha1-adrenoceptor subtype proteins in different tissues of neonatal and adult rats. *Can. J. Physiol. Pharmacol.* **2000**, *78*, 237–243. [CrossRef]
136. Piascik, M.T.; Guarino, R.D. The specific contribution of the novel alpha-1d adrenoceptor to the contraction of vascular smooth muscle. *J. Pharmacol. Exp. Ther.* **1995**, *275*, 1583–1589.
137. Yang, M.; Reese, J. Murine alpha1-adrenoceptor subtypes. I. Radioligand binding studies. *J. Pharmacol. Exp. Ther.* **1998**, *286*, 841–847. [PubMed]
138. Yang, M.; Verfurth, F. Is alpha1d-adrenoceptor protein detectable in rat tissues? *Naunyn Schmiedebergs Arch. Pharmacol.* **1997**, *355*, 438–446. [CrossRef] [PubMed]
139. Hague, C.; Chen, Z. Alpha(1)-adrenergic receptor subtypes: Non-identical triplets with different dancing partners? *Life Sci.* **2003**, *74*, 411–418. [CrossRef] [PubMed]
140. Gonzalez-Cabrera, P.J.; Gaivin, R.J. Genetic profiling of alpha 1-adrenergic receptor subtypes by oligonucleotide microarrays: Coupling to interleukin-6 secretion but differences in stat3 phosphorylation and gp-130. *Mol. Pharmacol.* **2003**, *63*, 1104–1116. [CrossRef] [PubMed]
141. Hein, P.; Michel, M.C. Signal transduction and regulation: Are all alpha1-adrenergic receptor subtypes created equal? *Biochem. Pharmacol.* **2007**, *73*, 1097–1106. [CrossRef] [PubMed]

142. Osborne, N.N. Binding of (-)[3h]noradrenaline to bovine membrane of the retina. Evidence for the existence of alpha 2-receptors. *Vis. Res.* **1982**, *22*, 1401–1407. [CrossRef]
143. Convents, A.; De Backer, J.P. Characterization of alpha 2-adrenergic receptors of calf retina membranes by [3h]-rauwolscine and [3h]-rx 781094 binding. *Biochem. Pharmacol.* **1987**, *36*, 2497–2503. [CrossRef]
144. Matsuo, T.; Cynader, M.S. Localization of alpha-2 adrenergic receptors in the human eye. *Ophthalmic Res.* **1992**, *24*, 213–219. [CrossRef]
145. Harrison, J.K.; Angelo, D.D. Pharmacological characterization of rat alpha 2-adrenergic receptors. *Mol. Pharmacol.* **1991**, *40*, 407.
146. Venkataraman, V.; Duda, T. Molecular and pharmacological identity of the α2d-adrenergic receptor subtype in bovine retina and its photoreceptors. *Mol. Cell. Biochem.* **1996**, *159*, 129–138. [CrossRef]
147. Bylund, D.B. *Adrenoceptors*; IUPHAR Media: London, UK, 1998; pp. 58–74.
148. Kalapesi, F.B.; Coroneo, M.T. Human ganglion cells express the alpha-2 adrenergic receptor: Relevance to neuroprotection. *Br. J. Ophthalmol.* **2005**, *89*, 758–763. [CrossRef]
149. Woldemussie, E.; Wijono, M. Localization of alpha 2 receptors in ocular tissues. *Vis. Neurosci.* **2007**, *24*, 745–756. [CrossRef] [PubMed]
150. Wheeler, L.A.; Gil, D.W. Role of alpha-2 adrenergic receptors in neuroprotection and glaucoma. *Surv. Ophthalmol.* **2001**, *45*, S290–S294. [CrossRef]
151. Gilsbach, R.; Hein, L. Are the pharmacology and physiology of α2adrenoceptors determined by α2-heteroreceptors and autoreceptors respectively? *Br. J. Pharmacol.* **2012**, *165*, 90–102. [CrossRef] [PubMed]
152. Maier, C.; Steinberg, G.K. Neuroprotection by the alpha 2-adrenoreceptor agonist dexmedetomidine in a focal model of cerebral ischemia. *Anesthesiology* **1993**, *79*, 306–312. [CrossRef]
153. Ma, D.; Rajakumaraswamy, N. Alpha2-adrenoceptor agonists: Shedding light on neuroprotection? *Br. Med. Bull.* **2004**, *71*, 77–92. [CrossRef]
154. Dong, C.-J.; Guo, Y. A2 adrenergic modulation of nmda receptor function as a major mechanism of rgc protection in experimental glaucoma and retinal excitotoxicity. *Investig. Ophthalmol. Vis. Sci.* **2008**, *49*, 4515–4522. [CrossRef]
155. Donello, J.E.; Padillo, E.U. Alpha(2)-adrenoceptor agonists inhibit vitreal glutamate and aspartate accumulation and preserve retinal function after transient ischemia. *J. Pharmacol. Exp. Ther.* **2001**, *296*, 216–223.
156. Vidal-Sanz, M.; Lafuente, M.a.P. Retinal ganglion cell death induced by retinal ischemia: Neuroprotective effects of two alpha-2 agonists. *Surv. Ophthalmol.* **2001**, *45*, S261–S267. [CrossRef]
157. WoldeMussie, E.; Ruiz, G. Neuroprotection of retinal ganglion cells by brimonidine in rats with laser-induced chronic ocular hypertension. *Investig. Ophthalmol. Vis.Sci.* **2001**, *42*, 2849–2855.
158. Katsimpris, J.M.; Siganos, D. Efficacy of brimonidine 0.2% in controlling acute postoperative intraocular pressure elevation after phacoemulsification. *J. Cataract Refract. Surg.* **2003**, *29*, 2288–2294. [CrossRef] [PubMed]
159. Greenfield, D.S.; Liebmann, J.M. Brimonidine: A new alpha2-adrenoreceptor agonist for glaucoma treatment. *J. Glaucoma* **1997**, *6*, 250–258. [CrossRef] [PubMed]
160. Reitsamer, H.A.; Posey, M. Effects of a topical alpha2 adrenergic agonist on ciliary blood flow and aqueous production in rabbits. *Exp. Eye Res.* **2006**, *82*, 405–415. [CrossRef] [PubMed]
161. Evans, D.W.; Hosking, S.L. Contrast sensitivity improves after brimonidine therapy in primary open angle glaucoma: A case for neuroprotection. *Br. J. Ophthalmol.* **2003**, *87*, 1463–1465. [CrossRef] [PubMed]
162. Shim, M.S.; Kim, K.Y.; Ju, W.K. Role of cyclic amp in the eye with glaucoma. *BMB Rep.* **2017**, *50*, 60–70.
163. Krupin, T.; Liebmann, J.M. A randomized trial of brimonidine versus timolol in preserving visual function: Results from the low-pressure glaucoma treatment study. *Am. J. Ophthalmol.* **2011**, *151*, 671–681. [CrossRef]
164. Kim, H.S.; Chang, Y.I. Alteration of retinal intrinsic survival signal and effect of alpha2-adrenergic receptor agonist in the retina of the chronic ocular hypertension rat. *Vis. Neurosci.* **2007**, *24*, 127–139. [CrossRef]
165. Dong, C.J.; Guo, Y. Alpha2 adrenergic receptor-mediated modulation of cytosolic ca++ signals at the inner plexiform layer of the rat retina. *Investig. Ophthalmol. Vis. Sci.* **2007**, *48*, 1410–1415. [CrossRef]
166. Han, Y.; Wu, S.M. Nmda-evoked [ca2+]i increase in salamander retinal ganglion cells: Modulation by pka and adrenergic receptors. *Vis. Neurosci.* **2002**, *19*, 249–256. [CrossRef]

167. Zhou, X.; Zhang, T. Brimonidine enhances inhibitory postsynaptic activity of off- and on-type retinal ganglion cells in a wistar rat chronic glaucoma model. *Exp. Eye Res.* **2019**, *189*, 107833. [CrossRef]
168. Wen, R.; Cheng, T. Alpha 2-adrenergic agonists induce basic fibroblast growth factor expression in photoreceptors in vivo and ameliorate light damage. *J. Neurosci.* **1996**, *16*, 5986–5992. [CrossRef] [PubMed]
169. Fujita, Y.; Sato, A. Brimonidine promotes axon growth after optic nerve injury through erk phosphorylation. *Cell Death Dis.* **2013**, *4*, e763. [CrossRef] [PubMed]
170. Li, T.; Yang, S. Modulation of α-adrenoceptor signalling protects photoreceptors after retinal detachment by inhibiting oxidative stress and inflammation. *Br. J. Pharmacol.* **2019**, *176*, 801–813. [CrossRef] [PubMed]
171. Guo, X.; Namekata, K. Brimonidine suppresses loss of retinal neurons and visual function in a murine model of optic neuritis. *Neurosci. Lett.* **2015**, *592*, 27–31. [CrossRef]
172. Wikberg-Matsson, A.; Simonsen, U. Potent α2a-adrenoceptor–mediated vasoconstriction by brimonidine in porcine ciliary arteries. *Investig. Ophthalmol. Vis. Sci.* **2001**, *42*, 2049–2055.
173. Kaya, S.; Kolodjaschna, J. Effect of the α2-adrenoceptor antagonist yohimbine on vascular regulation of the middle cerebral artery and the ophthalmic artery in healthy subjects. *Microvasc. Res.* **2011**, *81*, 117–122. [CrossRef]
174. Weigert, G.; Resch, H. Intravenous administration of clonidine reduces intraocular pressure and alters ocular blood flow. *Br. J. Ophthalmol.* **2007**, *91*, 1354–1358. [CrossRef]
175. Elena, P.-P.; Denis, P. Beta adrenergic binding sites in the human eye: An autoradiographic study. *J. Ocul. Pharmacol. Ther.* **1990**, *6*, 143–149. [CrossRef]
176. Granneman, J.G. The putative beta4-adrenergic receptor is a novel state of the beta1-adrenergic receptor. *Am. J. Physiol. Endocrinol. Metab.* **2001**, *280*, E199–E202. [CrossRef]
177. Madamanchi, A. Beta-adrenergic receptor signaling in cardiac function and heart failure. *McGill J. Med. MJM An Int. Forum Adv. Med. Sci. Stud.* **2007**, *10*, 99–104.
178. Ferrari-Dileo, G. Beta 1 and beta 2 adrenergic binding sites in bovine retina and retinal blood vessels. *Investig. Ophthalmol. Vis. Sci.* **1988**, *29*, 695–699. [PubMed]
179. Mori, A.; Miwa, T. Pharmacological evidence for the presence of functional β3-adrenoceptors in rat retinal blood vessels. *Naunyn-Schmiedeberg's Arch. Pharmacol.* **2010**, *382*, 119–126. [CrossRef] [PubMed]
180. Walker, R.J.; Steinle, J.J. Role of β-adrenergic receptors in inflammatory marker expression in müller cells. *Investig. Ophthalmol. Vis. Sci.* **2007**, *48*, 5276–5281. [CrossRef] [PubMed]
181. Steinle, J.J.; Booz, G.W. Beta 3-adrenergic receptors regulate retinal endothelial cell migration and proliferation. *J. Biol. Chem.* **2003**, *278*, 20681–20686. [CrossRef]
182. Lindgren, I.; Altimiras, J. Chronic prenatal hypoxia sensitizes beta-adrenoceptors in the embryonic heart but causes postnatal desensitization. *Am. J. Physiol. Regul. Integr. Comp. Physiol.* **2009**, *297*, R258–R264. [CrossRef]
183. Dal Monte, M.; Martini, D. Beta-adrenoreceptor agonism influences retinal responses to hypoxia in a model of retinopathy of prematurity. Investig. *Ophthalmol. Vis. Sci.* **2012**, *53*, 2181–2192. [CrossRef]
184. Aiello, L.P.; Avery, R.L. Vascular endothelial growth factor in ocular fluid of patients with diabetic retinopathy and other retinal disorders. *N. Engl. J. Med.* **1994**, *331*, 1480–1487. [CrossRef]
185. Chen, J.; Smith, L.E.H. Retinopathy of prematurity. *Angiogenesis* **2007**, *10*, 133–140. [CrossRef]
186. Ristori, C.; Filippi, L. Role of the adrenergic system in a mouse model of oxygen-induced retinopathy: Antiangiogenic effects of beta-adrenoreceptor blockade. *Investig. Ophthalmol. Vis. Sci.* **2011**, *52*, 155–170. [CrossRef]
187. Jiang, Y.; Zhang, Q. Beta-adrenergic receptor agonist decreases vegf levels through altered enos and pkc signaling in diabetic retina. *Growth Factors (Chur. Switz.)* **2015**, *33*, 1–8. [CrossRef]
188. Yun, J.-H.; Jeong, H.-S. B-adrenergic receptor agonists attenuate pericyte loss in diabetic retinas through akt activation. *FASEB J.* **2018**, *32*, 2324–2338. [CrossRef] [PubMed]
189. Wiley, L.A.; Rupp, G.R. Sympathetic innervation regulates basement membrane thickening and pericyte number in rat retina. *Investig. Ophthalmol. Vis. Sci.* **2005**, *46*, 744–748. [CrossRef] [PubMed]
190. Steinle, J.J.; Chin, V.C. Beta-adrenergic receptor stimulation modulates inos protein levels through p38 and erk1/2 signaling in human retinal endothelial cells. *Exp. Eye Res.* **2008**, *87*, 30–34. [CrossRef] [PubMed]
191. Steinle, J.J. Sympathetic neurotransmission modulates expression of inflammatory markers in the rat retina. *Exp. Eye Res.* **2007**, *84*, 118–125. [CrossRef]
192. Wallukat, G. The beta-adrenergic receptors. *Herz* **2002**, *27*, 683–690. [CrossRef]

193. Willets, J.M.; Challiss, R.A.J. Non-visual grks: Are we seeing the whole picture? *Trends Pharmacol. Sci.* **2003**, *24*, 626–633. [CrossRef]
194. Kelly, E.; Bailey, C.P. Agonist-selective mechanisms of gpcr desensitization. *Br. J. Pharmacol.* **2008**, *153*, S379–S388. [CrossRef]
195. Lymperopoulos, A.; Bathgate, A. Pharmacogenomics of the heptahelical receptor regulators g-protein-coupled receptor kinases and arrestins: The known and the unknown. *Pharmacogenomics* **2012**, *13*, 323–341. [CrossRef]
196. Pierce, K.L.; Lefkowitz, R.J. Classical and new roles of β-arrestins in the regulation of g-protein-coupled receptors. *Nat. Rev. Neurosci.* **2001**, *2*, 727–733. [CrossRef]
197. Lorenz, W.; Inglese, J. The receptor kinase family: Primary structure of rhodopsin kinase reveals similarities to the beta-adrenergic receptor kinase. *Proc. Natl. Acad. Sci. USA* **1991**, *88*, 8715–8719. [CrossRef]
198. Benovic, J.L.; Strasser, R.H. Beta-adrenergic receptor kinase: Identification of a novel protein kinase that phosphorylates the agonist-occupied form of the receptor. *Proc. Natl. Acad. Sci. USA* **1986**, *83*, 2797–2801. [CrossRef] [PubMed]
199. Lymperopoulos, A. Arrestins in the cardiovascular system: An update. *Prog. Mol. Biol. Transl. Sci.* **2018**, *159*, 27–57. [PubMed]
200. Kühn, H.; Hall, S.W. Light-induced binding of 48-kda protein to photoreceptor membranes is highly enhanced by phosphorylation of rhodopsin. *FEBS Lett.* **1984**, *176*, 473–478. [CrossRef]
201. Gurevich, V.V.; Chen, Q. Arrestins: Introducing signaling bias into multifunctional proteins. *Prog. Mol. Biol. Transl. Sci.* **2018**, *160*, 47–61.
202. Alloway, P.G.; Dolph, P.J. A role for the light-dependent phosphorylation of visual arrestin. *Prog. Mol. Biol. Transl. Sci.* **1999**, *96*, 6072. [CrossRef]
203. Hanyaloglu, A.C.; Zastrow, M.v. Regulation of gpcrs by endocytic membrane trafficking and its potential implications. *Annu. Rev. Pharmacol. Toxicol.* **2008**, *48*, 537–568. [CrossRef]
204. Dal Monte, M.; Cammalleri, M. Protective effects of β1/2 adrenergic receptor deletion in a model of oxygen-induced retinopathy. *Investig. Ophthalmol. Vis. Sci.* **2015**, *56*, 59–73. [CrossRef]
205. Martini, D.; Monte, M.D. Antiangiogenic effects of β2 -adrenergic receptor blockade in a mouse model of oxygen-induced retinopathy. *J. Neurochem.* **2011**, *119*, 1317–1329. [CrossRef]
206. Jiang, Y.; Zhang, Q. B2-adrenergic receptor knockout mice exhibit a diabetic retinopathy phenotype. *PLoS ONE* **2013**, *8*, e70555. [CrossRef]
207. Mori, A.; Sekito, A. Stimulation of β1- and β2-adrenoceptors dilates retinal blood vessels in rats. *Naunyn-Schmiedeberg's Arch. Pharmacol.* **2017**, *390*, 527–533. [CrossRef]
208. Mori, A.; Nakahara, T. Role of β3-adrenoceptors in regulation of retinal vascular tone in rats. *Naunyn-Schmiedeberg's Arch. Pharmacol.* **2011**, *384*, 603–608. [CrossRef] [PubMed]
209. Mori, A.; Taniai, A. Involvement of gi protein–dependent bkca channel activation in β2-adrenoceptor-mediated dilation of retinal arterioles in rats. *Naunyn-Schmiedeberg's Arch. Pharmacol.* **2020**, *393*, 2043–2052. [CrossRef] [PubMed]
210. Dal Monte, M.; Filippi, L. Beta3-adrenergic receptors modulate vascular endothelial growth factor release in response to hypoxia through the nitric oxide pathway in mouse retinal explants. *Naunyn-Schmiedeberg's Arch. Pharmacol.* **2013**, *386*, 269–278. [CrossRef] [PubMed]
211. Oikawa, F.; Nakahara, T. Protective effects of the β3-adrenoceptor agonist cl316243 against n-methyl-d-aspartate-induced retinal neurotoxicity. *Naunyn-Schmiedeberg's Arch. Pharmacol.* **2012**, *385*, 1077–1081. [CrossRef] [PubMed]
212. Jean-Luc, B. Beta3-adrenoreceptors in cardiovasular diseases: New roles for an "old" receptor. *Curr. Drug Deliv.* **2013**, *10*, 64–66.
213. Leineweber, K.; Büscher, R. B-adrenoceptor polymorphisms. *Naunyn-Schmiedeberg's Arch. Pharmacol.* **2004**, *369*, 1–22. [CrossRef] [PubMed]
214. Zalewska, M.; Siara, M. G protein-coupled receptors: Abnormalities in signal transmission, disease states and pharmacotherapy. *Acta Pol. Pharm.* **2014**, *71*, 229–243.
215. Dishy, V.; Sofowora, G.G. The effect of common polymorphisms of the β2-adrenergic receptor on agonist-mediated vascular desensitization. *N. Engl. J. Med.* **2001**, *345*, 1030–1035. [CrossRef]
216. Prokosch, V.; Panagis, L. A2-adrenergic receptors and their core involvement in the process of axonal growth in retinal explants. *Investig. Ophthalmol. Vis. Sci.* **2010**, *51*, 6688–6699. [CrossRef]

217. Wilhelm, B.; Lüdtke, H. Efficacy and tolerability of 0.2% brimonidine tartrate for the treatment of acute non-arteritic anterior ischemic optic neuropathy (naion): A 3-month, double-masked, randomised, placebo-controlled trial. *Graefe's Arch. Clin. Exp. Ophthalmol.* **2006**, *244*, 551–558.
218. Merin, S.; Obolensky, A. A pilot study of topical treatment with an alpha2-agonist in patients with retinal dystrophies. *J. Ocul. Pharmacol. Ther.* **2008**, *24*, 80–86. [CrossRef] [PubMed]
219. Filippi, L.; Cavallaro, G. Propranolol 0.1% eye micro-drops in newborns with retinopathy of prematurity: A pilot clinical trial. *Pediatric Res.* **2017**, *81*, 307–314. [CrossRef] [PubMed]

2

Cellular Reparative Mechanisms of Mesenchymal Stem Cells for Retinal Diseases

Suet Lee Shirley Ding [1], Suresh Kumar [2,3] and Pooi Ling Mok [1,3,*]

[1] Department of Biomedical Science, Faculty of Medicine and Health Sciences, University Putra Malaysia, 43400 UPM Serdang, Selangor, Malaysia; suetlee.ding@gmail.com
[2] Department of Medical Microbiology and Parasitology, Faculty of Medicine and Health Sciences, Universiti Putra Malaysia, 43400 UPM Serdang, Selangor, Malaysia; sureshkudsc@gmail.com
[3] Genetics and Regenerative Medicine Research Centre, Universiti Putra Malaysia, 43400 UPM Serdang, Selangor, Malaysia
* Correspondence: rachelmok2005@gmail.com;

Abstract: The use of multipotent mesenchymal stem cells (MSCs) has been reported as promising for the treatment of numerous degenerative disorders including the eye. In retinal degenerative diseases, MSCs exhibit the potential to regenerate into retinal neurons and retinal pigmented epithelial cells in both in vitro and in vivo studies. Delivery of MSCs was found to improve retinal morphology and function and delay retinal degeneration. In this review, we revisit the therapeutic role of MSCs in the diseased eye. Furthermore, we reveal the possible cellular mechanisms and identify the associated signaling pathways of MSCs in reversing the pathological conditions of various ocular disorders such as age-related macular degeneration (AMD), retinitis pigmentosa, diabetic retinopathy, and glaucoma. Current stem cell treatment can be dispensed as an independent cell treatment format or with the combination of other approaches. Hence, the improvement of the treatment strategy is largely subjected by our understanding of MSCs mechanism of action.

Keywords: mesenchymal stem cells; retinal degenerative diseases; MSC differentiation; paracrine activity; anti-inflammatory; immunomodulatory; anti-angiogenesis

1. Introduction

In the human eye, visual transmission begins when the light entered is being refracted to the posterior lining of the eye, referred to as the retina [1]. The retina is a conserved structure made up of five distinctive cellular layers of cell bodies and neuropils, comprising of photoreceptors, bipolar, horizontal, amacrine, and ganglion cells; and a supporting glial cell known as Müller glia (Figure 1) [1]. The light signal is first captured by the photoreceptors, which is then distributed along the Outer Nuclear Layer (ONL) of the retina [1]. The photoreceptors share a distinct structure consisting of an array of light-sensing rod and cone photoreceptor cell types, in which they are distinguishable by the light-sensitive, photo-pigment rhodopsin, and opsin, respectively [2]. These membranous photo-pigment proteins are tightly organized in a disc-like membrane to carry out signal transduction in the form of action potential [2]. Individually, the photoreceptors respond to light photon at a specific range of wavelength to achieve hyperpolarization state in the photoreceptor cell's membrane potential [3]. The photoreceptors convert light signal into electrical impulses and relay these impulses to bipolar cells [4]. The intensity of the relayed impulses were regulated by horizontal cells located in the outer plexiform layer [3]. The synaptic inputs were further relayed to ganglion cells and through the optic nerve into the visual cortex of the brain [4]. This process is known as photo-transduction in which failure will result in visual impairment.

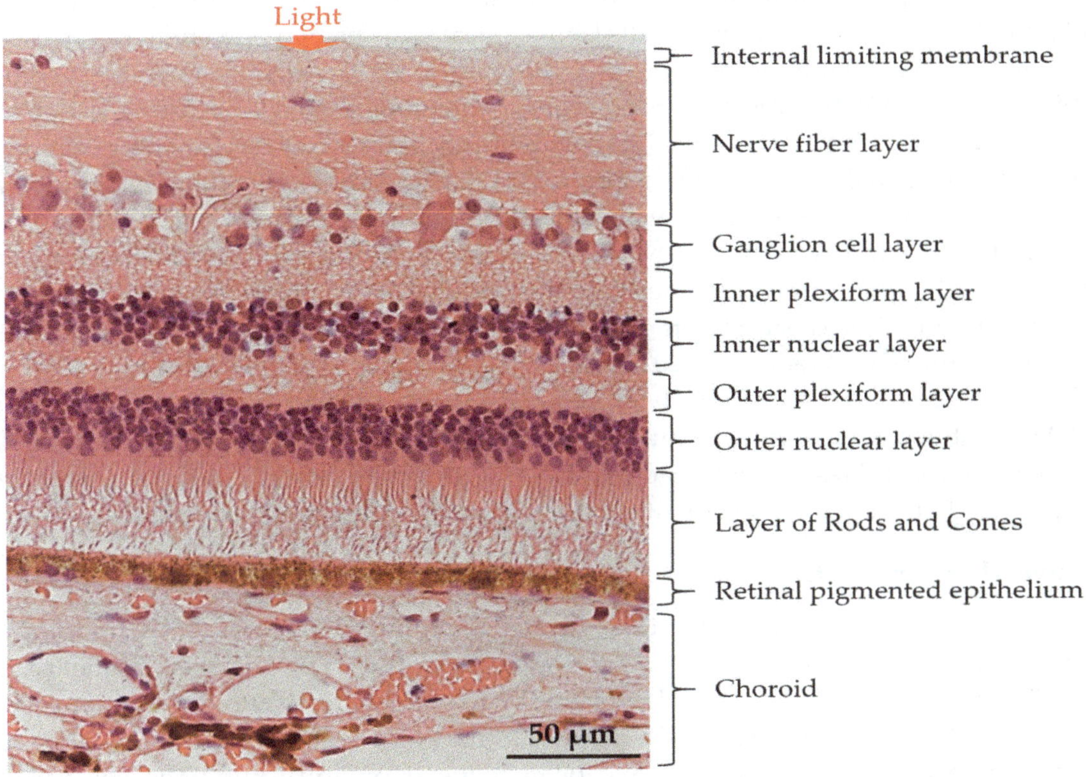

Figure 1. The basic retinal structure. Histological appearance of choroid and retinal layers. The retina is arranged in different layers of cells, from Retinal Pigment Epithelium (RPE), Outer Nuclear Layer (ONL), Outer Plexiform Layer (OPL), Inner Nuclear Layer (INL), Inner Plexiform Layer (IPL), and ganglion cell layer. The retinal layer harbors five retinal neuronal cells, primarily, the rod- and cone-photoreceptors, the Müller glia, the horizontal cell, the bipolar cell, the amacrine cell, and the Retinal Ganglion Cell (RGC). The arrow indicates the light transmission into the retina.

2. Current Therapeutic Approach for Retinal Diseases and Its Limitations

Ocular disorder is a universal health condition affecting either the anterior or posterior lining of the eye [6]. Over the years, expanding efforts have been carried out globally by the World Health Organization (WHO) to minimize visual impairment or blindness [6]. Treatment to reduce pathological condition affecting the posterior eye (majority in the retina) deserves greater attention due to the limited accessibility to treatment [6,7].

Retinal degenerative diseases are a group of heterogeneous conditions which include Age-related Macular Degeneration (AMD), retinitis pigmentosa, and diabetic retinopathy [8–11]. Numerous factors, such as oxidative stress, genetic diseases, light-induced damage, chemical insults, vascular defects or aging, have been suggested to contribute to the development of retinal degeneration [10,12–14]. Progressive degeneration of the retinal neurons, predominantly in the photoreceptors, Retinal Ganglion Cells (RGCs), as well as in the Retinal Pigment Epithelium (RPE), could result in severe deterioration of visual function and in due course, permanent visual loss [15,16]. As the mammalian retina has limited self-regenerative nature, visual impairment due to retinal degeneration is difficult to treat [17].

To date, therapeutic options such as surgical and pharmacological interventions are more suitable for patients with early diagnosis to minimize or reduce existing pathological retinal degenerative conditions from further deterioration [18,19]. In addition, some visual prostheses, such as Argus II, which is a cell-free retinal implant that acts on the RGCs to stimulate visual transmission in patients with retinitis pigmentosa or AMD, is costly and users reported difficulties in visual output interpretation [20,21]. In the meantime, results from clinical trials using Food and Drug Administration (FDA) approved anti-Vascular Endothelial Growth Factor (VEGF) drugs, such as Bevacizumab (Avastin) and Ranibizumab (Lucentis), have been reported as promising means to improve visual acuity and maintain retinal anatomy in patients associated with intraocular microvascular complications, such as diabetic retinopathy, retinal vein occlusion, and AMD [22,23]. Anti-VEGF antibodies could selectively bind to VEGF receptors present on the vascularized intraocular tissues—such as the conjunctiva, iris, retina, and RPE—and will therefore prevent massive release of pro-inflammatory cytokines responsible for pathologic intraocular neovascularization [24,25]. Nonetheless, these therapeutic approaches require multiple dosing regimens and repeated delivery via intravitreal injection in order to sustain visual acuity [26]. Wells et al., 2016 also evidenced patients were more prone to Anti-Platelet Trialists' Collaboration (APTC) events such as nonfatal strokes and vascular deaths following treatment with anti-VEGF antibodies [23]. In the course of exploring possible therapeutic alternatives, increasing evidence of research with Mesenchymal Stem Cells (MSCs), a type of adult stem cells, may prove to be a promising candidate for cell replacement therapy for retinal degenerative diseases.

3. Alternative Therapeutic Strategies for Retinal Repair Using Stem Cell-Based Approach

Much effort has been applied to the development of cell replacement therapies to functionally restore and replace lost or damaged tissues or organs that lack intrinsic tissue regenerative responses [27]. Stem cells are a type of cell with high self-renewability and differentiation capability, which are mostly favored to be used as a candidate for cell replacement therapy [28]. In retinal degenerative diseases, research works have been focused on improving the cell recovery and regeneration of terminally-differentiated retinal neuronal cells through delivery of unmodified or modified stem cells by genetic, chemical, or mechanical manipulation [29–32].

Embryonic Stem Cells (ESCs) hold an astonishing multi-germ layer differentiation potential that can be directed to form almost any cell type of the body [33]. Several clinical trials have advanced to evaluate the efficiency and safety of RPE-derived human ESCs (hESCs) on patients suffering from AMD (NCT01674829) or Stargardt's Macular Dystrophy (NCT01345006) [34]. The results of the first clinical study was not reported, however, the latter indicated that the patients benefitted from the transplantation and acquired general and peripheral visions by 8–20 points [34]. The investigators further suggested that RPE-derived hESCs could be a potential therapeutic cells that posed no evidence of unfavorable proliferation, immune-rejection, or uneventful systemic and ocular pathological conditions for a period of 22 months following to subretinal transplantation [34]. In another recent study, preliminary data on Phase I/II trial (NCT01344993) reported that patients affected by AMD demonstrated improvement in visual acuity after a year following allogeneic transplantation of pigmented epithelial cells derived from hESCs without any evidence of adverse effect or tumor formation related to the transplanted cells [34]. The results demonstrated that 13 out of the 18 patients showed reconstitution in the RPE structure and improvement in the functional activity [35]. The promising results have led to registration of more new and similar clinical investigations (NCT03046407, NCT02286089, and NCT02755428) to test the efficiency and safety of using RPE-derived hESCs for treatment of AMD. Despite this, their use often evokes ethical issues and requires combination treatment with immunosuppressive drugs to avoid immune rejection towards allogeneic transplant [29,36].

Alternatively, reprogramming somatic cells to a pluripotent state, termed as induced Pluripotent Stem Cells (iPSCs), has ultimately circumvented the risk to graft rejection and avoided ethical controversies in the use of human embryo [37]. The discovery in iPSC technology has regained embryonic-like property in a wide range of human somatic cells with Yamanaka pluripotent transcription factors, consisting of Octamer-binding protein 3/4 (Oct3/4), SRY-box (SOX2), Krüppel-like factor 4 (Klf4), and c-Myc [38]. Several studies have later revealed that cell reprogramming are independent of oncogenic factors, such as c-Myc and Klf4 [39,40], and using only human iPSCs transplanted into patients with exudative macular degeneration showed encouraging outcome in which patients who received iPSC-derived RPE sheet were hindered from further deterioration in visual acuity. However, in 2015, a disconcerting finding of gene mutation in the re-programmed cells prior to the transplantation has led to the termination of subsequent works in the study [39]. It is well documented that the tumorigenic potential in iPSCs, similar to those in ESCs, is the major clinical hurdle for cell-therapies. The risk of cell de-differentiation, genomic instability, and the presence of undifferentiated somatic cells in reprogrammed cells are highly susceptible to malignant transformation [41].

Epigenetic alteration in autologous iPSC-derived cells is capable of provoking T cell or Natural Killer (NK) cell dependent immune rejection prior to teratoma formation [42]. It was suggested that a minute shift in gene expression of transplanted iPSCs will be recognized as foreign antigen by the host defense mechanism to arrest possible tumor development [42,43]. In addition, Kawamura et al., 2016 further implied that the absence of host's immune surveillance predisposed to the risk of tumorigenicity, whereby iPSC-derived cells were witnessed to form tumor in immunosuppressed allogeneic transplantation model [42]. These results were comparable to what Hsieh et al., 2016 reported in iPSC-conditioned medium [44]. It was also evident that tumor growth may be driven by pluripotent-associated genes [45]. Currently, extensive efforts are being directed to reducing the chance of tumor formation in transplanted ESC and iPSC grafts [46]. As for the seemingly favorable clinical studies, the immunogenicity in iPSCs and the unpredictable risks in the late-onset oncogenic tendencies of the transplanted cells in humans have yet to be ascertained [35,47].

In order to overcome the risk of stem cell rejection during allogeneic or autologous transplantation, the quest continues to focus into stem cells isolated from multipotent, adult stromal cells, referred as MSCs. For cells to be considered as MSCs, they phenotypically express a distinct set of cell surface markers for CD105, CD90, and CD73 but lack CD79α, CD45, CD34, CD19, CD14, CD11b, and Human Leukocyte Antigen class II (HLA-II) [48]. In addition, these cells are able to undergo in vitro tri-lineage differentiation into osteogenic, adipogenic, and chondrogenic, as defined by the International Society for Cellular Therapies (ISCT) guideline for MSCs [48]. Owing to the lack of ethical concerns related to its use, MSCs can be found abundantly in the adult tissues, such as bone marrow, adipose tissue, and dental pulp, as well as in the fetal tissues and fluids, including the umbilical cord-tissue, -blood, and -amniotic fluid [49–54]. In addition to their wide distribution, MSCs are also known to possess minimal susceptibility to malignant transformation and are capable of avoiding immune cell recognition, hence providing a potential platform for allogeneic and autologous cell transplants [55].

Collectively, MSCs have been widely employed in various acute and chronic neurodegenerative conditions, including central-peripheral neuropathy, stroke, spinal cord injury, as well as ocular degenerative disorders [56–59]. From the accumulative pre-clinical studies (Table 1) and clinical trials (Table 2), administration of MSCs have revealed significant restoration of the visual system (Figure 2) through MSC-mediated therapeutic mechanisms involving (i) cell differentiation and trans-differentiation processes to replace loss or damaged cells, (ii) paracrine action for cell repair and revival, (iii) modulation of host's immune responses at inflamed site, and (iv) anti-angiogenic trophic action in certain ocular disorders (Figure 3) [48,54,60].

Table 1. Recent pre-clinical studies MSCs for the treatment of retinal diseases.

Disease Target	Source of MSCs	Experimental Design (Route of Delivery; Cell Concentration)	Research Outcomes	References
AMD	Rat bone marrow	Subretinal; 1.0×10^6 cells/eye	Integrated MSCs enhanced retinal cell survivability, architecture, and functionality of induced retinal degeneration rat model through MSC differentiation and replacement of loss RPE.	[61]
Diabetic retinopathy	Rat bone marrow	Intravitreal; 1.0×10^5 cells/μL	MSCs were found to integrate mostly in the diabetic eyes with reduction in retinal gliosis followed by an increased in retinal function.	[62]
	Mouse adipose tissue	Intravitreal; 1.0×10^5 cells/μL	MSCs regenerated into retinal astrocytes and RGC, and protected RGC from oxidative damage through secretion of MSC factors comprising of NGF, bFGF, and GDNF.	[51]
Retinal ischemia	Human bone marrow	Intravitreal; Not available	Administration of hypoxic-conditioned medium from MSCs in rat model of retinal ischemia promoted RGC survivability and restored retinal function through MSC paracrine effect.	[50]
	Not available	Intraocular; 1.0×10^4 cells/μL	Engrafted MSCs improved RGC survivability after retinal ischemic injury in a mouse model.	[63]
Retinal degeneration	Human bone marrow	Subretinal and intravitreal; 5.0×10^6 cells/μL	MSCs increased photoreceptor cell survivability from degeneration and sustained retinal function in retinal degenerating rat model.	[64]
		Epiretinally; 5×10^4 cells/μL		[65]
		Subretinal; 2.5×10^4 cells/μL		[66]
	Human umbilical cord blood	Subretinal; Not available	A significant preservation of degenerating rat retinal photoreceptors, function, and architecture through secretion of MSC neurotrophic factors, such as IL-6, FGF2, and BDNF.	[67]
Glaucoma	Rat bone marrow	In vitro co-culture system; Not available	In vitro co-cultured of MSCs with hypoxic-induced rat RGC exerted anti-apoptotic effect on RGC via reduction in caspase-3 activity.	[68]
	Human dental pulp, bone marrow, and adipose tissue	Intravitreal; 3.0×10^4 cells/μL	MSCs derived from human dental pulp and bone marrow increased RGC survivability and restored retinal function in ocular-induced hypertensive rat model.	[53]

MSCs, Mesenchymal Stem Cells; RPE, Retinal Pigment Epithelium; RGC, Retinal Ganglion Cell; NGF, Nerve Growth Factor; bFGF, basic Fibroblast Growth Factor; GDNF, Glial Cell Line-Derived Neurotrophic Factor; IL-6, Interleukin-6; FGF2, Fibroblast Growth Factor 2; BDNF, Brain-Derived Neurotrophic Factor.

Table 2. Current clinical trials using MSCs for the treatment of retinal diseases.

	Application	Source of MSCs	Experimental Design		Clinical Phases	Clinical Trials Identifier (ClinicalTrials.gov)
			Route of Delivery	Concentration of Stem cells		
i.	AMD	Umbilical tissue	Subretinal	6.0×10^4 cells–3.0×10^5 cells	Phase 1/2a	NCT01226628
		Bone marrow	Intravitreal	Not available	Phase 1/2	NCT02016508
		Bone marrow	Intravitreal	3.4×10^6 cells/0.1 mL	Phase 1	NCT01736059
		Bone marrow	Intravitreal	10.0×10^6 cells/0.1 mL	Phase 1/2	NCT01518127
ii.	Retinitis pigmentosa	Bone marrow	Intravitreal	3.4×10^6 cells/0.1 mL	Phase 1	NCT01736059
		Bone marrow	Intravitreal	1.0×10^6 cells/0.1 mL	Phase 1	NCT01531348
		Bone marrow	Intravitreal	10.0×10^6 cells/0.1 mL	Phase 2	NCT01560715
		Bone marrow	Intravitreal	3.4×10^6 cells/0.1 mL	Phase 1	NCT01736059
		Bone marrow	Intravitreal	10.0×10^6 cells/0.1 mL	Phase 1	NCT01068561
iii.	Diabetic retinopathy	Bone marrow	Intravitreal	3.4×10^6 cells/0.1 mL	Phase 1	NCT01736059
iv.	Ischemic retinopathy	Bone marrow	Intravitreal	10.0×10^6 cells/0.1 mL	Phase 1/2	NCT01518842

Phase 2a defines a pilot clinical trial for the evaluation of efficacy (and safety) in selective groups of patient subjects with associated disease or condition to be treated, diagnosed, or prevented.

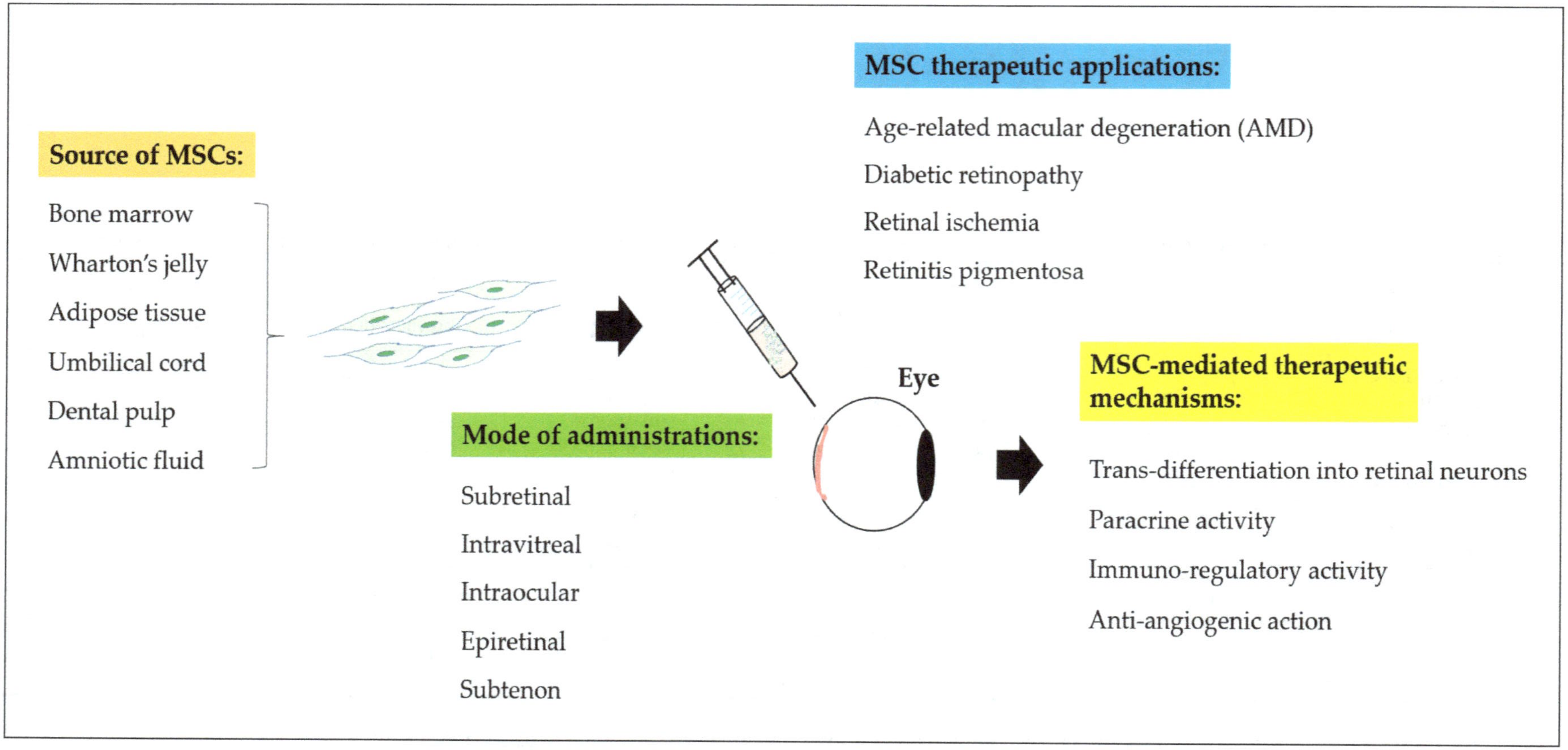

Figure 2. A schematic representation of Mesenchymal Stem Cells (MSCs) therapeutic strategies in retinal degenerative diseases. Different sources of MSC such as bone marrow, Wharton's jelly, adipose tissue, umbilical cord, dental pulp, and amniotic fluid have been discovered. Multiple routes of administration including subretinal, intravitreal, intraocular, epiretinal or subtenon injections can be implemented to deliver MSCs into the posterior lining of the eye. Delivery of MSCs into patients affected with posterior eye diseases including Age-related Macular Degeneration (AMD), diabetic retinopathy, retinal ischemia, and retinitis pigmentosa can be restored through trans-differentiation, paracrine activity, immuno-regulatory function, and anti-angiogenic action of MSCs.

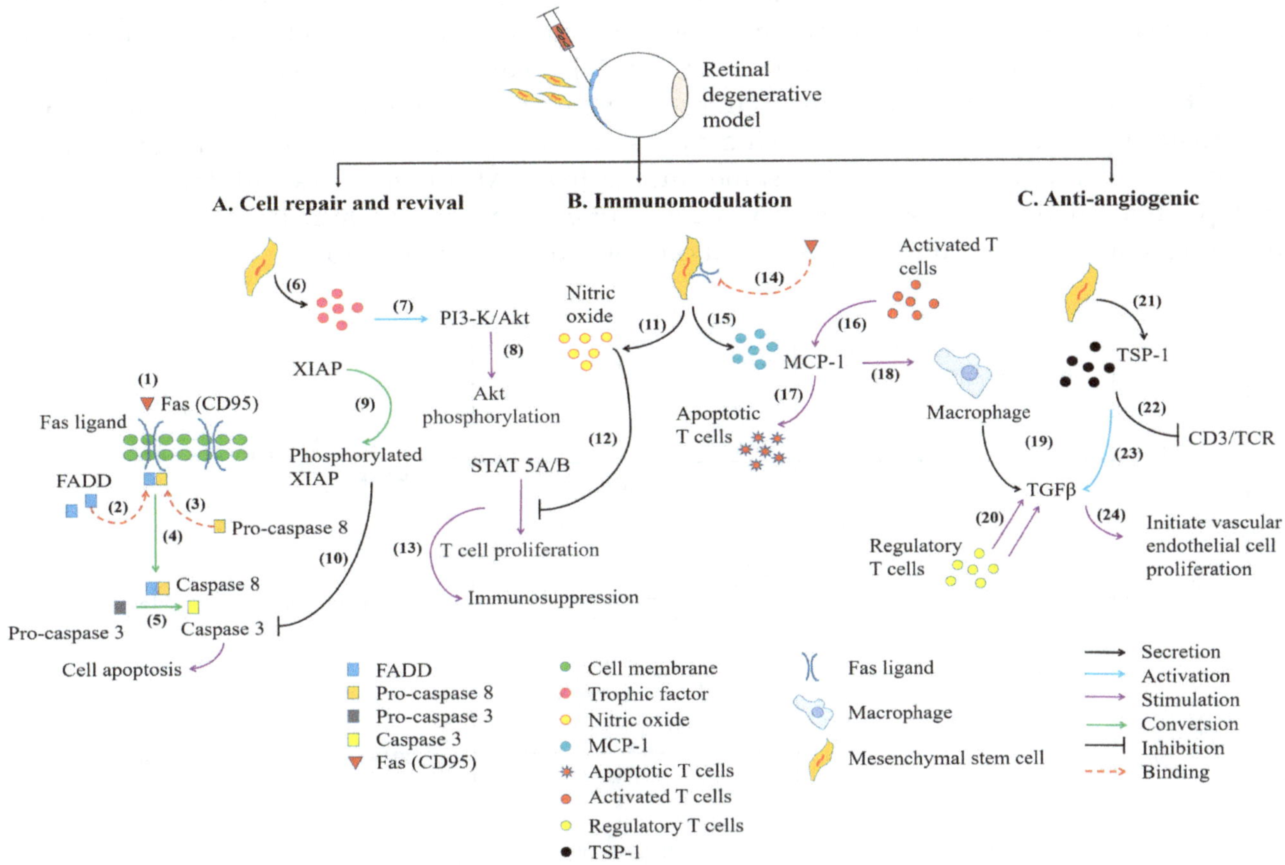

Figure 3. The signaling pathways involved in MSC-mediated therapeutic strategies in the eye. The cell death machinery involves (**1–2**) the binding of Fas/Fas ligand, which assembles Fas-Associated protein with Death Domain (FADD) to form a docking site for pro-caspase 8. This event initiates the (**3–4**) crosslinking of pro-caspase 8 to FADD and activates caspase 8. Activated caspase 8 (**5**) induces the conversion of pro-caspase 3 into caspase 3 which are essential for the initiation of cell apoptosis. The MSCs cellular reparative action can be exerted (**6–7**) by the release of its beneficial trophic factors, including IL-6 which could further promote the migration of MSCs towards site of injury. The binding of IL-6 on MSCs will activate Phosphatidylinositol-3-Kinase (PI3-K)/Akt signaling pathway. (**8–10**) The phosphorylated Akt then induces X-linked Inhibitor of Apoptosis Protein (XIAP) phosphorylation leading to inhibition of caspase 3 activity. The immunomodulatory action of MSCs can be depicted through (**11–13**) MSCs secretion of nitric oxide, which hampers Signal Transducer Activator-of-Transcription 5 (STAT5) phosphorylation and progressively leads to attenuation of T cell proliferation. The alleviation of T cell activity can be modulated through (**14–15**) the expression of Fas ligand on MSC cell surface. This creates binding site for Fas protein, in which induces MSCs secretion of Monocyte Chemotactic Protein-1 (MCP-1) protein. (**16–17**) The secreted proteins subsequently attract and induced apoptosis of activated T cells. (**18–20**) Accumulation of apoptotic T cells further stimulate macrophage to release Transforming Growth Factor-beta (TGF-β) and subsequently recruit regulatory T cells. The regulatory T cells could also convert cytotoxic T cells into regulatory T cells. In addition, (**21–22**) MSCs also secrete Thrombospondin type-1 (TSP-1) proteins to suppress Cluster of Differentiation 3 (CD3)/T cell receptor-mediated T cell proliferation. (**23–24**) The released TSP-1 proteins activate TGF-β activity to initiate vascular endothelial cell remodeling. MSC cell differentiation is not mentioned in this figure.

4. MSCs and Its Differentiation for the Treatment of Retinal Diseases

Like all mammals, human retina habitually lacks the ability to regenerate cells [27]. Controlled expression of certain intrinsic and/or extrinsic components regulates mammalian cells from regeneration at certain developmental stages [69]. Opposing this theory, numerous investigations have reported on the regenerative potential of MSC into endodermal and ectodermal lineages, in both in vitro and in vivo models (Figure 4) [70,71]. This lineage-switching phenomenon is referred to as either dedifferentiation or trans-differentiation processes [61]. De-differentiation is an innate regenerative activity, involving the reversion of a terminally differentiated cell into undifferentiated progenitor cell of the same lineage [69]. Meanwhile, trans-differentiation is a two-step differentiation process that involves the dedifferentiation of terminally-differentiated cells and subsequent differentiation into specialized cells of a different lineage [69].

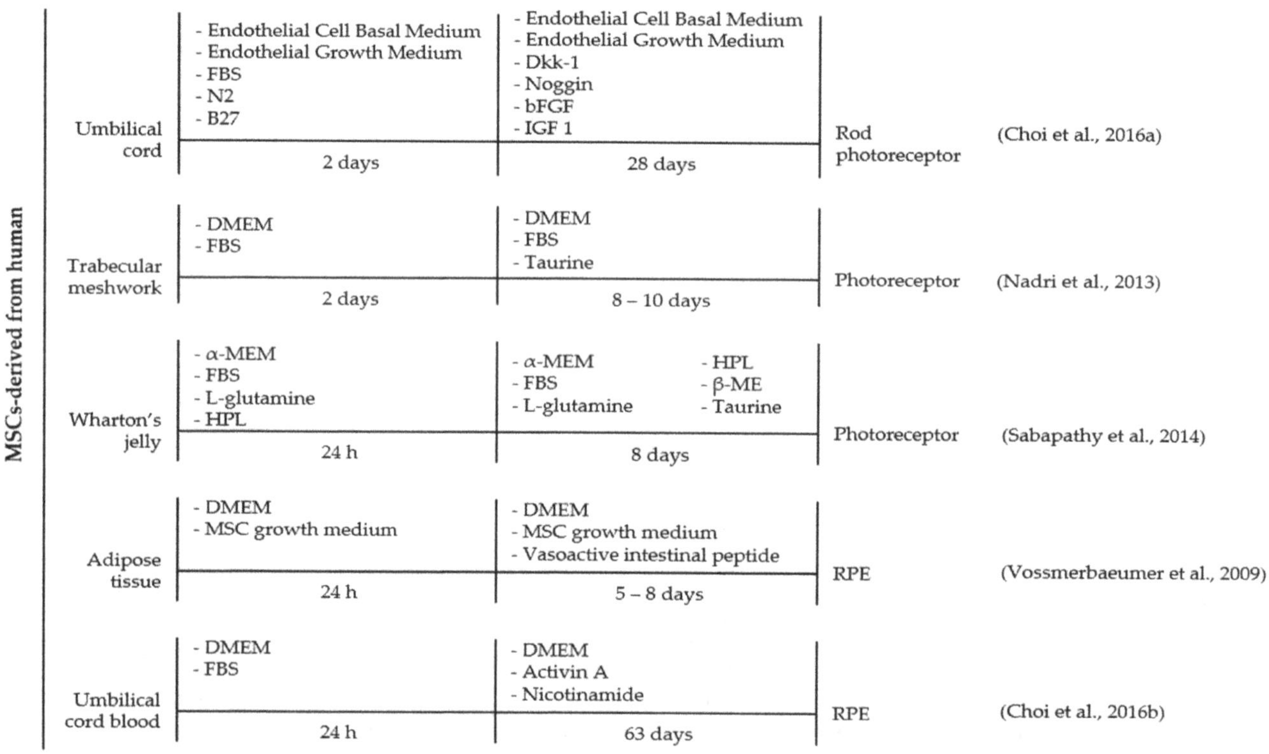

Figure 4. A timeline representation of strategies used to direct human MSCs differentiation into retinal neurons and retinal pigmented epithelial cells, in vitro. Generation of retinal cell from MSCs involve the manipulation of stem cell fate by cytokines, growth factors, or inhibitory peptides. MSCs derived from different tissue origins including bone marrow, dental pulp, umbilical cord, trabecular meshwork, Wharton's jelly, adipose tissue, and umbilical cord blood have previously demonstrated successful differentiation potential into retinal cells. The vast differentiation potential of MSCs into retinal cells includes photoreceptor, amacrine cell, RGC, and RPE-like cells that requires addition of specific cytokines, growth factors or inhibitory peptides. The differentiation factors are comprised of either taurine, activin A, basic Fibroblast Growth Factor (bFGF), β-mercaptoethanol (β-ME), Dickkopf Wnt signaling pathway inhibitor-1 (Dkk-1), noggin, insulin growth factor 1 (IGF 1), Human Platelet Lysate (HPL), and Vasoactive Intestinal Peptide. FBS, Fetal Bovine Serum; DMEM, Dulbecco's Modified Eagle Medium; α-MEM, alpha Minimal Essential Medium; B27, B27 supplement; and N2, N2 supplement.

A schematic diagram illustrated various protocols explored on MSCs of different origins to direct cell differentiation into retinal-like lineages, including photoreceptors and RPE cells (Figure 4). It was observed that MSCs can be induced to differentiate independently with taurine [72] or VIP [73] days or through a combination of selective induction cocktails [71,74,75] comprised of Dkk-1, Noggin, bFGF, and IGF 1 [71]; taurine, HPL, and β-ME [74]; or nicotinamide and activin A [71,75]. Meanwhile, using a different protocol on MSCs of similar source were found to develop into retinal neurons or RPE as early as 8 days [73] up to 63 days [75]. The discrepancy in the timeline encourages future optimization to achieve an immediate differentiation capacity at a minimal cost. It is also worth noting that the discrepancy between different protocols may also be influenced by the source [76,77] and isolation method of MSC [78], ontogenetic age [79,80], and others. Previous study observed MSCs derived from the umbilical cord expressed markers for pluripotent stem cells such as Octamer-binding protein 4 (Oct4), ATP-Binding Cassette sub-family G member 2 (ABCG2), Nanog homeobox (Nanog), and SOX2 that are crucial for neurogenic differentiation [78]. On the contrary, a study by Hu et al. evinced a distinct difference in neurogenic potential between human MSCs derived from adipose tissue and umbilical cord [81]. The author showed that cells derived from adipose tissue demonstrated greater efficiency into neuron-like cells up to 45% under retinoic acid induction medium [81]. The inconsistency data suggested the need to further examine the differentiation potential of MSCs from different sources to enable precise selection of MSCs for future regenerative study.

There has also been a debate raised over the poor lineage-switching potential in MSCs and only a marginal population of MSCs was observed to successfully differentiate into the desired cell [82]. One possible explanation has been suggested on the presence of "rare cell" that occupies the residential MSCs niche, termed as multilineage-differentiating stress-enduring (MUSE) cells, in which they represent the subpopulation of successfully differentiated MSCs [82,83]. MUSE cells are pluripotent somatic stem cells that are found intimately tied to the fibroblasts or MSCs of all tissues or organs, while they intrinsically displayed phenotypic markers of ESCs, iPSCs, and MSCs, such as Stage-Specific Embryonic Antigen-3 (SSEA-3), Tumor Resistance Antigen 1-60 (TRA-1-60), Nanog, Oct3/4, and SOX2 [83,84]. These cells displayed a comparable efficiency as ESCs in cell differentiation into multigerm lineages of mesodermal, endodermal, and ectodermal, and devoid of propensity into teratoma formation [83]. Since, MUSE cells are generally present in scarce number, selective isolation and expansion of pure MUSE cell population would elevate the chances to direct differentiation into retinal neurons or RPE and further enhance the efficiency of stem cell-based therapy in various human ocular degenerative disorders.

5. Paracrine Activity of MSCs Aids Retinal Cell Repair and Revival

One representative example of MSC paracrine support was provided by a recent study, whereby MSC homing response contributed to visual improvement with profound photoreceptor cells survivability in degenerating Royal College of Surgeons (RCS) rat retina [85]. The study outcome was attributed by trophic peptides released from MSCs to stimulate phagocytic activity of RPE on lethal accumulation of photoreceptor remnants [85]. Besides that, MSC transplantation was found to reduce substantial damage in the posterior lining of the eye and promote cell regeneration through paracrine release of Hypoxia-Inducible Factor-1α (HIF-1α) and axonal Growth-Associated Protein-43 (GAP–43), respectively [49].

The therapeutic effect of MSCs was also identified from the neurotrophic action of Ciliary Neurotrophic Factor (CNTF) and Brain-Derived Neurotrophic Factor (BDNF) secreted from MSCs in an oxidative-induced RGCs culture, and have led to the downregulation of pro-inflammatory cytokines, such as Tumor Necrosis Factor-α (TNF-α) and Interleukin-1β (IL-1β) release [86]. Mead et al., 2014 previously evidenced that MSCs exerted protective action in axotomized rat RGCs and promoted neurite formation, through paracrine release of Prostaglandin E2 Receptor (PGE2R) and IL-6-mediated growth factors, such as Platelet-Derived Growth Factor (PDGF) and Nerve Growth Factor (NGF) [87]. A similar trial was also reported that neurotrophic factors, such as NGF, bFGF, and Glial Cell Line-Derived Neurotrophic Factor (GDNF), released from adipose tissue-derived MSCs were found to preserve retinal ganglion cell survivability and reduced oxidative stress damage in the retina [51]. Furthermore, integrated MSCs were detected to differentiate into retinal astrocytes, RGCs, and pericytes in a diabetic-induced mice model [51]. The study outcome was further postulated in an induced diabetic retinopathy rat model, whereby successfully engrafted MSCs demonstrated selective protection against retinal gliosis along with the restoration of retinal vascular integrity and functionality and simultaneously differentiated into Müller glia [62]. These pre-clinical studies have confidently shown the promising use of MSCs in retinal degenerative disorders, most importantly, administration of MSCs were also found to illustrate infinite differentiation potential beyond its mesodermal origin.

Apart from the secretory cytokines and growth factors, there has been increasing evidence reported on the therapeutic potential of extracellular vesicles released from the MSCs [88,89]. Based on their distinct biological composition, extracellular vesicles can be classified into microvesicles, microparticles or exosomes, in which they play a crucial role in modulating cell-to-cell communication in a paracrine manner [88,90]. Considerable attention has been focused on MSC-derived exosomes, as these molecules are well-enriched with enzymes, which carry out protective responses in ocular degenerative disorders [88]. It was previously identified that the intravitreal delivery of exosomes-derived from MSCs exhibited restorative and protective actions in mouse models of retinal laser injury [91]. The author reported that transplanted exosomes were found to inhibit inflammatory-mediated cytokines infiltration, including Monocyte Chemotactic Protein-1 (MCP-1), TNF-α, and Intercellular Adhesion Molecule-1 (ICAM-1), hence, dampened macrophage- and T cell-mediated immune responses [91].

6. MSCs Alleviates Inflammation in Retinal Diseases

The human eye is a sophisticated organ that holds innate property in modulating immune responses in the ocular microenvironment. It has been described that parenchymal cells in the eye—particularly from the iris, ciliary body, and RPE cells—are able to suppress the intraocular immune reactivity, which makes the eye an immune-privileged site [92,93]. This innate feature in the eye is associated with the presence of immune modulators such as Fas ligand (CD95), Programmed Death Ligand (PDL)-1, Cytotoxic T-Lymphocyte Antigen 2 (CTLA-2), and CTLA-4 [93]. In addition, the presence of blood-aqueous barrier and Blood-Retina Barrier (BRB) that lack lymphatic drainage system could further limit possible migration of immune cells across the eye [93].

Dysregulation of the intraocular immune system is a pathological condition commonly manifested in AMD, glaucoma, diabetic retinopathy, and uveitis [94]. It is represented by a profound release of pro-inflammatory cytokines, chemokines, Matrix Metalloproteinases (MMPs), that progressively results in the loss of endothelium tight junction proteins, destruction, and leakage of BRB, hence, facilitating the infiltration of immune cells [95]. It is also believed that the privileged status of the eye may be compromised when predisposed to autoimmune reaction against self-antigens, for instance, uveal melanin, arrestin, interphotoreceptor retinoid-binding protein (IRBP), and recoverin, which are expressed in the retina, lens, and cornea [93,96]. This, in turn, will trigger subset of antigen-activated Cluster of Differentiation 4 (CD4) T cells to release transcription factors that are essential for downstream activation of autoimmune-associated T helper cell proliferation, such as IL-12 and Interferon-γ (IFN-γ) for T helper type 1 (T_h1) cells and IL-6, IL-21, IL-23, and Transforming Growth Factor-β (TGF-β) for T_h17 cells [96].

Sufficient number of studies have shown the capability of MSCs as a potent immunotherapeutic candidate to modulate both the innate and adaptive immune responses and suppress immunoreactivity in a broad range of diseases, including the eye [16,53]. Their immune evasive status could be attributed to the absence of activated T cells-associated ligands for HLA-I and co-stimulatory molecules from HLA-II, including CD40, CD80, and CD86, which are responsible in triggering graft rejection through T cell activation [55]. Also, these cells are capable to downregulate allogeneic lymphocyte proliferation and stimulate T regulatory cells expression [55,97]. Henceforth, MSCs are likely to obviate the major hurdles seen in cell therapy with ESCs and iPSCs [59,98]. In addition to their great potential, MSCs also have the advantages of fewer ethical concerns and less immune rejection. For example, Lee et al., 2015 has recently illustrated a significant preservation of the local niche of an inflammation-mediated murine eye model after periorbital delivery of MSCs [99]. The study showed that the restorative effect was accompanied by downregulation of pro-inflammatory cytokines activities and CD4 T cells infiltration [99]. Meanwhile, comparable study reported that MSCs were able to promote suppressive role of regulatory T cells and Forkhead Box P3 (FOXP3) transcription factor on T cell response via paracrine release of TGF-β from MSCs [100–102].

It has been reviewed that degeneration of RGC axons is a secondary phenomenon that occurs in patients with glaucoma that can be caused by retinal neovascularization or excessive accumulation of glutamate in the retina [103,104]. Based on an experimental study on glaucomatous rat model, the author reported an improvement in RGCs survivability following to intravitreal MSC transplantation [105]. The successfully integrated MSCs were found to reside into the ganglion cell layer and the INL, in which they influenced the host's immune response by suppressing pro-inflammatory cytokines production for interferon-γ and TNF-α via activation of IL-1 Receptor Antagonist (IL-1RA) and PGE2R [85].

7. MSCs Modulates Angiogenic Activity in Retinal Diseases

Sprouting of new blood vessels from pre-existing vessels through the angiogenesis process has been recognized in several types of ocular disorders, including diabetic retinopathy, retinopathy of prematurity, retinal vein occlusion, AMD, and glaucoma [8,16,54,106]. The occurrence of intraocular angiogenesis is further orchestrated by the increase of proangiogenic factors, mainly VEGF in the retinal neurons and RPE cells [95]. Untreated condition in the patients can lead to massive degradation in the basal endothelium membrane, neovascularization, and functional disruption of the neurosensors in the retina [107].

Among the vast potential of MSCs, substantial pre-clinical and clinical studies have equally validated on the therapeutic potential of MSCs in restoration of ocular neovascularization. In a recent study, subconjunctival injection bone marrow-derived MSCs into chemically-induced rat cornea where was found to encourage corneal wound healing and stabilized neovascularization lesion through suppression of VEGF, Matrix Metalloproteinase 9 (MMP-9), and Toll-Like Receptors (TLRs), which presumably contributes to the downregulation of pro-inflammatory cytokine production [108]. In an oxygen-induced retinopathy mouse model, intraperitoneal transplantation of human placental amniotic membrane-derived MSCs efficiently homed to and engrafted onto the injured site with profound release of angiogenic factor, Transforming Growth Factor-β1 (TGF-β1) from MSCs [54]. Astonishingly, upregulation of TGF-β1 level significantly decreased endothelial cell proliferation devoid of neovascularization while restoring retinal angiogenesis [54].

It is noteworthy that metabolic dysregulation in diabetic patients involves an uncontrollable increase in blood glucose (hyperglycemia) and cholesterol (hyperlipidemia) levels which stimulate VEGF secretion and ultimately contribute to the pathological alteration in the retinal vasculature integrity [107]. Ezquer et al., 2016 previously reported no apparent changes in pro-angiogenic expression observed upon administration of MSC in diabetic-induced mice model [51]. In this study, the author reported that MSCs exerted cytoprotective action through secretion of platelet-derived anti-angiogenic factor, Thrombospondin Type-1 (TSP-1), which is also produced primarily from the ocular surface epithelium, including the RPE, choroid, and Müller glial cells [51,109–111]. TSP-1 is a glycoprotein that has been found to modulate MSC functions including anti-angiogenic, anti-inflammatory, as well as immunomodulatory and immune-privileged activities in a healthy ocular microenvironment [51]. This data was further supported by a study conducted on an induced diabetic retinopathy rat model, whereby administration of bone marrow derived-MSCs demonstrated selective protection against retinal gliosis, increased vascular integrity, and retinal function [62]. At the same time, treated diabetic eyes demonstrated selective MSCs integration and differentiation into Müller glia, in comparison to the healthy sham eyes [62]. In another study conducted on diabetic-induced mice model, there was no sign of neovascularization, destruction of retinal vasculature, RGC loss or increase in pro-angiogenic factors upon intravitreal administration of adipose-derived MSCs [51].

In a preceding study [106], MSCs secreted a wide range of growth factors and cytokines as well as other proteolytic and angiogenic proteins—including VEGF, bFGF, TGF-β1, Stromal Cell-Derived Factor 1 (SDF-1), cathepsin, MMPs, and Plasminogen Activator Inhibitor 1 (PAI-1)—in response to tissue repair. The expression of these secretory proteins from MSCs were highly correlated to the onset of pathological neovascularization in the eye. A study by Hou et al., 2010 previously demonstrated that bone marrow-derived MSCs selectively migrated and engrafted into choroidal neovascularization lesions and further exaggerated the pathological condition [112]. A similar response has been reported on the secretory profile of diabetic rat bone marrow-derived MSCs were capable to induce angiogenic potential in in vitro endothelial cells culture via upregulation of secretion of local angiogenic mediators, such as Insulin-Like Growth Factor 1 (IGF-1) and Latent Transforming Growth Factor B Binding Protein type 1 (LTβP-1) [113]. Nevertheless, it was reported that subsequent expression of VEGF was found ameliorated, with an undetectable level of inflammatory proteins, such as TNF-α and FGF [113]. The suppression of inflammatory response could be contributed to the release of anti-angiogenic factors, such as TSP-1, from MSCs [51]. Chu et al., 2013 also observed similar suppression in VEGF activity, which was attributed to indirect inhibition of TSP-1 on VEGF receptor, via binding to CD36 and subsequent recruitment of SHP-1 onto VEGF target [114].

8. Conclusions

The limitation of self-reparative and regenerative capacity of retinal cells has opened up a new avenue for mesenchymal stem cell-based therapy for the treatment of ocular disorders including age-related macular degeneration, diabetic retinopathy, retinopathy of prematurity, and glaucoma. Mesenchymal stem cells have emerged as a valuable tool in cell replacement therapy due to the lack of ethical issues, easy isolation, and expansion and its privilege to escape from immune cell surveillance. MSCs have shown promising outcomes in cell regeneration through several mechanisms involving differentiation competency to replace loss or injured cells either by in vitro culture with selective growth factor or by the influence of local microenvironment regulatory inputs. We have also recapitulated the influence of paracrine network in MSCs that govern its reparative response through the release of restorative trophic factors and cytokines and further engaged on the modulatory signaling action of MSC in immune cells, specifically on T cell response. Lastly, the trophic factors or cytokines could also exert anti-angiogenic property involved in the restoration of ocular vasculopathies.

Acknowledgments: This research was completely supported by the grant from the Ministry of Science, Technology and Innovation (MOSTI), Malaysia through the Science Fund, under the grant number 5450817. This work was also supported by the Fundamental Research Grants Scheme (FRGS), Ministry of Education, Malaysia (Grant No.: 5524401), and the Putra Grants of Universiti Putra Malaysia, Malaysia (Grant No.: 9436300 and 9503900).

Author Contributions: Suet Lee Shirley Ding composed this manuscript and prepared the figures; Suresh Kumar analyzed, edited, and commented on both the manuscript and figures; Pooi Ling Mok conceived the manuscript design, analyzed, edited, and approved the manuscript. All authors reviewed the manuscript.

1. Athanasiou, D.; Aguilà, M.; Bevilacqua, D.; Novoselov, S.S.; Parfitt, D.A.; Cheetham, M.E. The cell stress machinery and retinal degeneration. *FEBS Lett.* **2013**, *587*, 2008–2017. [CrossRef] [PubMed]
2. Mannu, G.S. Retinal phototransduction. *Neurosciences* **2014**, *19*, 275–280. [PubMed]
3. Reed, B.T.; Behar-Cohen, F.; Krantic, S. Seeing early signs of Alzheimer's Disease through the lens of the eye. *Curr. Alzheimer Res.* **2016**, *14*, 6–17. [CrossRef]
4. Palczewski, K. Chemistry and biology of vision. *J. Biol. Chem.* **2012**, *287*, 1612–1619. [CrossRef] [PubMed]
5. Triviño, A.; de Hoz, R.; Rojas, B.; Gallego, B.I.; Ramírez, A.I.; Salazar, J.J.; Ramírez, J.M. Effects of Hypercholesterolaemia in the Retina. In *Ocular Diseases*; InTech: Rijeka, Croatia, 2012.
6. WHO (World Health Organization). WHO 2017. Available online: http://www.who.int/blindness/en/ (accessed on 8 June 2017).
7. Weng, Y.; Liu, J.; Jin, S.; Guo, W.; Liang, X.; Hu, Z. Nanotechnology-based strategies for treatment of ocular disease. *Acta Pharm. Sin. B* **2017**, *7*, 281–291. [CrossRef] [PubMed]
8. Hernández, C.; Dal Monte, M.; Simó, R.; Casini, G. Neuroprotection as a therapeutic target for diabetic retinopathy. *J. Diabetes Res.* **2016**, *2016*, 9508541. [CrossRef] [PubMed]

9. Narayan, D.S.; Wood, J.P.M.; Chidlow, G.; Casson, R.J. A review of the mechanisms of cone degeneration in retinitis pigmentosa. *Acta Ophthalmol.* **2016**, *94*, 748–754. [CrossRef] [PubMed]
10. Shaw, P.X.; Stiles, T.; Douglas, C.; Ho, D.; Fan, W.; Du, H.; Xiao, X. Oxidative stress, innate immunity, and age-related macular degeneration. *AIMS Mol. Sci.* **2016**, *3*, 196–221. [CrossRef] [PubMed]
11. Weinreb, R.N.; Aung, T.; Medeiros, F.A. The Pathophysiology and Treatment of Glaucoma. *JAMA* **2014**, *311*, 1901–1911. [CrossRef] [PubMed]
12. Van Norren, D.; Vos, J.J. Light damage to the retina: An historical approach. *Eye* **2016**, *30*, 169–172. [CrossRef] [PubMed]
13. Cejkova, J.; Trosan, P.; Cejka, C.; Lencova, A.; Zajicova, A.; Javorkova, E.; Kubinova, S.; Sykova, E.; Holan, V. Suppression of alkali-induced oxidative injury in the cornea by mesenchymal stem cells growing on nanofiber scaffolds and transferred onto the damaged corneal surface. *Exp. Eye Res.* **2013**, *116*, 312–323. [CrossRef] [PubMed]
14. Semeraro, F.; Cancarini, A.; dell'Omo, R.; Rezzola, S.; Romano, M.R.; Costagliola, C. Diabetic retinopathy: Vascular and inflammatory disease. *J. Diabetes Res.* **2015**, *2015*, 582060. [CrossRef] [PubMed]
15. Chader, G.J.; Young, M. Preface: Sight restoration through stem cell therapy. *Investig. Ophthalmol. Vis. Sci.* **2016**, *57*, ORSFa1–ORSFa5. [CrossRef] [PubMed]
16. Shirley Ding, S.L.; Leow, S.N.; Munisvaradass, R.; Koh, E.H.; Bastion, M.L.C.; Then, K.Y.; Kumar, S.; Mok, P.L. Revisiting the role of erythropoietin for treatment of ocular disorders. *Eye* **2016**, *30*, 1293–1309. [CrossRef] [PubMed]
17. Klassen, H. Stem cells in clinical trials for treatment of retinal degeneration. *Expert Opin. Biol. Ther.* **2015**, *16*, 7–14. [CrossRef] [PubMed]
18. Villegas, V.M.; Aranguren, L.A.; Kovach, J.L.; Schwartz, S.G.; Flynn, H.W., Jr. Current advances in the treatment of neovascular age-related macular degeneration. *Expert Opin. Drug Deliv.* **2016**, *14*, 273–282. [CrossRef] [PubMed]
19. Ferrara, N.; Adamis, A.P. Ten years of anti-vascular endothelial growth factor therapy. *Nat. Rev. Drug Discov.* **2016**, *15*, 385–403. [CrossRef] [PubMed]
20. Greenemeier, L. FDA approves first retinal implant. *Nature* **2013**, *15*, 26–28. [CrossRef]
21. Da Cruz, L.; Dorn, J.D.; Humayun, M.S.; Dagnelie, G.; Handa, J.; Barale, P.O.; Sahel, J.A.; Stanga, P.E.; Hafezi, F.; Safran, A.B.; et al. Five-year safety and performance results from the Argus II Retinal Prosthesis System Clinical Trial. *Ophthalmology* **2016**, *123*, 2248–2254. [CrossRef] [PubMed]
22. Rayess, N.; Houston, S.K.S.; Gupta, O.P.; Ho, A.C.; Regillo, C.D. Treatment outcomes after 3 years in neovascular age-related macular degeneration using a treat-and-extend regimen. *Am. J. Ophthalmol.* **2015**, *159*, 3–8.e1. [CrossRef] [PubMed]
23. Wells, J.A.; Glassman, A.R.; Ayala, A.R.; Jampol, L.M.; Bressler, N.M.; Bressler, S.B.; Brucker, A.J.; Ferris, F.L.; Hampton, G.R.; Jhaveri, C.; et al. Aflibercept, Bevacizumab, or Ranibizumab for Diabetic Macular Edema two-year results from a comparative effectiveness randomized clinical trial. *Ophthalmology* **2016**, *123*, 1351–1359. [CrossRef] [PubMed]
24. Boyer, D.S.; Hopkins, J.J.; Sorof, J.; Ehrlich, J.S. Anti-vascular endothelial growth factor therapy for diabetic macular edema. *Ther. Adv. Endocrinol. Metab.* **2013**, *4*, 151–169. [CrossRef] [PubMed]
25. Ferrara, N. VEGF and intraocular neovascularization: From discovery to therapy. *Transl. Vis. Sci. Technol.* **2016**, *5*, 10. [CrossRef] [PubMed]
26. Solomon, S.D.; Lindsley, K.; Vedula, S.S.; Krzystolik, M.G.; Hawkins, B.S. Anti-vascular endothelial growth factor for neovascular age-related macular degeneration. *Cochrane Database Syst. Rev.* **2014**, *8*, CD005139.
27. Eguizabal, C.; Montserrat, N.; Veiga, A.; Belmonte, J.I. Dedifferentiation, transdifferentiation, and reprogramming: Future directions in regenerative medicine. *Semin. Reprod. Med.* **2013**, *31*, 82–94. [CrossRef] [PubMed]
28. Christodoulou, I.; Kolisis, F.N.; Papaevangeliou, D.; Zoumpourlis, V. Comparative evaluation of human mesenchymal stem cells of fetal (Wharton's Jelly) and adult (adipose tissue) origin during prolonged in vitro expansion: Considerations for cytotherapy. *Stem Cells Int.* **2013**, *2013*, 246134. [CrossRef] [PubMed]
29. Assawachananont, J.; Mandai, M.; Okamoto, S.; Yamada, C.; Eiraku, M.; Yonemura, S.; Sasai, Y.; Takahashi, M. Transplantation of embryonic and induced pluripotent stem cell-derived 3D retinal sheets into retinal degenerative mice. *Stem Cell Rep.* **2014**, *2*, 662–674. [CrossRef] [PubMed]

30. Rezanejad, H.; Soheili, Z.S.; Haddad, F.; Matin, M.M.; Samiei, S.; Manafi, A.; Ahmadieh, H. In vitro differentiation of adipose-tissue-derived mesenchymal stem cells into neural retinal cells through expression of human *PAX6* (5a) gene. *Cell Tissue Res.* **2014**, *356*, 65–75. [CrossRef] [PubMed]
31. Ng, T.K.; Yung, J.S.Y.; Choy, K.W.; Cao, D.; Leung, C.K.S.; Cheung, H.S.; Pang, C.P. Transdifferentiation of periodontal ligament-derived stem cells into retinal ganglion-like cells and its microRNA signature. *Sci. Rep.* **2015**, *5*, 16429. [CrossRef] [PubMed]
32. Worthington, K.S.; Green, B.J.; Rethwisch, M.; Wiley, L.A.; Tucker, B.A.; Guymon, C.A.; Salem, A.K. Neuronal differentiation of induced pluripotent stem cells on surfactant templated chitosan hydrogels. *Biomacromolecules* **2016**, *17*, 1684–1695. [CrossRef] [PubMed]
33. Nicoară, S.D.; Şuşman, S.; Tudoran, O.; Bărbos, O.; Chereches, G.; Aştilean, S.; Potara, M.; Soriţău, O. Novel strategies for the improvement of stem cells' transplantation in degenerative retinal diseases. *Stem Cells Int.* **2016**, *2016*, 1236721. [CrossRef] [PubMed]
34. Schwartz, S.D.; Regillo, C.D.; Lam, B.L.; Eliott, D.; Rosenfeld, P.J.; Gregori, N.Z.; Hubschman, J.P.; Davis, J.L.; Heilwell, G.; Spirn, M.; et al. Human embryonic stem cell-derived retinal pigment epithelium in patients with age-related macular degeneration and Stargardt's macular dystrophy: Follow-up of two open-label phase 1/2 studies. *Lancet* **2015**, *385*, 509–516. [CrossRef]
35. Schwartz, S.D.; Tan, G.; Hosseini, H.; Nagiel, A. Subretinal transplantation of embryonic stem cell-derived retinal pigment epithelium for the treatment of macular degeneration: An assessment at 4 years. *Investig. Ophthalmol. Vis. Sci.* **2016**, *57*, ORSFc1–ORSFc9. [CrossRef] [PubMed]
36. Seki, T.; Fukuda, K. Methods of induced pluripotent stem cells for clinical application. *World J. Stem Cells* **2015**, *7*, 116–125. [CrossRef] [PubMed]
37. Takahashi, K.; Yamanaka, S. Induced pluripotent stem cells in medicine and biology. *Development* **2013**, *140*, 2457–2461. [CrossRef] [PubMed]
38. Osakada, F.; Ikeda, H.; Mandai, M.; Wataya, T.; Watanabe, K.; Yoshimura, N.; Akaike, A.; Sasai, Y.; Takahashi, M. Toward the generation of rod and cone photoreceptors from mouse, monkey and human embryonic stem cells. *Nat. Biotechnol.* **2008**, *26*, 215–224. [CrossRef] [PubMed]
39. Alexander, P.; Thomson, H.A.J.; Luff, A.J.; Lotery, A.J. Retinal pigment epithelium transplantation: Concepts, challenges, and future prospects. *Eye* **2015**, *29*, 992–1002. [CrossRef] [PubMed]
40. Li, Y.; Li, X.; Zhao, H.; Feng, R.; Zhang, X.; Tai, D.; An, G.; Wen, J.; Tan, J. Efficient induction of pluripotent stem cells from menstrual blood. *Stem Cells Dev.* **2013**, *22*, 1147–1158. [CrossRef] [PubMed]
41. Nakano-Okuno, M.; Borah, B.R.; Nakano, I. Ethics of iPSC-Based clinical research for age-related macular degeneration: Patient-centered risk-benefit analysis. *Stem Cell Rev. Rep.* **2014**, *10*, 743–752. [CrossRef] [PubMed]
42. Kawamura, A.; Miyagawa, S.; Fukushima, S.; Kawamura, T.; Kashiyama, N.; Ito, E.; Masuda, S.; Toda, K.; Hatazawa, J.; Morii, E. Teratocarcinomas arising from allogeneic induced pluripotent stem cell-derived cardiac tissue constructs provoked host immune rejection in mice. *Sci. Rep.* **2016**, *6*, 19464. [CrossRef] [PubMed]
43. Itakura, G.; Kobayashi, Y.; Nishimura, S.; Iwai, H.; Takano, M.; Iwanami, A.; Toyama, Y.; Okano, H.; Nakamura, M. Controlling immune rejection is a fail-safe system against potential tumorigenicity after human iPSC-derived neural stem cell transplantation. *PLoS ONE* **2015**, *10*, e0116413. [CrossRef] [PubMed]
44. Hsieh, C.-T.; Luo, Y.-H.; Chien, C.-S.; Wu, C.-H.; Tseng, P.-C.; Chiou, S.-H.; Lee, Y.C.; Whang-Peng, J.; Chen, Y.M. Induced pluripotent stem cell–conditioned medium suppressed melanoma tumorigenicity through the enhancement of natural-killer cellular immunity. *J. Immunother.* **2016**, *39*, 153–159. [CrossRef] [PubMed]
45. Scheiner, Z.S.; Talib, S.; Feigal, E.G. The potential for immunogenicity of autologous induced pluripotent stem cell-derived therapies. *J. Biol. Chem.* **2014**, *289*, 4571–4577. [CrossRef] [PubMed]
46. Zarbin, M. Cell-based therapy for degenerative retinal disease. *Trends Mol. Med.* **2016**, *22*, 115–134. [CrossRef] [PubMed]
47. Song, W.K.; Park, K.M.; Kim, H.J.; Lee, J.H.; Choi, J.; Chong, S.Y.; Shim, S.H.; del Priore, L.V.; Lanza, R. Treatment of macular degeneration using embryonic stem cell-derived retinal pigment epithelium: Preliminary results in Asian patients. *Stem Cell Rep.* **2015**, *4*, 860–872. [CrossRef] [PubMed]
48. Mok, P.L.; Leong, C.F.; Cheong, S.K. Cellular mechanisms of emerging applications of mesenchymal stem cells. *Malays. J. Pathol.* **2013**, *35*, 17–32. [PubMed]

49. Chung, S.; Rho, S.; Kim, G.; Kim, S.-R.; Baek, K.-H.; Kang, M.; Lew, H. Human umbilical cord blood mononuclear cells and chorionic plate-derived mesenchymal stem cells promote axon survival in a rat model of optic nerve crush injury. *Int. J. Mol. Med.* **2016**, *37*, 1170–1180. [CrossRef] [PubMed]
50. Roth, S.; Dreixler, J.C.; Mathew, B.; Balyasnikova, I.; Mann, J.R.; Boddapoti, V.; Xue, L.; Lesniak, M.S. Hypoxic-Preconditioned bone marrow stem cell medium significantly improves outcome after retinal ischemia in rats. *Investig. Ophthalmol. Vis. Sci.* **2016**, *57*, 3522–3532. [CrossRef] [PubMed]
51. Ezquer, M.; Urzua, C.A.; Montecino, S.; Leal, K.; Conget, P.; Ezquer, F. Intravitreal administration of multipotent mesenchymal stromal cells triggers a cytoprotective microenvironment in the retina of diabetic mice. *Stem Cell Res. Ther.* **2016**, *7*, 42. [CrossRef] [PubMed]
52. Leow, S.N.; Luu, C.D.; Nizam, M.H.H.; Mok, P.L.; Ruhaslizan, R.; Wong, H.S.; Halim, W.H.W.A.; Ng, M.H.; Ruszymah, B.H.I.; Chowdhury, S.R.; et al. Safety and efficacy of human Wharton's Jelly-derived mesenchymal stem cells therapy for retinal degeneration. *PLoS ONE* **2015**, *10*, e0128973. [CrossRef] [PubMed]
53. Mead, B.; Hill, L.J.; Blanch, R.J.; Ward, K.; Logan, A.; Berry, M.; Leadbeater, W.; Scheven, B.A. Mesenchymal stromal cell-mediated neuroprotection and functional preservation of retinal ganglion cells in a rodent model of glaucoma. *Cytotherapy* **2016**, *18*, 487–496. [CrossRef] [PubMed]
54. Kim, K.S.; Park, J.M.; Kong, T.H.; Kim, C.; Bae, S.H.; Kim, H.W.; Moon, J. Retinal angiogenesis effects of TGF-β1 and paracrine factors secreted from human placental stem cells in response to a pathological environment. *Cell Transplant.* **2016**, *25*, 1145–1157. [CrossRef] [PubMed]
55. Zhao, Q.; Ren, H.; Han, Z. Mesenchymal stem cells: Immunomodulatory capability and clinical potential in immune diseases. *J. Cell. Immunother.* **2016**, *2*, 3–20. [CrossRef]
56. Cejka, C.; Holan, V.; Trosan, P.; Zajicova, A.; Javorkova, E.; Cejkova, J. The favorable effect of mesenchymal stem cell treatment on the antioxidant protective mechanism in the corneal epithelium and renewal of corneal optical properties changed after alkali burns. *Oxid. Med. Cell. Longev.* **2016**, *2016*, 5843809. [CrossRef] [PubMed]
57. Schafer, R.; Spohn, G.; Baer, P.C. Mesenchymal stem/stromal cells in regenerative medicine: Can preconditioning strategies improve therapeutic efficacy? *Transfus. Med. Hemother.* **2016**, *43*, 256–267. [CrossRef] [PubMed]
58. Zeng, X.; Ma, Y.H.; Chen, Y.F.; Qiu, X.C.; Wu, J.L.; Ling, E.A.; Zeng, Y.S. Autocrine fibronectin from differentiating mesenchymal stem cells induces the neurite elongation in vitro and promotes nerve fiber regeneration in transected spinal cord injury. *J. Biomed. Mater. Res. A* **2016**, *104*, 1902–1911. [CrossRef] [PubMed]
59. Nakano, M.; Nagaishi, K.; Konari, N.; Saito, Y.; Chikenji, T.; Mizue, Y.; Fujimiya, M. Bone marrow-derived mesenchymal stem cells improve diabetes-induced cognitive impairment by exosome transfer into damaged neurons and astrocytes. *Sci. Rep.* **2016**, *6*, 24805. [CrossRef] [PubMed]
60. Zhao, P.-T.; Zhang, L.-J.; Shao, H.; Bai, L.-L.; Yu, B.; Su, C.; Dong, L.J.; Liu, X.; Li, X.R.; Zhang, X.M. Therapeutic effects of mesenchymal stem cells administered at later phase of recurrent experimental autoimmune uveitis. *Int. J. Ophthalmol.* **2016**, *9*, 1381–1389. [PubMed]
61. Guan, Y.; Cui, L.; Qu, Z.; Lu, L.; Wang, F.; Wu, Y.; Zhang, J.; Gao, F.; Tian, H.; Xu, L.; et al. Subretinal transplantation of rat MSCs and erythropoietin gene modified rat MSCs for protecting and rescuing degenerative retina in rats. *Curr. Mol. Med.* **2013**, *13*, 1419–1431. [CrossRef] [PubMed]
62. Çerman, E.; Akkoç, T.; Eraslan, M.; Şahin, Ö.; Özkara, S.; Aker, F.V.; Subaşı, C.; Karaöz, E.; Akkoç, T. Retinal electrophysiological effects of intravitreal bone marrow derived mesenchymal stem cells in streptozotocin induced diabetic rats. *PLoS ONE* **2016**, *11*, e0156495.
63. Gramlich, O.W.; Burand, A.J.; Brown, A.J.; Deutsch, R.J.; Kuehn, M.H.; Ankrum, J.A. Cryopreserved mesenchymal stromal cells maintain potency in a retinal ischemia/reperfusion injury model: Toward an off-the-shelf therapy. *Sci. Rep.* **2016**, *6*, 26463. [CrossRef] [PubMed]
64. Tzameret, A.; Sher, I.; Belkin, M.; Treves, A.J.; Meir, A.; Nagler, A.; Levkovitch-Verbin, H.; Barshack, I.; Rosner, M.; Rotenstreich, Y. Transplantation of human bone marrow mesenchymal stem cells as a thin subretinal layer ameliorates retinal degeneration in a rat model of retinal dystrophy. *Exp. Eye Res.* **2014**, *118*, 135–144. [CrossRef] [PubMed]
65. Tzameret, A.; Sher, I.; Belkin, M.; Treves, A.J.; Meir, A.; Nagler, A.; Levkovitch-Verbin, H.; Rotenstreich, Y.; Solomon, A.S. Epiretinal transplantation of human bone marrow mesenchymal stem cells rescues retinal and vision function in a rat model of retinal degeneration. *Stem Cell Res.* **2015**, *15*, 387–394. [CrossRef] [PubMed]

66. Lu, B.; Wang, S.; Girman, S.; McGill, T.; Ragaglia, V.; Lund, R. Human adult bone marrow-derived somatic cells rescue vision in a rodent model of retinal degeneration. *Exp. Eye Res.* **2010**, *91*, 449–455. [CrossRef] [PubMed]
67. Lund, R.D.; Wang, S.; Lu, B.; Girman, S.; Holmes, T.; Sauvé, Y.; Messina, D.J.; Harris, I.R.; Kihm, A.J.; Harmon, A.M.; et al. Cells isolated from umbilical cord tissue rescue photoreceptors and visual functions in a rodent model of retinal disease. *Stem Cells* **2009**, *25*, 602–611. [CrossRef]
68. Yuan, J.; Yu, J.X. Gender difference in the neuroprotective effect of rat bone marrow mesenchymal cells against hypoxia-induced apoptosis of retinal ganglion cells. *Neural Regen. Res.* **2016**, *11*, 846–853. [CrossRef] [PubMed]
69. Jopling, C.; Boue, S.; Izpisua Belmonte, J.C. Dedifferentiation, transdifferentiation and reprogramming: Three routes to regeneration. *Nat. Rev. Mol. Cell Biol.* **2011**, *12*, 79–89. [CrossRef] [PubMed]
70. Katagiri, H.; Kushida, Y.; Nojima, M.; Kuroda, Y.; Wakao, S.; Ishida, K.; Endo, F.; Kume, K.; Takahara, T.; Nitta, H.; et al. A distinct subpopulation of bone marrow mesenchymal stem cells, muse cells, directly commit to the replacement of liver components. *Am. J. Transplant.* **2016**, *16*, 468–483. [CrossRef] [PubMed]
71. Choi, S.W.; Shin, J.; Kim, J.; Shin, T.-H.; Seo, Y. Direct cell fate conversion of human somatic stem cells into cone and rod photoreceptor-like cells by inhibition of microRNA-203. *Oncotarget* **2016**, *7*, 42139–42149. [CrossRef] [PubMed]
72. Nadri, S.; Yazdani, S.; Arefian, E.; Gohari, Z.; Eslaminejad, M.B.; Kazemi, B.; Soleimani, M. Mesenchymal stem cells from trabecular meshwork become photoreceptor-like cells on amniotic membrane. *Neurosci. Lett.* **2013**, *541*, 43–48. [CrossRef] [PubMed]
73. Vossmerbaeumer, U.; Ohnesorge, S.; Kuehl, S.; Haapalahti, M.; Kluter, H.; Jonas, J.B.; Thierse, H.J.; Bieback, K. Retinal pigment epithelial phenotype induced in human adipose tissue-derived mesenchymal stromal cells. *Cytotherapy* **2009**, *11*, 177–188. [CrossRef] [PubMed]
74. Sabapathy, V.; Sundaram, B.; Vm, S.; Mankuzhy, P.; Kumar, S. Human wharton's jelly mesenchymal stem cells plasticity augments scar-free skin wound healing with hair growth. *PLoS ONE* **2014**, *9*, e93726. [CrossRef] [PubMed]
75. Choi, S.W.; Kim, J.-J.; Seo, M.-S.; Park, S.-B.; Shin, T.-H.; Shin, J.-H.; Seo, Y.; Kim, H.S.; Kang, K.S. Inhibition by miR-410 facilitates direct retinal pigment epithelium differentiation of umbilical cord blood-derived mesenchymal stem cells. *J. Vet. Sci.* **2016**, *18*, 59–65. [CrossRef] [PubMed]
76. Hass, R.; Kasper, C.; Böhm, S.; Jacobs, R. Different populations and sources of human mesenchymal stem cells (MSC): A comparison of adult and neonatal tissue-derived MSC. *Cell Commun. Signal.* **2011**, *9*, 12. [CrossRef] [PubMed]
77. Choi, Y.S.; Park, Y.-B.; Ha, C.-W.; Kim, J.A.; Heo, J.-C.; Han, W.-J.; Oh, S.Y.; Choi, S.J. Different characteristics of mesenchymal stem cells isolated from different layers of full term placenta. *PLoS ONE* **2017**, *12*, e0172642. [CrossRef] [PubMed]
78. Divya, M.S.; Roshin, G.E.; Divya, T.S.; Rasheed, V.A.; Santhoshkumar, T.R.; Elizabeth, K.E.; James, J.; Pillai, R.M. Umbilical cord blood-derived mesenchymal stem cells consist of a unique population of progenitors co-expressing mesenchymal stem cell and neuronal markers capable of instantaneous neuronal differentiation. *Stem Cell Res. Ther.* **2012**, *3*, 57. [CrossRef] [PubMed]
79. Trivanović, D.; Jauković, A.; Popović, B.; Krstić, J.; Mojsilović, S.; Okić-Djordjević, I.; Kukolj, T.; Obradović, H.; Santibanez, J.F.; Bugarski, D. Mesenchymal stem cells of different origin: Comparative evaluation of proliferative capacity, telomere length and pluripotency marker expression. *Life Sci.* **2015**, *141*, 61–73. [CrossRef] [PubMed]
80. Jones, G.N.; Moschidou, D.; Puga-Iglesias, T.-I.; Kuleszewicz, K.; Vanleene, M.; Shefelbine, S.J.; Bou-Gharios, G.; Fisk, N.M.; David, A.L.; de Coppi, P.; et al. Ontological differences in first compared to third trimester human fetal placental chorionic stem cells. *PLoS ONE* **2012**, *7*, e43395. [CrossRef] [PubMed]
81. Hu, L.; Hu, J.; Zhao, J.; Liu, J.; Ouyang, W.; Yang, C.; Gong, N.; Du, L.; Khanal, A.; Chen, L. Side-by-side comparison of the biological characteristics of human umbilical cord and adipose tissue-derived mesenchymal stem cells. *Biomed. Res. Int.* **2013**, *2013*, 438243. [CrossRef] [PubMed]
82. Dezawa, M. Muse cells provide the pluripotency of mesenchymal stem cells: Direct contribution of muse cells to tissue regeneration. *Cell Transplant.* **2016**, *25*, 849–861. [CrossRef] [PubMed]

83. Simerman, A.A.; Phan, J.D.; Dumesic, D.A.; Chazenbalk, G.D. Muse cells: Nontumorigenic pluripotent stem cells present in adult tissues—A paradigm shift in tissue regeneration and evolution. *Stem Cells Int.* **2016**, *2016*, 1463258. [CrossRef] [PubMed]
84. Kanno, H. Regenerative therapy for neuronal diseases with transplantation of somatic stem cells. *World J. Stem Cells* **2013**, *5*, 163–171. [CrossRef] [PubMed]
85. Bakondi, B.; Girman, S.; Lu, B.; Wang, S. Multimodal delivery of isogenic mesenchymal stem cells yields synergistic protection from retinal degeneration and vision loss. *Stem Cells Transl. Med.* **2017**, *6*, 444–457. [CrossRef] [PubMed]
86. Cui, Y.; Xu, N.; Xu, W.; Xu, G. Mesenchymal stem cells attenuate hydrogen peroxide-induced oxidative stress and enhance neuroprotective effects in retinal ganglion cells. *Vitr. Cell. Dev. Biol. Anim.* **2016**, *53*, 328–335. [CrossRef] [PubMed]
87. Mead, B.; Logan, A.; Berry, M.; Leadbeater, W.; Scheven, B.A. Paracrine-mediated neuroprotection and neuritogenesis of axotomised retinal ganglion cells by human dental pulp stem cells: Comparison with human bone marrow and adipose-derived mesenchymal stem cells. *PLoS ONE* **2014**, *9*, e109305. [CrossRef] [PubMed]
88. Lai, R.C.; Yeo, R.W.Y.; Lim, S.K. Mesenchymal stem cell exosomes. *Semin. Cell Dev. Biol.* **2015**, *40*, 82–88. [CrossRef] [PubMed]
89. Burrello, J.; Monticone, S.; Gai, C.; Gomez, Y.; Kholia, S.; Camussi, G. Stem cell-derived extracellular vesicles and immune-modulation. *Front. Cell Dev. Biol.* **2016**, *4*, 83. [CrossRef] [PubMed]
90. Wyse, R.D.; Dunbar, G.L.; Rossignol, J. Use of genetically modified mesenchymal stem cells to treat neurodegenerative diseases. *Int. J. Mol. Sci.* **2014**, *15*, 1719–1745. [CrossRef] [PubMed]
91. Yu, B.; Shao, H.; Su, C.; Jiang, Y.; Chen, X.; Bai, L.; Zhang, Y.; Li, Q.; Zhang, X.; Li, X. Exosomes derived from MSCs ameliorate retinal laser injury partially by inhibition of MCP-1. *Sci. Rep.* **2016**, *6*, 34562. [CrossRef] [PubMed]
92. Nussenblatt, R.B.; Lee, R.W.J.; Chew, E.; Wei, L.; Liu, B.; Sen, H.N.; Dick, A.D.; Ferris, F.L. Immune responses in age-related macular degeneration and a possible long-term therapeutic strategy for prevention. *Am. J. Ophthalmol.* **2014**, *158*, 5–11. [CrossRef] [PubMed]
93. Forrester, J.V.; Xu, H. Good news-bad news: The yin and yang of immune privilege in the eye. *Front. Immunol.* **2012**, *3*, 338. [CrossRef] [PubMed]
94. Perez, V.L.; Caspi, R.R. Immune mechanisms in inflammatory and degenerative eye disease. *Trends Immunol.* **2015**, *36*, 354–363. [CrossRef] [PubMed]
95. Klaassen, I.; Van Noorden, C.J.F.; Schlingemann, R.O. Molecular basis of the inner blood-retinal barrier and its breakdown in diabetic macular edema and other pathological conditions. *Prog. Retin. Eye Res.* **2013**, *34*, 19–48. [CrossRef] [PubMed]
96. Caspi, R.R. A look at autoimmunity and inflammation in the eye. *J. Clin. Investig.* **2010**, *120*, 3073–3083. [CrossRef] [PubMed]
97. Gao, F.; Chiu, S.M.; Motan, D.A.L.; Zhang, Z.; Chen, L.; Ji, H.-L.; Tse, H.F.; Fu, Q.L.; Lian, Q. Mesenchymal stem cells and immunomodulation: Current status and future prospects. *Cell Death Dis.* **2016**, *7*, e2062. [CrossRef] [PubMed]
98. Steinberg, G.K.; Kondziolka, D.; Wechsler, L.R.; Lunsford, L.D.; Coburn, M.L.; Billigen, J.B.; Kim, A.S.; Johnson, J.N.; Bates, D.; King, B.; et al. Clinical outcomes of transplanted modified bone marrow-derived mesenchymal stem cells in stroke: A phase 1/2a study. *Stroke* **2016**, *47*, 1817–1824. [CrossRef] [PubMed]
99. Lee, M.J.; Ko, A.Y.; Ko, J.H.; Lee, H.J.; Kim, M.K.; Wee, W.R.; Khwarg, S.I.; Oh, J.Y. Mesenchymal stem/stromal cells protect the ocular surface by suppressing inflammation in an experimental dry eye. *Mol. Ther.* **2015**, *23*, 139–146. [CrossRef] [PubMed]
100. Tasso, R.; Ilengo, C.; Quarto, R.; Cancedda, R.; Caspi, R.R.; Pennesi, G. Mesenchymal stem cells induce functionally active T-regulatory lymphocytes in a paracrine fashion and ameliorate experimental autoimmune uveitis. *Investig. Ophthalmol. Vis. Sci.* **2012**, *53*, 786–793. [CrossRef] [PubMed]
101. Zhang, L.; Zheng, H.; Shao, H.; Nian, H.; Zhang, Y.; Bai, L.; Su, C.; Liu, X.; Dong, L.; Li, X.; et al. Long-term therapeutic effects of mesenchymal stem cells compared to dexamethasone on recurrent experimental autoimmune uveitis of rats. *Investig. Ophthalmol. Vis. Sci.* **2014**, *55*, 5561–5571. [CrossRef] [PubMed]

102. Jia, Z.; Jiao, C.; Zhao, S.; Li, X.; Ren, X.; Zhang, L.; Han, Z.C.; Zhang, X. Immunomodulatory effects of mesenchymal stem cells in a rat corneal allograft rejection model. *Exp. Eye Res.* **2012**, *102*, 44–49. [CrossRef] [PubMed]
103. Davis, B.M.; Crawley, L.; Pahlitzsch, M.; Javaid, F.; Cordeiro, M.F. Glaucoma: The retina and beyond. *Acta Neuropathol.* **2016**, *132*, 807–826. [CrossRef] [PubMed]
104. Munemasa, Y.; Kitaoka, Y. Molecular mechanisms of retinal ganglion cell degeneration in glaucoma and future prospects for cell body and axonal protection. *Front. Cell. Neurosci.* **2012**, *6*, 60. [CrossRef] [PubMed]
105. Emre, E.; Yüksel, N.; Duruksu, G.; Pirhan, D.; Subaşi, C.; Erman, G.; Karaöz, E. Neuroprotective effects of intravitreally transplanted adipose tissue and bone marrow-derived mesenchymal stem cells in an experimental ocular hypertension model. *Cytotherapy* **2015**, *17*, 543–559. [CrossRef] [PubMed]
106. Gao, F.; Hou, H.; Liang, H.; Weinreb, R.N.; Wang, H.; Wang, Y. Bone marrow-derived cells in ocular neovascularization: Contribution and mechanisms. *Angiogenesis* **2016**, *19*, 107–118. [CrossRef] [PubMed]
107. Das, U.N. Diabetic macular edema, retinopathy and age-related macular degeneration as inflammatory conditions. *Arch. Med. Sci.* **2016**, *12*, 1142–1157. [CrossRef] [PubMed]
108. Ghazaryan, E.; Zhang, Y.; He, Y.; Liu, X.; Li, Y.; Xie, J.; Su, G. Mesenchymal stem cells in corneal neovascularization: Comparison of different application routes. *Mol. Med. Rep.* **2016**, *14*, 3104–3112. [CrossRef] [PubMed]
109. Yafai, Y.; Eichler, W.; Iandiev, I.; Unterlauft, J.-D.; Jochmann, C.; Wiedemann, P.; Bringmann, A. Thrombospondin-1 is produced by retinal glial cells and inhibits the growth of vascular endothelial cells. *Ophthalmic Res.* **2014**, *52*, 81–88. [CrossRef] [PubMed]
110. Farnoodian, M.; Kinter, J.B.; Yadranji Aghdam, S.; Zaitoun, I.; Sorenson, C.M.; Sheibani, N. Expression of pigment epithelium-derived factor and thrombospondin-1 regulate proliferation and migration of retinal pigment epithelial cells. *Physiol. Rep.* **2015**, *3*, e12266. [CrossRef] [PubMed]
111. Contreras-Ruiz, L.; Regenfuss, B.; Mir, F.A.; Kearns, J.; Masli, S. Conjunctival inflammation in thrombospondin-1 deficient mouse model of Sjögren's syndrome. *PLoS ONE* **2013**, *8*, e75937. [CrossRef] [PubMed]
112. Hou, H.-Y.; Liang, H.-L.; Wang, Y.-S.; Zhang, Z.-X.; Wang, B.-R.; Shi, Y.-Y.; Dong, X.; Cai, Y. A therapeutic strategy for choroidal neovascularization based on recruitment of mesenchymal stem cells to the sites of lesions. *Mol. Ther.* **2010**, *18*, 1837–1845. [CrossRef] [PubMed]
113. Ribot, J.; Caliaperoumal, G.; Paquet, J.; Boisson-Vidal, C.; Petite, H.; Anagnostou, F. Type 2 diabetes alters mesenchymal stem cell secretome composition and angiogenic properties. *J. Cell. Mol. Med.* **2016**. [CrossRef] [PubMed]
114. Chu, L.Y.; Ramakrishnan, D.P.; Silverstein, R.L. Thrombospondin-1 modulates VEGF signaling via CD36 by recruiting SHP-1 to VEGFR2 complex in microvascular endothelial cells. *Blood* **2013**, *122*, 1822–1832. [CrossRef] [PubMed]

3

Metabolic and Redox Signaling of the Nucleoredoxin-Like-1 Gene for the Treatment of Genetic Retinal Diseases

Emmanuelle Clérin [1], Myriam Marussig [2], José-Alain Sahel [1,3] and Thierry Léveillard [1,*]

1 Department of Genetics, Sorbonne Université, INSERM, CNRS, Institut de la Vision, 17 rue Moreau, F-75012 Paris, France; emmanuelle.clerin@inserm.fr (E.C.); J.sahel@gmail.com (J.-A.S.)
2 SparingVision, 55 rue de Lyon, 75012 Paris, France; myriam.marussig@sparingvision.com
3 CHNO des Quinze-Vingts, DHU Sight Restore, INSERM-DGOS CIC 1423, 28 rue de Charenton, F-75012 Paris, France
* Correspondence: thierry.leveillard@inserm.fr;

Abstract: The loss of cone photoreceptor function in retinitis pigmentosa (RP) severely impacts the central and daily vision and quality of life of patients affected by this disease. The loss of cones follows the degeneration of rods, in a manner independent of the causing mutations in numerous genes associated with RP. We have explored this phenomenon and proposed that the loss of rods triggers a reduction in the expression of rod-derived cone viability factor (RdCVF) encoded by the nucleoredoxin-like 1 (*NXNL1*) gene which interrupts the metabolic and redox signaling between rods and cones. After providing scientific evidence supporting this mechanism, we propose a way to restore this lost signaling and prevent the cone vision loss in animal models of RP. We also explain how we could restore this signaling to prevent cone vision loss in animal models of the disease and how we plan to apply this therapeutic strategy by the administration of both products of *NXNL1* encoding the trophic factor RdCVF and the thioredoxin enzyme RdCVFL using an adeno-associated viral vector. We describe in detail all the steps of this translational program, from the design of the drug, its production, biological validation, and analytical and preclinical qualification required for a future clinical trial that would, if successful, provide a treatment for this incurable disease.

Keywords: retinitis pigmentosa; cone photoreceptor; central vision; rod-derived cone viability factor; aerobic glycolysis; thioredoxin signaling; gene therapy; adeno-associated viral vector; chemical manufacturing; clinical trial

1. Introduction

Inherited retinal degenerations (IRDs) are genetically and clinically heterogeneous blinding diseases that are now emerging as clinical targets for gene therapies [1–3]. The fervor of these ongoing efforts is motivated by the recent successful treatment of the *RPE65*-related form of Leber congenital amaurosis (LCA), a severe blinding disease, by a recombinant adeno-associated viral (AAV) vector that corrects the genetic deficit in those patients [4]. RPE65 is a success story, biblical in impact [5]. RPE65 was discovered in 1993 as a protein of 65 kDa expressed specifically by the retinal pigmented epithelium (RPE) [6]. The same group reported in 1997 that loss of function mutations in the gene encoding for RPE65 cause certain forms of LCA (*LCA2*) [7], and in 1998 that RPE65 is essential for the trans-isomerization of all-trans retinal esters, as they accumulate in the RPE of the *Rpe65-/-* mouse [8]. The booster of the story was the existence of a large animal model of *LCA2*, a briard dog discovered the same year [9]. A consortium of veterinarians, clinicians, and gene therapists reported the benefit of the subretinal injection of an AAV serotype 2 encoding for RPE65 in that dog model in 2001 [10].

Lancelot, one briard dog whose vision in the treated eye was restored, was photographed in front of the American congress during a meeting that restored the hope of future success of gene therapy after years of doubt [11–13]. This encouraged three independent research groups to initiate first in man studies that led to success during phases I of clinical trials, as reported on 2008 [14–16]. Nevertheless, the benefit of the treatment over long periods was controversial [17]. The group led by Jean Bennett made critical improvement of the treatment by showing the absence of advert effects associated with the treatment of the contralateral eye of the patients [18], while the two other groups reported the absence of benefit for the treated patients on the long-term [19–21]. The lack of persistence of the benefit of the treatment in some patients was interpreted in light of the natural history of the disease [22,23]. The absence of conversion of all-*trans*-retinol to 11-*cis*-retinal due to a mutation in the *RPE65* gene interrupts the resupply of functional, light-sensitive opsin proteins in photoreceptors [24]. The administration of a functional copy of *RPE65* by corrective gene therapy restores this deficit for vision. However, *LCA2* patients have retinal degeneration and loss of photoreceptors starting in the first decade of life [25]. The aggregation of short-wavelength cone opsins likely caused rapid cone degeneration through an endoplasmic reticulum stress pathway in an animal model with a genetic deficit of lecithin-retinol acyltransferase (LRAT), another LCA gene involved in the recycling of 11-*cis*-retinal in the RPE [26]. Consequently, if the disease has progressed to a certain stage, the restoration of the function of RPE65 is not able to stop photoreceptor degeneration. The results of a randomized phase 3 trial funded by Spark Therapeutics about the benefits of the subretinal injection of AAV2-hRPE65v2 developed by Jean Bennett were reported on July 2017. That study includes patients for which vision was preserved for three years [27]. The U.S. Food and Drug Administration (FDA) approved gene therapy using AAV2-hRPE65v2 (Luxturna®) for the treatment of patients with biallelic *RPE65* mutations in December 2017, followed by the European Medicines Agency (EMA) on November 2018 [4]. Spark Therapeutics announced that the company will follow the treated patients over 15 years.

Jean Bennet and her team were first of the rope [28]. Many other recessive inherited retinal degenerations could be treated by restoring the gene function altered by the mutations by introducing a normal copy of that gene, and this is what is happening [3]. The only negative argument against this approach is the very high cost for the society of having to correct more than one hundred genes one by one [29]. Issues of cost versus benefits will become increasingly important as a wave of costly new therapies tested in small patient populations are developed and approved (see [30] and Supplementary Table S1).

For dominant forms of IRDs, the situation is more complex like for the dominant mutations of the splicing factor gene *PRPF31* [31]. Surprisingly, most familial pedigrees contain affected and non-affected carrier individuals. This is explained by variable haploinsufficiency [32]. Those families are composed of members of different genetic compositions. For one subject, the dominant mutation in *PRPF31* on one chromosome is paired with a wild-type allele on the second chromosome with expression above a threshold. The residual protein level is sufficient for normal retinal function and this subject is asymptomatic. For another member of this pedigree, the dominant mutation in *PRPF31* on one chromosome is paired with a wild-type allele on the second chromosome with expression below this threshold. The residual protein level is not sufficient for normal retinal function and this subject is symptomatic. In this case the administration in the retina of a normal copy of the *PRPF31* gene should allow crossing this threshold of expression transforming patients into asymptomatic carriers.

The situation is even much more complex in the case of mutations in the rhodopsin gene, the first gene identified to cause retinitis pigmentosa (RP) [33]. Dominant mutations result in either gain-of-function or dominant negative functions [34]. They were stratified into six classes based on the molecular properties, with deficits of transport to the outer segment (class I), folding (class II), endocytosis (class III), protein stability (class IV), or alternatively increased activation rate for transducin (class V) and constitutive activation (class VI). Stimulating the unfolded protein response was shown to benefit rod function in a dominant rat model carrying a class II mutation [35]. The first therapeutic attempt in a rodent model of the disease used an engineered ribozyme, a catalytic RNA that specifically triggers the destruction of the mRNA encoding a class II P23H mutant rhodopsin mRNA [36]. Hammerhead ribozymes are able to induce site-specific cleavage of RNA, with ribozymes including two different oligoribonucleotides with regions of complementarity [37]. One obvious limitation of such approach is that the catalytic ribozyme is designed to target a specific mutation, while more than 150 point mutations in rhodopsin have been shown to cause RP [38]. Within the United States, the majority of rhodopsin mutations causing the disease is attributable to a single sequence variation at codon 23, suggesting a founder effect, but it is rare in Europe [39–41]. Diseases associated with mutations in this codon result in a relatively mild clinical phenotype [42,43]. To circumvent the large number of mutations, RNA interference-based mutation-independent approach was validated in various models RP with dominant mutations in the rhodopsin gene [44,45]. The strategy combines silencing the expression of the rhodopsin gene, both the mutant and normal rhodopsin genes, and simultaneously providing mRNA that encodes for the wild-type rhodopsin that is engendered to be resistant to the interfering RNA used by using the genetic code degeneration [46]. Botta et al. used the ability of the transcription factor Krüppel-like factor 15 (KLF15) to recognize a DNA element within the rhodopsin promoter to silence the expression of autosomal dominant mutant rhodopsin after delivery of an AAV vector–mediated ectopic expression of KLF15 in rod photoreceptors [47].

Recent progress in genome editing using clustered regularly interspaced short palindromic repeat/Cas9 (CRISPR/Cas9) technology led to the development of therapeutic approaches of RP by in vivo genome editing [48,49]. Targeting in vivo the neural retina-specific leucine zipper (*NRL*) gene in rods using CRISPR-Cas9 technology was also used to repress rod differentiation to circumvent the deleterious effect of mutations of genes expressed specifically by rods [50]. Other mutation-independent approaches were studied aiming at preventing an event common to all forms of rod cell death, starting by targeting apoptosis since it is the final fate for rods in animal models and for patients suffering of RP [51,52]. Overexpression of histone deacetylase 4 (HDAC4) or even its N-terminal domain suppresses multiple cell death and prolongs rod survival in an autosomal recessive model of RP, the *rd1* mice [53]. Administration of ciliary neurotrophic factor (CNTF) protects photoreceptors of murine models of RP [54], but was not confirmed in the first clinical trial [55]. Downregulation of microglia activation using either the microRNA miR-204 [56] or fractalkine, a soluble form of the chemokine CX3CL1 prevent and photoreceptor cell death in several mouse models of RP [57]. Oxidative damage was successfully targeted by delivering the transcription factor nuclear factor, erythroid 2 like 2 (NFE2L2), known as NRF2, that regulates hundreds of genes that preserve photoreceptors against oxidative stress [58]. Iron may be involved in oxidative damage since intraperitoneally-injected transferrin prevents photoreceptor degeneration in *rd10* mice [59]. Other approaches have been used to sustain photoreceptor metabolic needs [60,61].

One main limitation of these approaches targeting rods is that patients suffering of RP are often identified by ophthalmologists after consultation at a stage where rod photoreceptors are already dead. Rod degeneration leads to night blindness so, for patients living in an urban setting, night vision problems may not be apparent until the retinal disease is in an advanced stage. Consequently, preventing the degeneration of rods will not be beneficial to these patients.

2. Rod-Derived Cone Viability Factor

The diagnosis of RP has probably existed historically for hundreds, if not thousands of years, but was recognized as a complicated form of night blindness only after the invention of the ophthalmoscope in 1851. In RP, there is a progression from night blindness which originates from the death of rod photoreceptors by apoptosis, to the dysfunction of cone photoreceptors concentrated at the center of the retina, the fovea. This secondary event leads to complete blindness [62,63]. On the other hand, congenital stationary night blindness (CSNB) does not lead to the loss of central vision. The most remarkable CSNB pedigree comprising 2121 people goes back to Jean Nougaret, a butcher of the 17th century (1637–1719) of Vendémian in the Hérault. In 1831, a fifth-generation descendant demanded an exemption from military service because of his poor night vision. Unfortunately for him, the examination found that the young man could read by candlelight, so in photopic conditions that involve the function of cones, and the doctor concluded by a simulation and found it good for seven years of service. It was only in 1838 that the family transmission of his night blindness was demonstrated by Belgian ophthalmologist Florent Cunier, freeing him from military duty [64]. In 1996, a missense mutation in the gene encoding the rod transducin alpha subunit (*GNAT1*) responsible for the pathology of the Nougaret family was identified in eleventh-generation members [65]. This entertaining story has its importance today since some persons within this large pedigree, uncertain of being affected, were shown to be as night-blind as their relatives through the same *GNAT1* mutation [66]. The night vision disturbance of CSNB is overlooked because it is highly subjective especially for individuals living in an urban or well-lit environment [67]. This led Professor Alan Wright to declare that keeping the cones alive will help some 1.5 million people worldwide to see, as well as Jean Nougaret and his descendants [68]. More recently Professor Henry Kaplan restated that if therapy can prevent or reverse the onset of cone degeneration within the macula most patients would be immeasurably helped and able to live normal lives [69]. This strategy is medically applicable since, in patients and in a dog model of RP, visual discriminance can be achieved with a very limited number of functional cones [70,71].

What causes the dysfunction and ultimately the death of cones remained obscure for years [72]. The identification of the first mutation causing RP in human left the scientific community perplexed. After having localized the gene on a short interval of the long arm of chromosome 3, a dominant mutation in the gene encoding for the rhodopsin, the visual pigment of rods, was identified [73–75]. Electroretinogram (ERG) measurements of affected members of this pedigree confirmed that RP progresses from an early abnormal rod response to a subsequent altered cone response. In advanced cases, RP is associated with a complete loss of rods, with a few remaining foveal cones with shortened and disorganized outer segments [76]. The reason why a mutation in a gene expressed exclusively in rods can lead to widespread degeneration of both rods and cones in these patients was puzzling [77]. It was observed that cone outer segment function remains normal until >75% of the rod outer segment are lost [78].

This two-phase degeneration sequence was initially described in retinal degeneration (*rd1*) mice by Carter-Dawson et al. [79]. The *rd1* mouse carries a recessive mutation of the cGMP-dependent phosphodiesterase beta subunit gene, *Pde6b*, selectively expressed by rods [80]. Mutations in the human orthologue gene, *PDE6B*, are causing RP [81]. Specific ablation of rod photoreceptors in transgenic mice results in the failure of cone cells in elaborating their outer segments [82,83]. It was observed in various animal models of RP including rodents, pigs, dogs, and even toads [83–86]. The analysis of the kinetics of rod and cone cells death in several mouse models of RP excludes that dying rods are toxically damaging the cones [87]. Transplantation of a wild-type photoreceptor layer (97% rod photoreceptors in the mouse) in the subretinal space of the *rd1* mouse slows down the secondary degeneration of cones [88,89]. We showed that the effect is mediated by soluble molecules originating from the neural retina and not from the adjacent RPE [90]. Partial characterization of this trophic interaction demonstrated that the activity is carried by molecules having the apparent molecular weight compatible with that of proteins [91]. In the same study, we showed that the fraction is active on cone-enriched culture made from chicken embryo, a model originally developed by Ruben Adler [92]. The existence of cone-protecting proteins in the extracellular matrix surrounding the photoreceptors has been suggested using this biological system, where the photoreceptors spontaneously degenerate between seven and 10 days in culture [93]. The degeneration of rods in the *rd1* retina could result in the loss of expression of secreted protein factors necessary for cone survival. In RP patients, the secondary cone dysfunction leads to blindness since the cones are responsible not only for the vision of the colors, but also for all useful functions (perception of details, reading) of daylight vision [94].

The identification of proteins able to prevent the spontaneously cell degeneration in the cone-enriched culture was performed by high content screening [95]. The screened factors were produced by transient transfection of a retinal cDNA library in COS-1 cells. The conditioned media of the equivalent of 210,000 clones containing, among others, the secreted proteins were applied to primary cones from chicken and the viability was scored after seven days. A cDNA with an open reading frame of 109 amino acids was identified and the protein was named rod-derived cone viability factor (RdCVF). RdCVF is a splicing variant of the nucleoredoxin-like-1 (*NXNL1*) gene corresponding to intron retention and a conserved in-frame stop codon (OMIM # 608791) translated from a ~7 kb messenger RNA [96]. *NXNL1* expression is rod-dependent in the mouse and human retina and its promoter is regulated by the homeoprotein CRX [97–99]. The injection of recombinant RdCVF protein protects the cones of the *rd1* mouse from degenerating [95]. In a transgenic model of autosomal dominant RP with expression of the mutant rhodopsin protein under the control of a rod promoter, we showed that a synthetic human RdCVF protein prevents secondary cone degeneration that could be scored using photopic ERG which scores cone function [100]. The protection, observed over a period of three months, was associated with the preservation of the outer segments of the cones, the subcellular structure that carries the light sensitive molecules, the opsins [101,102]. Similar results were obtained by the administration of RdCVF through gene therapy [102]. More recently, we showed that cone function can be preserved in the *rd10* mouse, a second model of recessive RP, by delivering RdCVF using a recombinant AAV vector [103]. The effect of RdCVF is independent of the genetic origin of the disease, so a therapy aimed at preventing central vision loss should benefit to all RP patients whatever the mutation they carry in any of the 65 genes known to date [104].

A cell surface receptor for RdCVF was identified by far-Western blotting [96]. The single-pass transmembrane domain protein basigin (BSG) is expressed in two different isoforms. The protein BSG2 possesses two extracellular immunoglobulin (Ig) domains and is expressed widely in many organs where it is involved in addressing lactate transporters to the membrane. The protein BSG1, produced by alternative splicing, possesses a third Ig domain, and its expression is restricted to photoreceptors [104]. We found that RdCVF interacts specifically with a complex made of BSG1 and the glucose transporter GLUT1 (SLC2A1) at the surface of the cones. The increased glucose entry into the cones is metabolized by aerobic glycolysis [105]. The bifurcation from oxidative phosphorylation takes place after the production of pyruvate by glycolysis. The pyruvate (PYR) can be transported to the mitochondria by the mitochondrial pyruvate carrier (MPC) where it is metabolized by the tricarboxylic acid cycle (TCA) that is connected with the mitochondrial respiratory chain to produced ATP in aerobic conditions. The whole process is known as oxidative phosphorylation (OXPHO). The pyruvate can alternatively be metabolized to produce lactate (LACT) by lactate dehydrogenase (LDH). Lactate is then transported out of the cell by lactate transporters (MCTs). RdCVF stimulates aerobic glycolysis to provide triglycerides that are used by cones for the renewal of the outer segments. For reasons that are only partially known, aerobic glycolysis favors the diversification at mid-course of the glycolytic reaction of carbons from glucose at the level of dihydroxyacetone phosphate (DHAP). A certain proportion of DHAP is converted into glycerol-3-phosphate (G3P) by glycerol-3-phosphate dehydrogenase (G3PDH). G3P is the precursor of the hydrophilic head of phospholipids made with fatty acids, among which poly-unsaturated fatty acids (PUFA) are derived from nutrition. Recently, it was demonstrated experimentally that, for rods, aerobic glycolysis is necessary for rod outer segment renewal, a phenomenon parallel to that described for cones [106].

3. The Thioredoxin RdCVFL

Interestingly, the splicing of the unique intron of the *NXNL1* gene produces a second messenger RNA encoding for an enzymatically active thioredoxin, RdCVFL [107,108]. Both rods and cones of the mouse carrying a homologous recombination of the *Nxnl1* gene are affected, a deficit that progresses with age [109]. The lack of expression of the thioredoxin RdCVFL leads to increased oxidative damage. We observed a higher concentration of molecular adducts produced by lipid peroxidation in the retina of these mice. The phototransduction is initiated in the outer segment of photoreceptors made of stacks of lipid bilayers where the opsin molecule is enchased. These membranes are particularly enriched in PUFA which are prone to oxidation [110]. The retina of a mouse with a specific deletion of the *Nxnl1* in cones is more susceptible to oxidative damages since *Nxnl1* is also expressed by cones (3% of all photoreceptors in the mouse) [111]. Contrarily to the rods, there is no intron retention of the *Nxnl1* mRNA in the cones that express only the thioredoxin RdCVFL.

Reactive oxygen species (ROS) are produced in physiological conditions by leakage from the mitochondrial respiratory chain and inhibits key enzymes in the glycolytic pathway [112,113]. The thioredoxin system reduces oxidized thiol groups of cysteines in proteins among which glycolytic enzymes and restores their function [114]. The thioredoxin enzymes, among which RdCVFL must be reduced by thioredoxin reductase (TXNRD) since the catalytic cysteines become oxidized when the enzyme reduces its substrate [115]. TXNRD requires its co-factor NADPH produced by the pentose phosphate pathway (PPP) in its reduced form to function. Consequently, the reducing power of RdCVFL in cones is proportional to the uptake of glucose and the rederivation of the glycolytic flux to the PPP. ROS inhibition of glycolysis leads to the accumulation of glucose-6-phosphate (G6P), the first metabolite produced from glucose in the cell, which is redirected to the PPP producing two molecules of NADPH by reduction for TXNRD activity [116,117]. In this metabolic and redox signaling, the reducing power of RdCVFL relies on the metabolism of glucose by cones whose uptake is stimulated by RdCVF [118].

The combination of the non-cell autonomous action of RdCVF on metabolism with the cell-autonomous activity of RdCVFL on redox homeostasis is the rational of a current translational program aimed at preventing the loss of central vision, resulting from cone dysfunction, in RP patients independently of the causative mutations.

4. Design of the Therapeutic Molecule

The actions of both RdCVF and RdCVFL seem to be required for the maintenance of cone function throughout life, so that repeated injections of the recombinant proteins are precluded. As in the case of Luxturna®, the development of an AAV vector encoding for RdCVF and RdCVFL would provide a long-term protection of central vision in patients. These two therapeutic products are made by alternative splicing of the *NXNL1* gene in the rods, but our current knowledge of the regulation of splicing of this gene makes the use of a genomic construct hazardous. The combination of two distinct human cDNAs encoding for RdCVF (109 amino acids) and RdCVFL (212 amino acids) would be a rational approach. The configurations of two cassettes on opposite strands, with 5′ or 3′ ends pointing the external invert terminal repeats (ITRs), could result in the formation of palindromes that could interfere with encapsidation of the single strand DNA into the viral particle and are thought to be at risk for the development of the drug [119]. In a safer configuration, the two cDNA are arranged tandemly on the same strand. The reduction of tandem repeats sequence of the common part of the two cDNAs is obtained by modifying the used codons in order to make the vector more stable during its production [120]. Notice that this is a deviation of codon optimization since this method applies a codon optimization algorithm to a human cDNA sequence for making the translation of the protein more efficient in human cells [121]. The expression of these cDNAs is regulated by a promoter. Since RdCVF is acting in a non-cell autonomous manner, the cytomegalovirus (CMV) promoter fused to the chicken β-actin (CBA) promoter that drives the expression of the transgene in most cells is particularly suited [122,123] (Figure 1A). Such ubiquitous promoter has been used successfully in experiments aimed at protecting the cones in vivo [96,103]. The protective action of the thioredoxin RdCVFL is cell autonomous, so that its cDNA should be expressed by the cells that are protected, the photoreceptors, rods, and cones [111,124]. Since our strategy is to restore the metabolic and redox signaling in the retina of patients having lost their rods, a cone specific promoter appears as the most effective solution. In previous work, we have successfully used a hybrid promoter made of the locus control region (LCR) of the cone's red (L) and green (M) promoter fused to the proximal promoter region of the red opsin gene (OPN1L/MW) to deliver RdCVFL to the cones [125,126] (Figure 1B). In order to reduce the contribution of the promoter located 5′ in the construct to the expression of the transgene located in the 3′ position, it is advisable to introduce a transcription terminator element that will isolate both cassettes [127,128]. It is important to maintain the entire size of the construct including the external ITRs in the limit of what can be encapsidated efficiently in the AAV particle of 25 nm [129]. AAV can package a vector larger than its genome size, up to 5.2 kb, the packaging of larger or smaller loads is suboptimal and the transduction of cells less efficient [130–132]. AAV vector genomes never exceeding 5.2 kb in length can accommodate the RdCVF-RdCVFL expression cassettes. The two cassettes are introduced in a proviral plasmid whose size is largely superior to 5.2 kb in order to avoid reverse packaging of vector sequences during the production of the viral particles by the use of a long stuffer sequence [133]. In order to assure that this stuffer sequence is biologically inert, researchers in the field have used a fragment of the genome of bacteriophage lambda, while this sequence contains several short open reading frames [134]. These elements combined with possible reverse packaging may be viewed as a risk by regulatory authorities. One way to circumvent this possible problem is to identify inert sequences in the human genome; sequences that do not contain any signal or structural particularities. The possible encapsidation of prokaryotic sequences during recombinant adeno-associated virus production questions the resistance gene used to propagate the proviral plasmid [135]. To date, the use of the β-lactam antibiotic family, including ampicillin, is not acceptable for regulatory authorities, in order to avoid concerns for patients showing allergic reactivity to β-lactam antibiotics. Therefore, the kanamycin gene is commonly used. The proviral plasmid should be entirely sequenced on both strands after its assembly. Special care is devoted to the sequence of the ITRs because of their role in the production of active AAV particles, their instability, and the difficulties to access to the sequence due to the presence of DNA secondary structure [136]. The construct should be then validated by analyzing the expression of the two transgenes after transient transfection and viral infection of cells in vitro. This presents no difficulty for RdCVF that is expressed under the control of a ubiquitous promoter, but requires more effort for RdCVFL that is regulated by a cone-specific promoter [137].

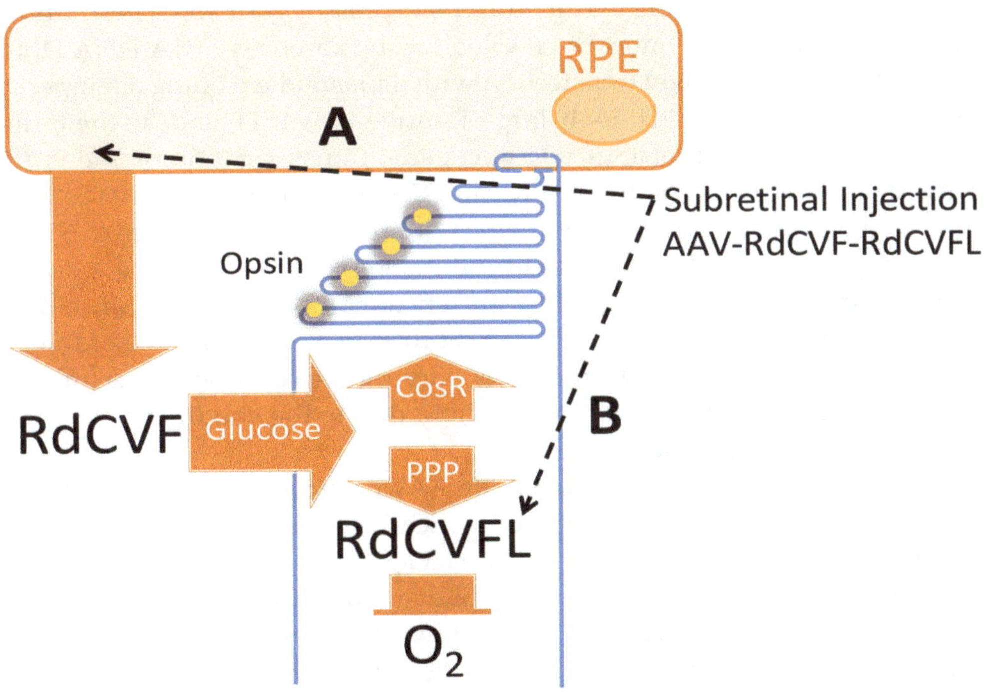

Figure 1. Subretinal injection of AAV-RdCVF-RdCVFL to prevent the loss of function of cones in retinitis pigmentosa, (**A**) Transduction of the drug (recombinant AAV) to the retinal pigmented epithelium, expression and secretion of RdCVF to stimulate glucose entry, cone outer segment renewal (CosR) and the pentose phosphate pathway (PPP). (**B**) Transduction of the drug (recombinant AAV) to the cones and stimulation of redox homeostasis through NADPH, reduced by the metabolism of glucose through the pentose phosphate pathway.

5. Chemical Manufacturing

As a prerequisite to the production of AAV particle to be used in a clinical trial, all plasmids must be produced under conditions consistent with current good manufacturing practice (GMP) [138]. They have to be free of transmissible spongiform encephalopathy and bovine spongiform encephalopathy. They must have a very low level of endotoxin, of residual host cell protein, and be of genomic DNA. Recombinant AAV particles are most commonly produced by co-transfection of three distinct plasmids in mammalian cells vectors: (1) the proviral plasmids containing RdCVF and RdCVFL and their regulatory sequences; (2) the AAV rep and *cap* genes provided in trans; and (3) helper functions from adenovirus for efficient replication of the recombinant genome [139]. The serotype of the AAV particles can be modulated by the use of a plasmid encoding the capsid proteins VP1, 2, and 3. While the transgene is more commonly constructed with ITR sequences from AAV serotype 2, the capsid proteins provided in trans can specify a distinct serotype of the particles, for example, serotype 5 [140,141]. Since RdCVF is acting in a non-cell autonomous manner, its administration does not need to target specific cells in the retina and it can even be administrated in the animal in systemic ways [96,103]. Thioredoxin RdCVFL acts in a cell-autonomous manner of photoreceptors, so the potent serotypes are those reported to transduce cones in the case of RP, as serotypes 5, 8, and 9 [111,142,143]. As an alternative to mammalian cells, a protocol using invertebrate cell lines from *Spodoptera frugiperda* (Sf9) infected with the baculovirus *Autographa californica* was also developed [144,145]. Since Sf9-produced AAV have altered capsid compositions and lower biological potencies, we will not discuss their use further [146]. The most established method for the production of AAV vectors is plasmid tri-transfection of human embryonic kidney (HEK)293 cells [147]. The HEK293 cell line has been generated by transfection of cultures of normal human embryonic kidney cells with sheared adenovirus 5 DNA containing the adenovirus E1A and E1B genes [148]. HEK293 cells express the oncogenic protein E1A that binds to the retinoblastoma protein encoding by the tumor suppressor gene *RB1* [149]. Consequently, the clinical batches of recombinant AAV must be checked for the absence of E1A DNA [150]. A subclone of HEK293 cells has been generated by transfection with a plasmid encoding a temperature-sensitive mutant of the simian virus (SV)40 [151]. SV40 large T antigen (SV40T) binds to the tumor suppressor p53 protein, and this association contributes to oncogenic transformation by the virus [152]. Thus, even if the productivity of AAV particles is higher in HEK293T than in HEK293 cells, it is advisable to use HEK293 to avoid additional potent problems with the presence of trace of SV40T DNA [153]. HEK293 are usually grown as adherent cells in the presence of fetal bovine serum that must be purchased from countries exempted of spongiform encephalopathy [154]. Since the productivity of AAV particles depends not only on the cells used but also of the sequence of the transgene, it is necessary to develop the manufacturing process by varying the conditions (plasmid quantities and ratio, duration of transfection, time of harvest, etc.) to define the conditions of what is called the upstream process to optimize the yield.

The downstream process is the purification of the AAV particles after their production by HEK293 or HEK293T cells. Isopycnic ultracentrifugation on cesium chloride (CsCl) gradient allows the separation of the particles with single-strand DNA packaged in it (full particles) from those without DNA (empty particles) due to the difference in their buoyant density [155]. Alternatively, the particles are purified using iodixanol-based density gradients with a ratio full/empty inferior to the CsCl gradient method. Since performing ultracentrifugation is a rupture in the chain of downstream processes it is complicated for producing clinical grade AAV. This is the reason for the development of alternative approaches using chromatography, a process that is performed in a pipeline from upstream to downstream process [156]. Affinity chromatography cannot distinguish between the full and empty capsids, but empirical assays led to the development of chromatographic methods to enrich for full particles [157]. The proportion of full, empty, and partially encapsidated particles is analyzed by analytical ultracentrifugation [158]. Another important aspect is the measurement of the titer of the preparation that is most commonly achieved by quantitative PCR (qPCR). Accurate titration is critical for ensuring correct and reproducible dosing in both preclinical and clinical settings. Attempts to standardize the protocol over platforms have shown little success [159]. A potential problem with qPCR is its dependence on a DNA standard curve that itself can be incorrectly calibrated. Currently, the method of choice is an absolute quantification using droplet digital PCR [160,161]. It remains that the titer of the AAV preparation that is biologically active in the proof-of-concept experiments in a research laboratory has to match that of the clinical-grade production, a task that requires the use of an AAV biological standard. This is complicated when the protocol of purification of AAV differs between the research laboratory and the clinical platform, for example, when the proof-of-concept of the therapeutic benefit has been obtained with research-grade AAV purified by ultracentrifugation on CsCl or an iodixanol gradient to clinical-grade AAV purified by methods more adapted to industrial production [147,162]. It is not only that the latter contains empty particles but potentially a certain proportion of partially encapsidated particles that can be scored as positive in the titration using droplet digital PCR but do not transduce the entire transgene. The quantity of full versus partially encapsidated particles can be assessed using alkaline gel electrophoresis [163].

When the full manufacturing process is fully optimized and the analytical tests for the limited quantities of host cell proteins, host cells, and plasmid DNA, and the absence of production of replicative particles are developed, a first production of the therapeutic AAV is made as a reference for any further comparison. Then, a second production following exactly the same methods provides the pilot material for the proof-of-concept of its activity in the animal model(s) of the disease.

6. Preclinical Studies

An important step in the transfer of the treatment of RP using the combination of RdCVF and RdCVFL is to provide a proof-of-concept in an animal mouse model of the disease using the pilot material of the clinical-grade AAV. We can use a mouse model of recessive RP, and the *rd10* mouse is considered to be the most appropriate to test the benefit on the combination of both products of the *NXNL1* gene [103,111]. This model is the most appropriate to test for the benefit of the combination of both products of the *NXNL1* gene. Interestingly, this model can be used to measure cone function using optometry, a behavior assay that relies on head tracking movement that is proportional to acuity and contrast sensitivity [164]. The effect of the treatment of *rd10* is evaluated by several temporal sequences of electroretinogram (ERG) measurements of cone function by photopic and flicker ERG and optometry assays [103,111,137]. At the end of each experiment, the density of the cones is measured using e-conome after the sacrifice of the animals [165]. In this model, those three measures are proportional and provide robustness to the results. The experiment setup is crucial at this stage of the project for several reasons. First, the kinetics of degeneration of photoreceptors in the *rd10* mouse is influenced by light [166]. To avoid any artifactual differences between the individually-treated animals, all the mice should be exposed to the same quantity of light over the entire duration of the experiment. This is achieved through horizontal illumination from light sources fixed on the wall, the only solution to ensure that homogeneity, which is controlled using luxmeters positioned in the rack supporting the cages of the animals. A second concern is the enrichment that retards photoreceptor degeneration in that model [167]. The most practical solution is to remove the enrichment when the experimental mice are born to ensure that they all become blind by post-natal day (PND) 50. A third problem is the difference in vision loss between gender [168]. It is necessary to use only one sex or, alternatively, to homogeneously distribute males and females in each group of animals. Since the onset of rod degeneration is at PND18 and that the onset of expression of the transgene is about one week long, the mice are injected at PND15 [103,111]. It is essential to use a group of *rd10* animals injected with a non-active AAV (usually encoding green fluorescent protein (GFP)] prepared with the same protocol as negative control [96]). Each mouse receives the treatment in one eye and the contralateral eye is sham operated to distinguish the possible effect of the surgery to be separated from that of the drug [100,169].

After the completion of that study, the clinical grade AAV is produced and used for toxicological and biodistribution studies under good laboratory practices (GLP) conditions. Since the products of the *NXNL1* gene are expressed in the retina of patients prior to the degeneration of photoreceptors, an immune response against the transgene products is not expected. Those studies are done according to regulatory guidelines [170–172] and the results are used to request the clinical trial authorization to regulatory bodies. While not mandatory, it is advisable to use non-human primates (NHPs), most often macaques, because among mammals only primates have a fovea [173]. Only laboratories with accreditation can perform such analyses with the objective of demonstrating the absence of toxicity at the therapeutic dose and minimal toxic effect at several times this dose to provide a safety margin. This is usually performed at two different time-points after treatment. Biodistribution studies document the spreading of the recombinant AAV particles into the whole organism which is quite limited after subretinal injection. In addition, the tolerance of the surgical procedure is validated. While it is reasonable that RdCVF will be secreted by RPE-infected cells from the site of injection to the cones within the fovea, the cell-autonomous mechanism of action of RdCVFL under the control of a cone-specific promoter implies that the cones are optimally transduced following subretinal or suprachoroid injection [111,174]. The suprachoroidal space is a potential route to the center of the retina. Subretinal injection creates a temporary bullous detachment, separating the photoreceptor outer segments from the RPE layer. Typically, the subretinal injection bleb resolves over the following few days in humans. Lateral spread adjacent to the initial subretinal injection site of transduction was observed in dogs as a result of a continued detachment of the retina as the bleb flattened out over the first thee3 days post injection [175]. Lateral spread could allow subretinal injection in the parafoveal region to produce transduction of the foveal cells while circumventing the deleterious effects of inducing a foveal detachment. The phenomenon was studied in the dog [175]. Two hundred fifty μl of AAV vector at 5×10^{11} vg/mL were injected in the subretinal space in the tapetal region, the *area centralis*, of the fundus of the dog retina. By estimating the size of that bleb using the human retina and the known distance separating the optic nerve head and the fovea it is possible to calculate the volume to be injected.

In order to liberate clinical batches of the drug, they must be qualified using a potency assay that demonstrates that the drug is biologically active. In a research laboratory this is performed using primary cells and animal models that cannot be used within an industrial process. At the early clinical stages, the expression of RdCVF and RdCVFL mRNA can be measured using quantitative RT-PCR and the proteins by sandwich ELISA, but both requires the transduction of an immortalized cell line, cells that can be handled in a confined environment. Since RdCVFL is under control of a cone opsin promoter, only retinoblastoma cell lines that originate from cone precursors are expressing this transgene after their transduction with the AAV expressing RdCVF and RdCVFL [176]. At more advanced stages, the biological activities of both transgenes requires the development of tests after the transduction of the drug in such cell lines.

7. Clinical Trial

One of the main aspect of a trial for RP treatment is to recruit a population of patients with a homogenous secondary degeneration of cones [41,177–184]. While the protection of cone function using RdCVF and RdCVFL is predicted to be independent of the causative mutation, in a first stage of a clinical trial recruiting a RP cohort representing a full diversity of mutation in the 65 causative genes reported so far (https://sph.uth.edu/retnet/) may result in an enormous phenotype heterogeneity that will mask any possible benefit for vision after statistical analysis. Since we have demonstrated the positive effects of cone vision of a rodent models of recessive and dominant RP, patients carrying a recessive mutation of the *PDE6B* gene (4% of all recessive RP) and those with dominant mutations in the *RHO* gene (25% of all dominant RP) are better suited for this phase of the project [101]. The cohort will enroll such patients without further stratification. A retrospective study of the visual phenotype of such of patients allow to predict, in addition to the absence of advert effects, what can be expected in terms of benefit and how long after treatment this benefit could be recorded. This study is done to document RP natural history on both anatomical and functional parameters. Even if the mode of action of RdCVF suggests that the cone outer segment could be reconstructed [96], in a more realistic assumption, the prevention of the deconstruction of the cone outer segment following rod cell-death is directly proportional to this rate of deconstruction and of cone vision loss during a given period of time. The retrospective study will be used to evaluate the patients that can benefit from the treatment based on criteria that include the identification of fast progressors. The same cohort will be enrolled in a prospective study for which a subset will received an injection in the macula and peri-macula area of the drug. Even if the first patients will receive a sub-optimal dose for security reasons, the total number of full AAV particles to be injected can be calculated from the efficient dose in the *rd10* mouse in the preclinical study to which must be applied a coefficient calculated by the difference in the number of cones in the mouse and human retina: 113,000 cones in the mouse and 6,400,000 cones in the human retina [165,185]. A low dose will be evaluated on a few severe patients, but an efficient dose will then be evaluated on a cohort of patients with moderate to severe RP. This cohort will exclude patients with no detectable ellipsoid zone that reflects the presence of cone outer segments by spectral domain optical coherence tomography (SD-OCT) [186,187].

The absence of adverse effects and the benefit of the treatment will be assessed by comparing the rate of loss of cone vision of the treated eyes to untreated eyes. The time necessary in the trial to see efficacy may be of several years by measuring visual acuity using kinetic perimetry but other parameters, such as an autofluorescent ring, may evolve faster [188,189]. This should encourage a multicentric and international phase III trial which will be standardized using data on the natural history of the cohorts at each site. An example of other possible complications is the prevalence of the P23H dominant mutation of the rhodopsin gene in North America, while the most prevalent mutation in Europe is P347L [40,41]. Patients with the P347L mutation have an early onset and severe disease, but patients with the P23H mutation are slow progressors [43,190]. This difference will have to be taken in consideration during the evaluation of the benefit of the treatment of RP patients with a recombinant AAV encoding for RdCVF and RdCVFL.

8. Conclusions

The dominance of rods in the retina of most mammals is the result of an evolutionary constraint known as nocturnal bottleneck [191]. The reasons explaining why, in RP, rods are affected before cones, even in cases of mutations in genes expressed by both types of photoreceptors, is presently unknown. The secondary loss of function of cones is observed irrespective of the type of mutations. The interruption of the metabolic and redox signaling between rods and cones though the loss of expression of RdCVF following rod cell death explains quite well the phenomenon which is initiated by the reduction of cone vision because of the shortening of the cone outer segments [117,118]. Even if this mechanism may not be unique [192], the administration of both products of the *NXNL1* gene provides the rational for a therapy aimed at preventing or delaying the loss of central vision in all genetic forms of RP.

9. Patents

This section is not mandatory, but may be added if there are patents resulting from the work reported in this manuscript.

Author Contributions: Conceptualization: J.-A.S. and T.L.; methodology: M.M. and E.C.; writing—review and editing: E.C., M.M., J.-A.S., and T.L. All authors have read and agree to the published version of the manuscript.

Acknowledgments: Frédéric Blond for proofreading the manuscript and Sophie Skorupka for advice on regulatory aspects.

Abbreviations

AAV	Adeno-associated viral vector
ATP	Adenosine triphosphate
BSG	Basigin
BSG1	Basigin-1 with three immunoglobulin domains
BSG2	Basigin-2 with two immunoglobulin domains
CBA	Chicken beta-actin
cGMP	Cyclic guanosine monophosphate
CMV	Cytomegalovirus
CNTF	Ciliary neurotrophic factor
COS-1	Immortalizing CV-1 cell line
CsCl	Cesium chloride
CSNB	Congenital stationary night blindness
CX3CL1	C-X3-C motif chemokine ligand 1 or fractalkine
DHAP	Dihydroxyacetone phosphate
EMA	European Medicines Agency
ERG	Electroretinogram
FDA	Food and Drug Administration
G3P	Glycerol-3-phosphate
G3PDH	Glycerol-3-phosphate dehydrogenase
G6P	Glucose-6-phosphate
GFP	Green fluorescent protein
GLP	Good laboratory practices
GLUT1	Glucose transporter SLC2A1
GMP	Good manufacturing practice
GNAT1	rod transducin alpha subunit
HEK293	Human embryonic kidney 293 cell line
HDAC4	Histone deacetylase 4
Ig	Immunoglobulin domain
ITRs	Invert terminal repeats
KLF15	Krüppel-like factor 15
LACT	Lactate
LCA	Leber congenital amaurosis
LCA2	Leber congenital amaurosis with a mutation in the RPE65 gene
LCR	Locus control region
LDH	Lactate dehydrogenase
LRAT	Lecithin-retinol acyltransferase
MTCs	Lactate transporters
MPC	Mitochondrial pyruvate carrier
NADPH	Nicotinamide adenine dinucleotide phosphate, reduced
NHPs	Non-human primates
NXNL1	Nucleoredoxin-like 1gene
OPN1L/MW	Long and middle wave opsin gene
OXPHO	Oxidative phosphorylation
PDE6B	Phosphodiesterase 6B
PPP	Pentose phosphate pathway
PRPF31	Pre-mRNA processing factor 31
PUFA	Poly-unsaturated fatty acids
PYR	Pyruvate

qPCR	Quantitative polymerase chain reaction
RB1	Tumor suppressor retinoblastoma 1
rd1	Retinal degeneration 1 mutant
RdCVF	Rod-derived cone viability factor
RdCVFL	Thioredoxin enzyme rod-derived cone viability factor long
ROS	Reactive oxygen species
RP	Retinitis pigmentosa
RPE	Retinal pigmented epithelium
RPE65	Retinal pigment epithelium protein of 65 kDa
SD-OCT	Spectral domain optical coherence tomography
SV40T	Simian virus 40 large T antigen
TCA	Tricarboxylic acid cycle
TXNRD	Thioredoxin reductase

References

1. Takahashi, V.K.L.; Takiuti, J.T.; Jauregui, R.; Tsang, S.H. Gene therapy in inherited retinal degenerative diseases, a review. *Ophthalmic Genet.* **2018**, *39*, 560–568. [CrossRef]
2. Kumaran, N.; Michaelides, M.; Smith, A.J.; Ali, R.R.; Bainbridge, J.W.B. Retinal gene therapy. *Br. Med. Bull.* **2018**, *126*, 13–25. [CrossRef] [PubMed]
3. Trapani, I.; Auricchio, A. Has retinal gene therapy come of age? From bench to bedside and back to bench. *Hum. Mol. Genet.* **2019**, *28*, R108–R118. [CrossRef] [PubMed]
4. Apte, R.S. Gene Therapy for Retinal Degeneration. *Cell* **2018**, *173*, 5. [CrossRef] [PubMed]
5. Kaiser, J. Clinical research. Gene therapists celebrate a decade of progress. *Science* **2011**, *334*, 29–30. [CrossRef]
6. Hamel, C.P.; Tsilou, E.; Pfeffer, B.A.; Hooks, J.J.; Detrick, B.; Redmond, T.M. Molecular cloning and expression of RPE65, a novel retinal pigment epithelium-specific microsomal protein that is post-transcriptionally regulated in vitro. *J. Biol. Chem.* **1993**, *268*, 15751–15757.
7. Marlhens, F.; Bareil, C.; Griffoin, J.M.; Zrenner, E.; Amalric, P.; Eliaou, C.; Liu, S.Y.; Harris, E.; Redmond, T.M.; Arnaud, B.; et al. Mutations in RPE65 cause Leber's congenital amaurosis. *Nat. Genet.* **1997**, *17*, 139–141. [CrossRef]
8. Redmond, T.M.; Yu, S.; Lee, E.; Bok, D.; Hamasaki, D.; Chen, N.; Goletz, P.; Ma, J.X.; Crouch, R.K.; Pfeifer, K. Rpe65 is necessary for production of 11-cis-vitamin A in the retinal visual cycle. *Nat. Genet.* **1998**, *20*, 344–351. [CrossRef]
9. Aguirre, G.D.; Baldwin, V.; Pearce-Kelling, S.; Narfstrom, K.; Ray, K.; Acland, G.M. Congenital stationary night blindness in the dog: Common mutation in the RPE65 gene indicates founder effect. *Mol. Vis.* **1998**, *4*, 23.
10. Acland, G.M.; Aguirre, G.D.; Ray, J.; Zhang, Q.; Aleman, T.S.; Cideciyan, A.V.; Pearce-Kelling, S.E.; Anand, V.; Zeng, Y.; Maguire, A.M.; et al. Gene therapy restores vision in a canine model of childhood blindness. *Nat. Genet.* **2001**, *28*, 92–95. [CrossRef]
11. Lehrman, S. Virus treatment questioned after gene therapy death. *Nature* **1999**, *401*, 517–518. [CrossRef] [PubMed]
12. Marshall, E. Gene therapy death prompts review of adenovirus vector. *Science* **1999**, *286*, 2244–2245. [CrossRef] [PubMed]
13. Barbour, V. The balance of risk and benefit in gene-therapy trials. *Lancet* **2000**, *355*, 384. [CrossRef]
14. Maguire, A.M.; Simonelli, F.; Pierce, E.A.; Pugh, E.N., Jr.; Mingozzi, F.; Bennicelli, J.; Banfi, S.; Marshall, K.A.; Testa, F.; Surace, E.M.; et al. Safety and efficacy of gene transfer for Leber's congenital amaurosis. *N. Engl. J. Med.* **2008**, *358*, 2240–2248. [CrossRef]
15. Bainbridge, J.W.; Smith, A.J.; Barker, S.S.; Robbie, S.; Henderson, R.; Balaggan, K.; Viswanathan, A.; Holder, G.E.; Stockman, A.; Tyler, N.; et al. Effect of gene therapy on visual function in Leber's congenital amaurosis. *N. Engl. J. Med.* **2008**, *358*, 2231–2239. [CrossRef]
16. Cideciyan, A.V.; Aleman, T.S.; Boye, S.L.; Schwartz, S.B.; Kaushal, S.; Roman, A.J.; Pang, J.J.; Sumaroka, A.; Windsor, E.A.; Wilson, J.M.; et al. Human gene therapy for RPE65 isomerase deficiency activates the retinoid cycle of vision but with slow rod kinetics. *Proc. Natl. Acad. Sci. USA* **2008**, *105*, 15112–15117. [CrossRef]

17. Ledford, H. Success against blindness encourages gene therapy researchers. *Nature* **2015**, *526*, 487–488. [CrossRef]
18. Bennett, J.; Ashtari, M.; Wellman, J.; Marshall, K.A.; Cyckowski, L.L.; Chung, D.C.; McCague, S.; Pierce, E.A.; Chen, Y.; Bennicelli, J.L.; et al. AAV2 gene therapy readministration in three adults with congenital blindness. *Sci. Transl. Med.* **2012**, *4*, 120ra15. [CrossRef]
19. Cideciyan, A.V.; Jacobson, S.G.; Beltran, W.A.; Sumaroka, A.; Swider, M.; Iwabe, S.; Roman, A.J.; Olivares, M.B.; Schwartz, S.B.; Komaromy, A.M.; et al. Human retinal gene therapy for Leber congenital amaurosis shows advancing retinal degeneration despite enduring visual improvement. *Proc. Natl. Acad. Sci. USA* **2013**, *110*, E517–E525. [CrossRef]
20. Jacobson, S.G.; Cideciyan, A.V.; Roman, A.J.; Sumaroka, A.; Schwartz, S.B.; Heon, E.; Hauswirth, W.W. Improvement and decline in vision with gene therapy in childhood blindness. *N. Engl. J. Med.* **2015**, *372*, 1920–1926. [CrossRef]
21. Bainbridge, J.W.; Mehat, M.S.; Sundaram, V.; Robbie, S.J.; Barker, S.E.; Ripamonti, C.; Georgiadis, A.; Mowat, F.M.; Beattie, S.G.; Gardner, P.J.; et al. Long-term effect of gene therapy on Leber's congenital amaurosis. *N. Engl. J. Med.* **2015**, *372*, 1887–1897. [CrossRef] [PubMed]
22. Boye, S.E.; Huang, W.C.; Roman, A.J.; Sumaroka, A.; Boye, S.L.; Ryals, R.C.; Olivares, M.B.; Ruan, Q.; Tucker, B.A.; Stone, E.M.; et al. Natural history of cone disease in the murine model of Leber congenital amaurosis due to CEP290 mutation: Determining the timing and expectation of therapy. *PLoS ONE* **2014**, *9*, e92928. [CrossRef] [PubMed]
23. Beltran, W.A.; Cideciyan, A.V.; Iwabe, S.; Swider, M.; Kosyk, M.S.; McDaid, K.; Martynyuk, I.; Ying, G.S.; Shaffer, J.; Deng, W.T.; et al. Successful arrest of photoreceptor and vision loss expands the therapeutic window of retinal gene therapy to later stages of disease. *Proc. Natl. Acad. Sci. USA* **2015**, *112*, E5844–E5853. [CrossRef] [PubMed]
24. Wright, C.B.; Redmond, T.M.; Nickerson, J.M. A History of the Classical Visual Cycle. *Prog. Mol. Biol. Transl. Sci.* **2015**, *134*, 433–448.
25. Caruso, R.C.; Aleman, T.S.; Cideciyan, A.V.; Roman, A.J.; Sumaroka, A.; Mullins, C.L.; Boye, S.L.; Hauswirth, W.W.; Jacobson, S.G. Retinal disease in Rpe65-deficient mice: Comparison to human leber congenital amaurosis due to RPE65 mutations. *Investig. Ophthalmol. Vis. Sci.* **2010**, *51*, 5304–5313. [CrossRef]
26. Zhang, T.; Zhang, N.; Baehr, W.; Fu, Y. Cone opsin determines the time course of cone photoreceptor degeneration in Leber congenital amaurosis. *Proc. Natl. Acad. Sci. USA* **2011**, *108*, 8879–8884. [CrossRef]
27. Russell, S.; Bennett, J.; Wellman, J.A.; Chung, D.C.; Yu, Z.F.; Tillman, A.; Wittes, J.; Pappas, J.; Elci, O.; McCague, S.; et al. Efficacy and safety of voretigene neparvovec (AAV2-hRPE65v2) in patients with RPE65-mediated inherited retinal dystrophy: A randomised, controlled, open-label, phase 3 trial. *Lancet* **2017**, *390*, 849–860. [CrossRef]
28. Frison-Roche, R. *Premier de Cordée: Roman*; J'ai Lu: Paris, France, 1941.
29. Darrow, J.J. Luxturna: FDA documents reveal the value of a costly gene therapy. *Drug Discov. Today* **2019**, *24*, 949–954. [CrossRef]
30. Blond, F.; Leveillard, T. Functional Genomics of the Retina to Elucidate its Construction and Deconstruction. *Int. J. Mol. Sci.* **2019**, *20*, 4922. [CrossRef]
31. Vithana, E.N.; Abu-Safieh, L.; Allen, M.J.; Carey, A.; Papaioannou, M.; Chakarova, C.; Al-Maghtheh, M.; Ebenezer, N.D.; Willis, C.; Moore, A.T.; et al. A human homolog of yeast pre-mRNA splicing gene, PRP31, underlies autosomal dominant retinitis pigmentosa on chromosome 19q13.4 (RP11). *Mol. Cell* **2001**, *8*, 375–381.
32. Rose, A.M.; Bhattacharya, S.S. Variant haploinsufficiency and phenotypic non-penetrance in PRPF31-associated retinitis pigmentosa. *Clin. Genet.* **2016**, *90*, 118–126. [CrossRef]
33. Dryja, T.P.; McGee, T.L.; Hahn, L.B.; Cowley, G.S.; Olsson, J.E.; Reichel, E.; Sandberg, M.A.; Berson, E.L. Mutations within the rhodopsin gene in patients with autosomal dominant retinitis pigmentosa. *N. Engl. J. Med.* **1990**, *323*, 1302–1307. [CrossRef] [PubMed]
34. Mendes, H.F.; van der Spuy, J.; Chapple, J.P.; Cheetham, M.E. Mechanisms of cell death in rhodopsin retinitis pigmentosa: Implications for therapy. *Trends Mol. Med.* **2005**, *11*, 177–185. [CrossRef]
35. Gorbatyuk, M.S.; Knox, T.; LaVail, M.M.; Gorbatyuk, O.S.; Noorwez, S.M.; Hauswirth, W.W.; Lin, J.H.; Muzyczka, N.; Lewin, A.S. Restoration of visual function in P23H rhodopsin transgenic rats by gene delivery of BiP/Grp78. *Proc. Natl. Acad. Sci. USA* **2010**, *107*, 5961–5966. [CrossRef]

36. Lewin, A.S.; Drenser, K.A.; Hauswirth, W.W.; Nishikawa, S.; Yasumura, D.; Flannery, J.G.; LaVail, M.M. Ribozyme rescue of photoreceptor cells in a transgenic rat model of autosomal dominant retinitis pigmentosa. *Nat. Med.* **1998**, *4*, 967–971. [CrossRef] [PubMed]
37. Phylactou, L.A.; Kilpatrick, M.W.; Wood, M.J. Ribozymes as therapeutic tools for genetic disease. *Hum. Mol. Genet.* **1998**, *7*, 1649–1653. [CrossRef] [PubMed]
38. Hauswirth, W.W.; Lewin, A.S. Ribozyme uses in retinal gene therapy. *Prog. Retin. Eye Res.* **2000**, *19*, 689–710. [CrossRef]
39. Malanson, K.M.; Lem, J. Rhodopsin-mediated retinitis pigmentosa. *Prog. Mol. Biol. Transl. Sci.* **2009**, *88*, 1–31.
40. Audo, I.; Manes, G.; Mohand-Said, S.; Friedrich, A.; Lancelot, M.E.; Antonio, A.; Moskova-Doumanova, V.; Poch, O.; Zanlonghi, X.; Hamel, C.P.; et al. Spectrum of rhodopsin mutations in French autosomal dominant rod-cone dystrophy patients. *Investig. Ophthalmol. Vis. Sci.* **2010**, *51*, 3687–3700. [CrossRef]
41. Fernandez-San Jose, P.; Blanco-Kelly, F.; Corton, M.; Trujillo-Tiebas, M.J.; Gimenez, A.; Avila-Fernandez, A.; Garcia-Sandoval, B.; Lopez-Molina, M.I.; Hernan, I.; Carballo, M.; et al. Prevalence of Rhodopsin mutations in autosomal dominant Retinitis Pigmentosa in Spain: Clinical and analytical review in 200 families. *Acta Ophthalmol.* **2015**, *93*, e38–e44. [CrossRef]
42. Oh, K.T.; Longmuir, R.; Oh, D.M.; Stone, E.M.; Kopp, K.; Brown, J.; Fishman, G.A.; Sonkin, P.; Gehrs, K.M.; Weleber, R.G. Comparison of the clinical expression of retinitis pigmentosa associated with rhodopsin mutations at codon 347 and codon 23. *Am. J. Ophthalmol.* **2003**, *136*, 306–313. [CrossRef]
43. Bonilha, V.L.; Rayborn, M.E.; Bell, B.A.; Marino, M.J.; Beight, C.D.; Pauer, G.J.; Traboulsi, E.I.; Hollyfield, J.G.; Hagstrom, S.A. Retinal histopathology in eyes from patients with autosomal dominant retinitis pigmentosa caused by rhodopsin mutations. *Graefe's Arch. Clin. Exp. Ophthalmol.* **2015**, *253*, 2161–2169.
44. O'Reilly, M.; Palfi, A.; Chadderton, N.; Millington-Ward, S.; Ader, M.; Cronin, T.; Tuohy, T.; Auricchio, A.; Hildinger, M.; Tivnan, A.; et al. RNA interference-mediated suppression and replacement of human rhodopsin in vivo. *Am. J. Hum. Genet.* **2007**, *81*, 127–135. [CrossRef]
45. Cideciyan, A.V.; Sudharsan, R.; Dufour, V.L.; Massengill, M.T.; Iwabe, S.; Swider, M.; Lisi, B.; Sumaroka, A.; Marinho, L.F.; Appelbaum, T.; et al. Mutation-independent rhodopsin gene therapy by knockdown and replacement with a single AAV vector. *Proc. Natl. Acad. Sci. USA* **2018**, *115*, E8547–E8556. [CrossRef] [PubMed]
46. Kiang, A.S.; Palfi, A.; Ader, M.; Kenna, P.F.; Millington-Ward, S.; Clark, G.; Kennan, A.; O'Reilly, M.; Tam, L.C.; Aherne, A.; et al. Toward a gene therapy for dominant disease: Validation of an RNA interference-based mutation-independent approach. *Mol. Ther. J. Am. Soc. Gene Ther.* **2005**, *12*, 555–561. [CrossRef] [PubMed]
47. Botta, S.; de Prisco, N.; Marrocco, E.; Renda, M.; Sofia, M.; Curion, F.; Bacci, M.L.; Ventrella, D.; Wilson, C.; Gesualdo, C.; et al. Targeting and silencing of rhodopsin by ectopic expression of the transcription factor KLF15. *JCI Insight* **2017**, *2*, e96560. [CrossRef] [PubMed]
48. Suzuki, K.; Tsunekawa, Y.; Hernandez-Benitez, R.; Wu, J.; Zhu, J.; Kim, E.J.; Hatanaka, F.; Yamamoto, M.; Araoka, T.; Li, Z.; et al. In vivo genome editing via CRISPR/Cas9 mediated homology-independent targeted integration. *Nature* **2016**, *540*, 144–149. [CrossRef] [PubMed]
49. Vagni, P.; Perlini, L.E.; Chenais, N.A.L.; Marchetti, T.; Parrini, M.; Contestabile, A.; Cancedda, L.; Ghezzi, D. Gene Editing Preserves Visual Functions in a Mouse Model of Retinal Degeneration. *Front. Neurosci.* **2019**, *13*, 945. [CrossRef] [PubMed]
50. Moreno, A.M.; Fu, X.; Zhu, J.; Katrekar, D.; Shih, Y.-R.V.; Marlett, J.; Cabotaje, J.; Tat, J.; Naughton, J.; Lisowski, L.; et al. In Situ Gene Therapy via AAV-CRISPR-Cas9-Mediated Targeted Gene Regulation. *Mol. Ther. J. Am. Soc. Gene Ther.* **2018**, *26*, 1818–1827. [CrossRef]
51. Samardzija, M.; Wenzel, A.; Thiersch, M.; Frigg, R.; Reme, C.; Grimm, C. Caspase-1 ablation protects photoreceptors in a model of autosomal dominant retinitis pigmentosa. *Investig. Ophthalmol. Vis. Sci.* **2006**, *47*, 5181–5190. [CrossRef]
52. Marigo, V. Programmed cell death in retinal degeneration: Targeting apoptosis in photoreceptors as potential therapy for retinal degeneration. *Cell Cycle* **2007**, *6*, 652–655. [CrossRef]
53. Guo, X.; Wang, S.B.; Xu, H.; Ribic, A.; Mohns, E.J.; Zhou, Y.; Zhu, X.; Biederer, T.; Crair, M.C.; Chen, B. A short N-terminal domain of HDAC4 preserves photoreceptors and restores visual function in retinitis pigmentosa. *Nat. Commun.* **2015**, *6*, 8005. [CrossRef]

54. Lipinski, D.M.; Barnard, A.R.; Singh, M.S.; Martin, C.; Lee, E.J.; Davies, W.I.L.; MacLaren, R.E. CNTF Gene Therapy Confers Lifelong Neuroprotection in a Mouse Model of Human Retinitis Pigmentosa. *Mol. Ther. J. Am. Soc. Gene Ther.* **2015**, *23*, 1308–1319. [CrossRef]
55. Birch, D.G.; Bennett, L.D.; Duncan, J.L.; Weleber, R.G.; Pennesi, M.E. Long-term Follow-up of Patients with Retinitis Pigmentosa Receiving Intraocular Ciliary Neurotrophic Factor Implants. *Am. J. Ophthalmol.* **2016**, *170*, 10–14. [CrossRef]
56. Karali, M.; Guadagnino, I.; Marrocco, E.; De Cegli, R.; Carissimo, A.; Pizzo, M.; Casarosa, S.; Conte, I.; Surace, E.M.; Banfi, S. AAV-miR-204 Protects from Retinal Degeneration by Attenuation of Microglia Activation and Photoreceptor Cell Death. *Mol. Ther. Nucleic Acids* **2019**, *19*, 144–156. [CrossRef]
57. Wang, S.K.; Xue, Y.; Rana, P.; Hong, C.M.; Cepko, C.L. Soluble CX3CL1 gene therapy improves cone survival and function in mouse models of retinitis pigmentosa. *Proc. Natl. Acad. Sci. USA* **2019**, *116*, 10140–10149. [CrossRef]
58. Xiong, W.; MacColl Garfinkel, A.E.; Li, Y.; Benowitz, L.I.; Cepko, C.L. NRF2 promotes neuronal survival in neurodegeneration and acute nerve damage. *J. Clin. Investig.* **2015**, *125*, 1433–1445. [CrossRef]
59. Picard, E.; Jonet, L.; Sergeant, C.; Vesvres, M.-H.; Behar-Cohen, F.; Courtois, Y.; Jeanny, J.-C. Overexpressed or intraperitoneally injected human transferrin prevents photoreceptor degeneration in rd10 mice. *Mol. Vis.* **2010**, *16*, 2612–2625.
60. Petit, L.; Punzo, C. mTORC1 sustains vision in retinitis pigmentosa. *Oncotarget* **2015**, *6*, 16786–16787. [CrossRef]
61. Zhang, L.; Du, J.; Justus, S.; Hsu, C.-W.; Bonet-Ponce, L.; Wu, W.-H.; Tsai, Y.-T.; Wu, W.-P.; Jia, Y.; Duong, J.K.; et al. Reprogramming metabolism by targeting sirtuin 6 attenuates retinal degeneration. *J. Clin. Investig.* **2016**, *126*, 4659–4673. [CrossRef]
62. Portera-Cailliau, C.; Sung, C.H.; Nathans, J.; Adler, R. Apoptotic photoreceptor cell death in mouse models of retinitis pigmentosa. *Proc. Natl. Acad. Sci. USA* **1994**, *91*, 974–978. [CrossRef]
63. Hartong, D.T.; Berson, E.L.; Dryja, T.P. Retinitis pigmentosa. *Lancet* **2006**, *368*, 1795–1809. [CrossRef]
64. Snyder, C. Jean Nougaret, the butcher from Provence, and his family. *Arch. Ophthalmol.* **1963**, *69*, 676–678. [CrossRef] [PubMed]
65. Dryja, T.P.; Hahn, L.B.; Reboul, T.; Arnaud, B. Missense mutation in the gene encoding the alpha subunit of rod transducin in the Nougaret form of congenital stationary night blindness. *Nat. Genet.* **1996**, *13*, 358–360. [CrossRef] [PubMed]
66. Rosenberg, T.; Haim, M.; Piczenik, Y.; Simonsen, S.E. Autosomal Dominant Stationary Night-Blindness—A Large Family Rediscovered. *Acta Ophthalmol.* **1991**, *69*, 694–702. [CrossRef] [PubMed]
67. Zeitz, C.; Robson, A.G.; Audo, I. Congenital stationary night blindness: An analysis and update of genotype-phenotype correlations and pathogenic mechanisms. *Prog. Retin. Eye Res.* **2015**, *45*, 58–110. [CrossRef]
68. Wright, A.F. A searchlight through the fog. *Nat. Genet.* **1997**, *17*, 132–134. [CrossRef]
69. Kaplan, H.J.; Wang, W.; Dean, D.C. Restoration of Cone Photoreceptor Function in Retinitis Pigmentosa. *Transl. Vis. Sci. Technol.* **2017**, *6*, 5. [CrossRef]
70. Geller, A.M.; Sieving, P.A. Assessment of foveal cone photoreceptors in Stargardt's macular dystrophy using a small dot detection task. *Vis. Res.* **1993**, *33*, 1509–1524. [CrossRef]
71. Petersen-Jones, S.M.; Occelli, L.M.; Winkler, P.A.; Lee, W.; Sparrow, J.R.; Tsukikawa, M.; Boye, S.L.; Chiodo, V.; Capasso, J.E.; Becirovic, E.; et al. Patients and animal models of CNGβ1-deficient retinitis pigmentosa support gene augmentation approach. *J. Clin. Investig.* **2017**, *128*, 190–206. [CrossRef]
72. Cronin, T.; Leveillard, T.; Sahel, J.A. Retinal degenerations: From cell signaling to cell therapy; pre-clinical and clinical issues. *Curr. Gene Ther.* **2007**, *7*, 121–129. [CrossRef]
73. Applebury, M.L. Molecular-Genetics—Insight into Blindness. *Nature* **1990**, *343*, 316–317. [CrossRef]
74. Daiger, S.P.; Humphries, M.M.; Giesenschlag, N.; Sharp, E.; McWilliam, P.; Farrer, J.; Bradley, D.; Kenna, P.; McConnell, D.J.; Sparkes, R.S.; et al. Linkage analysis of human chromosome 4: Exclusion of autosomal dominant retinitis pigmentosa (ADRP) and detection of new linkage groups. *Cytogenet. Cell Genet.* **1989**, *50*, 181–187. [CrossRef]
75. Dryja, T.P.; McGee, T.L.; Reichel, E.; Hahn, L.B.; Cowley, G.S.; Yandell, D.W.; Sandberg, M.A.; Berson, E.L. A point mutation of the rhodopsin gene in one form of retinitis pigmentosa. *Nature* **1990**, *343*, 364–366. [CrossRef]

76. Kolb, H.; Gouras, P. Electron microscopic observations of human retinitis pigmentosa, dominantly inherited. *Investig. Ophthalmol.* **1974**, *13*, 487–498.
77. Berson, E.L. Ocular findings in a form of retinitis pigmentosa with a rhodopsin gene defect. *Trans. Am. Ophthalmol. Soc.* **1990**, *88*, 355–388.
78. Cideciyan, A.V.; Hood, D.C.; Huang, Y.; Banin, E.; Li, Z.Y.; Stone, E.M.; Milam, A.H.; Jacobson, S.G. Disease sequence from mutant rhodopsin allele to rod and cone photoreceptor degeneration in man. *Proc. Natl. Acad. Sci. USA* **1998**, *95*, 7103–7108. [CrossRef]
79. Carter-Dawson, L.D.; LaVail, M.M.; Sidman, R.L. Differential effect of the rd mutation on rods and cones in the mouse retina. *Investig. Ophthalmol. Vis. Sci.* **1978**, *17*, 489–498.
80. Bowes, C.; Li, T.; Danciger, M.; Baxter, L.C.; Applebury, M.L.; Farber, D.B. Retinal degeneration in the rd mouse is caused by a defect in the beta subunit of rod cGMP-phosphodiesterase. *Nature* **1990**, *347*, 677–680. [CrossRef]
81. McLaughlin, M.E.; Sandberg, M.A.; Berson, E.L.; Dryja, T.P. Recessive mutations in the gene encoding the beta-subunit of rod phosphodiesterase in patients with retinitis pigmentosa. *Nat. Genet.* **1993**, *4*, 130–134. [CrossRef]
82. Usukura, J.; Khoo, W.; Abe, T.; Breitman, M.L.; Shinohara, T. Cone cells fail to develop normally in transgenic mice showing ablation of rod photoreceptor cells. *Cell Tissue Res.* **1994**, *275*, 79–90. [CrossRef]
83. McCall, M.A.; Gregg, R.G.; Merriman, K.; Goto, Y.; Peachey, N.S.; Stanford, L.R. Morphological and physiological consequences of the selective elimination of rod photoreceptors in transgenic mice. *Exp. Eye Res.* **1996**, *63*, 35–50. [CrossRef]
84. Scott, P.A.; de Castro, J.P.; DeMarco, P.J.; Ross, J.W.; Njoka, J.; Walters, E.; Prather, R.S.; McCall, M.A.; Kaplan, H.J. Progression of Pro23His Retinopathy in a Miniature Swine Model of Retinitis Pigmentosa. *Transl. Vis. Sci. Technol.* **2017**, *6*, 4. [CrossRef] [PubMed]
85. Mieziewska, K.; Van Veen, T.; Aguirre, G.D. Development and fate of interphotoreceptor matrix components during dysplastic photoreceptor differentiation: A lectin cytochemical study of rod-cone dysplasia 1. *Exp. Eye Res.* **1993**, *56*, 429–441. [CrossRef] [PubMed]
86. Choi, R.Y.; Engbretson, G.A.; Solessio, E.C.; Jones, G.A.; Coughlin, A.; Aleksic, I.; Zuber, M.E. Cone degeneration following rod ablation in a reversible model of retinal degeneration. *Investig. Ophthalmol. Vis. Sci.* **2011**, *52*, 364–373. [CrossRef]
87. Punzo, C.; Kornacker, K.; Cepko, C.L. Stimulation of the insulin/mTOR pathway delays cone death in a mouse model of retinitis pigmentosa. *Nat. Neurosci.* **2009**, *12*, 44–52. [CrossRef]
88. Mohand-Said, S.; Hicks, D.; Simonutti, M.; Tran-Minh, D.; Deudon-Combe, A.; Dreyfus, H.; Silverman, M.S.; Ogilvie, J.M.; Tenkova, T.; Sahel, J. Photoreceptor transplants increase host cone survival in the retinal degeneration (rd) mouse. *Ophthalmic Res.* **1997**, *29*, 290–297. [CrossRef]
89. Mohand-Said, S.; Hicks, D.; Dreyfus, H.; Sahel, J.A. Selective transplantation of rods delays cone loss in a retinitis pigmentosa model. *Arch. Ophthalmol.* **2000**, *118*, 807–811. [CrossRef]
90. Mohand-Said, S.; Deudon-Combe, A.; Hicks, D.; Simonutti, M.; Forster, V.; Fintz, A.C.; Leveillard, T.; Dreyfus, H.; Sahel, J.A. Normal retina releases a diffusible factor stimulating cone survival in the retinal degeneration mouse. *Proc. Natl. Acad. Sci. USA* **1998**, *95*, 8357–8362. [CrossRef]
91. Fintz, A.C.; Audo, I.; Hicks, D.; Mohand-Said, S.; Leveillard, T.; Sahel, J. Partial characterization of retina-derived cone neuroprotection in two culture models of photoreceptor degeneration. *Investig. Ophthalmol. Vis. Sci.* **2003**, *44*, 818–825. [CrossRef]
92. Adler, R.; Hatlee, M. Plasticity and differentiation of embryonic retinal cells after terminal mitosis. *Science* **1989**, *243*, 391–393. [CrossRef]
93. Hewitt, A.T.; Lindsey, J.D.; Carbott, D.; Adler, R. Photoreceptor survival-promoting activity in interphotoreceptor matrix preparations: Characterization and partial purification. *Exp. Eye Res.* **1990**, *50*, 79–88. [CrossRef]
94. Weleber, R.G.; Gregory-Evans, K. Retinitis Pigmentosa and Allied Disorders A2—Ryan, Stephen, J. In *Retina*, 4th ed.; Chapter 17; Hinton, D.R., Schachat, A.P., Wilkinson, C.P., Eds.; Mosby: Edinburgh, UK, 2006; pp. 395–498.
95. Leveillard, T.; Mohand-Said, S.; Lorentz, O.; Hicks, D.; Fintz, A.C.; Clerin, E.; Simonutti, M.; Forster, V.; Cavusoglu, N.; Chalmel, F.; et al. Identification and characterization of rod-derived cone viability factor. *Nat. Genet.* **2004**, *36*, 755–759. [CrossRef]

96. Ait-Ali, N.; Fridlich, R.; Millet-Puel, G.; Clerin, E.; Delalande, F.; Jaillard, C.; Blond, F.; Perrocheau, L.; Reichman, S.; Byrne, L.C.; et al. Rod-derived cone viability factor promotes cone survival by stimulating aerobic glycolysis. *Cell* **2015**, *161*, 817–832. [CrossRef]
97. Lambard, S.; Reichman, S.; Berlinicke, C.; Niepon, M.L.; Goureau, O.; Sahel, J.A.; Leveillard, T.; Zack, D.J. Expression of rod-derived cone viability factor: Dual role of CRX in regulating promoter activity and cell-type specificity. *PLoS ONE* **2010**, *5*, e13075. [CrossRef]
98. Reichman, S.; Kalathur, R.K.; Lambard, S.; Ait-Ali, N.; Yang, Y.; Lardenois, A.; Ripp, R.; Poch, O.; Zack, D.J.; Sahel, J.A.; et al. The homeobox gene CHX10/VSX2 regulates RdCVF promoter activity in the inner retina. *Hum. Mol. Genet.* **2010**, *19*, 250–261. [CrossRef]
99. Delyfer, M.N.; Raffelsberger, W.; Mercier, D.; Korobelnik, J.F.; Gaudric, A.; Charteris, D.G.; Tadayoni, R.; Metge, F.; Caputo, G.; Barale, P.O.; et al. Transcriptomic analysis of human retinal detachment reveals both inflammatory response and photoreceptor death. *PLoS ONE* **2011**, *6*, e28791. [CrossRef]
100. Yang, Y.; Mohand-Said, S.; Danan, A.; Simonutti, M.; Fontaine, V.; Clerin, E.; Picaud, S.; Leveillard, T.; Sahel, J.A. Functional cone rescue by RdCVF protein in a dominant model of retinitis pigmentosa. *Mol. Ther. J. Am. Soc. Gene Ther.* **2009**, *17*, 787–795. [CrossRef]
101. Leveillard, T.; Sahel, J.A. Rod-derived cone viability factor for treating blinding diseases: From clinic to redox signaling. *Sci. Transl. Med.* **2010**, *2*, 26ps16. [CrossRef]
102. Sahel, J.A.; Leveillard, T.; Picaud, S.; Dalkara, D.; Marazova, K.; Safran, A.; Paques, M.; Duebel, J.; Roska, B.; Mohand-Said, S. Functional rescue of cone photoreceptors in retinitis pigmentosa. *Graefe's Arch. Clin. Exp. Ophthalmol.* **2013**, *251*, 1669–1677.
103. Byrne, L.C.; Dalkara, D.; Luna, G.; Fisher, S.K.; Clerin, E.; Sahel, J.A.; Leveillard, T.; Flannery, J.G. Viral-mediated RdCVF and RdCVFL expression protects cone and rod photoreceptors in retinal degeneration. *J. Clin. Investig.* **2015**, *125*, 105–116. [CrossRef]
104. Ochrietor, J.D.; Moroz, T.P.; van Ekeris, L.; Clamp, M.F.; Jefferson, S.C.; deCarvalho, A.C.; Fadool, J.M.; Wistow, G.; Muramatsu, T.; Linser, P.J. Retina-specific expression of 5A11/Basigin-2, a member of the immunoglobulin gene superfamily. *Investig. Ophthalmol. Vis. Sci.* **2003**, *44*, 4086–4096; RetNet Retinal Information Network. Available online: https://sph.uth.edu/retnet/sum-dis.htm (accessed on 10 October 2019).
105. Leveillard, T. Cancer metabolism of cone photoreceptors. *Oncotarget* **2015**, *6*, 32285–32286. [CrossRef]
106. Chinchore, Y.; Begaj, T.; Wu, D.; Drokhlyansky, E.; Cepko, C.L. Glycolytic reliance promotes anabolism in photoreceptors. *eLife* **2017**, *6*, e25946. [CrossRef]
107. Chalmel, F.; Leveillard, T.; Jaillard, C.; Lardenois, A.; Berdugo, N.; Morel, E.; Koehl, P.; Lambrou, G.; Holmgren, A.; Sahel, J.A.; et al. Rod-derived Cone Viability Factor-2 is a novel bifunctional-thioredoxin-like protein with therapeutic potential. *BMC Mol. Biol.* **2007**, *8*, 74. [CrossRef]
108. Brennan, L.A.; Lee, W.; Kantorow, M. TXNL6 is a novel oxidative stress-induced reducing system for methionine sulfoxide reductase a repair of alpha-crystallin and cytochrome C in the eye lens. *PLoS ONE* **2010**, *5*, e15421. [CrossRef]
109. Cronin, T.; Raffelsberger, W.; Lee-Rivera, I.; Jaillard, C.; Niepon, M.L.; Kinzel, B.; Clerin, E.; Petrosian, A.; Picaud, S.; Poch, O.; et al. The disruption of the rod-derived cone viability gene leads to photoreceptor dysfunction and susceptibility to oxidative stress. *Cell Death Differ.* **2010**, *17*, 1199–1210. [CrossRef]
110. Sahel, J. Metabolic and redox signaling in the retina. *Cell. Mol. Life Sci. CMLS* **2016**, *74*, 3649–3665.
111. Mei, X.; Chaffiol, A.; Kole, C.; Yang, Y.; Millet-Puel, G.; Clerin, E.; Ait-Ali, N.; Bennett, J.; Dalkara, D.; Sahel, J.A.; et al. The Thioredoxin Encoded by the Rod-Derived Cone Viability Factor Gene Protects Cone Photoreceptors Against Oxidative Stress. *Antioxid. Redox Signal.* **2016**, *24*, 909–923. [CrossRef]
112. Anastasiou, D.; Poulogiannis, G.; Asara, J.M.; Boxer, M.B.; Jiang, J.K.; Shen, M.; Bellinger, G.; Sasaki, A.T.; Locasale, J.W.; Auld, D.S.; et al. Inhibition of pyruvate kinase M2 by reactive oxygen species contributes to cellular antioxidant responses. *Science* **2011**, *334*, 1278–1283. [CrossRef]
113. Hildebrandt, T.; Knuesting, J.; Berndt, C.; Morgan, B.; Scheibe, R. Cytosolic thiol switches regulating basic cellular functions: GAPDH as an information hub? *Biol. Chem.* **2015**, *396*, 523–537. [CrossRef]
114. Lopez-Grueso, M.J.; Gonzalez-Ojeda, R.; Requejo-Aguilar, R.; McDonagh, B.; Fuentes-Almagro, C.A.; Muntane, J.; Barcena, J.A.; Padilla, C.A. Thioredoxin and glutaredoxin regulate metabolism through different multiplex thiol switches. *Redox Biol.* **2019**, *21*, 101049. [CrossRef]

115. Ren, X.; Zou, L.; Lu, J.; Holmgren, A. Selenocysteine in mammalian thioredoxin reductase and application of ebselen as a therapeutic. *Free Radic. Biol. Med.* **2018**, *127*, 238–247. [CrossRef]
116. Camacho, E.T.; Brager, D.; Elachouri, G.; Korneyeva, T.; Millet-Puel, G.; Sahel, J.A.; Leveillard, T. A Mathematical Analysis of Aerobic Glycolysis Triggered by Glucose Uptake in Cones. *Sci. Rep.* **2019**, *9*, 4162. [CrossRef]
117. Leveillard, T.; Sahel, J.A. Metabolic and redox signaling in the retina. *Cell. Mol. Life Sci. CMLS* **2017**, *74*, 3649–3665. [CrossRef]
118. Leveillard, T.; Ait-Ali, N. Cell Signaling with Extracellular Thioredoxin and Thioredoxin-Like Proteins: Insight into Their Mechanisms of Action. *Oxidative Med. Cell. Longev.* **2017**, *2017*, 8475125. [CrossRef]
119. Domenger, C.; Grimm, D. Next-generation AAV vectors-do not judge a virus (only) by its cover. *Hum. Mol. Genet.* **2019**, *28*, R3–R14. [CrossRef]
120. Martinez-Fernandez De La Camara, C.; Cehajic-Kapetanovic, J.; MacLaren, R.E. RPGR gene therapy presents challenges in cloning the coding sequence. *Expert Opin. Biol. Ther.* **2019**, *9*, 63–71. [CrossRef]
121. Bell, P.; Wang, L.; Chen, S.J.; Yu, H.; Zhu, Y.; Nayal, M.; He, Z.; White, J.; Lebel-Hagan, D.; Wilson, J.M. Effects of Self-Complementarity, Codon Optimization, Transgene, and Dose on Liver Transduction with AAV8. *Hum. Gene Ther. Methods* **2016**, *27*, 228–237. [CrossRef]
122. Dai, Y.; Roman, M.; Naviaux, R.K.; Verma, I.M. Gene therapy via primary myoblasts: Long-term expression of factor IX protein following transplantation in vivo. *Proc. Natl. Acad. Sci. USA* **1992**, *89*, 10892–10895. [CrossRef]
123. Miyazaki, J.; Takaki, S.; Araki, K.; Tashiro, F.; Tominaga, A.; Takatsu, K.; Yamamura, K. Expression vector system based on the chicken beta-actin promoter directs efficient production of interleukin-5. *Gene* **1989**, *79*, 269–277.
124. Elachouri, G.; Lee-Rivera, I.; Clerin, E.; Argentini, M.; Fridlich, R.; Blond, F.; Ferracane, V.; Yang, Y.; Raffelsberger, W.; Wan, J.; et al. Thioredoxin rod-derived cone viability factor protects against photooxidative retinal damage. *Free Radic. Biol. Med.* **2015**, *81*, 22–29. [CrossRef]
125. Zack, D.J.; Bennett, J.; Wang, Y.; Davenport, C.; Klaunberg, B.; Gearhart, J.; Nathans, J. Unusual topography of bovine rhodopsin promoter-lacZ fusion gene expression in transgenic mouse retinas. *Neuron* **1991**, *6*, 187–199. [CrossRef]
126. Mancuso, K.; Hauswirth, W.W.; Li, Q.; Connor, T.B.; Kuchenbecker, J.A.; Mauck, M.C.; Neitz, J.; Neitz, M. Gene therapy for red-green colour blindness in adult primates. *Nature* **2009**, *461*, 784–787. [CrossRef]
127. Tian, J.; Andreadis, S.T. Independent and high-level dual-gene expression in adult stem-progenitor cells from a single lentiviral vector. *Gene Ther.* **2009**, *16*, 874–884. [CrossRef]
128. Nojima, T.; Dienstbier, M.; Murphy, S.; Proudfoot, N.J.; Dye, M.J. Definition of RNA polymerase II CoTC terminator elements in the human genome. *Cell Rep.* **2013**, *3*, 1080–1092. [CrossRef]
129. Parrish, C.; Berns, K. Parvoviridae. In *Fields Virology*, 5th ed.; Lippincott Williams & Wilkins: Philadelphia, PA, USA, 2007; pp. 2437–2477.
130. Dong, J.Y.; Fan, P.D.; Frizzell, R.A. Quantitative analysis of the packaging capacity of recombinant adeno-associated virus. *Hum. Gene Ther.* **1996**, *7*, 2101–2112. [CrossRef]
131. Grieger, J.C.; Samulski, R.J. Packaging capacity of adeno-associated virus serotypes: Impact of larger genomes on infectivity and postentry steps. *J. Virol.* **2005**, *79*, 9933–9944. [CrossRef]
132. Wu, Z.; Yang, H.; Colosi, P. Effect of genome size on AAV vector packaging. *Mol. Ther. J. Am. Soc. Gene Ther.* **2010**, *18*, 80–86. [CrossRef]
133. Bennicelli, J.; Wright, J.F.; Komaromy, A.; Jacobs, J.B.; Hauck, B.; Zelenaia, O.; Mingozzi, F.; Hui, D.; Chung, D.; Rex, T.S.; et al. Reversal of blindness in animal models of leber congenital amaurosis using optimized AAV2-mediated gene transfer. *Mol. Ther. J. Am. Soc. Gene Ther.* **2008**, *16*, 458–465. [CrossRef]
134. Cheng, S.W.; Court, D.L.; Friedman, D.I. Transcription termination signals in the nin region of bacteriophage lambda: Identification of Rho-dependent termination regions. *Genetics* **1995**, *140*, 875–887.
135. Chadeuf, G.; Ciron, C.; Moullier, P.; Salvetti, A. Evidence for encapsidation of prokaryotic sequences during recombinant adeno-associated virus production and their in vivo persistence after vector delivery. *Mol. Ther. J. Am. Soc. Gene Ther.* **2005**, *12*, 744–753. [CrossRef]
136. Wang, X.S.; Qing, K.; Ponnazhagan, S.; Srivastava, A. Adeno-associated virus type 2 DNA replication in vivo: Mutation analyses of the D sequence in viral inverted terminal repeats. *J. Virol.* **1997**, *71*, 3077–3082. [CrossRef]

137. Kole, C.; Klipfel, L.; Yang, Y.; Ferracane, V.; Blond, F.; Reichman, S.; Millet-Puel, G.; Clerin, E.; Ait-Ali, N.; Pagan, D.; et al. Otx2-Genetically Modified Retinal Pigment Epithelial Cells Rescue Photoreceptors after Transplantation. *Mol. Ther. J. Am. Soc. Gene Ther.* **2018**, *26*, 219–237. [CrossRef]
138. Schmeer, M.; Buchholz, T.; Schleef, M. Plasmid DNA Manufacturing for Indirect and Direct Clinical Applications. *Hum. Gene Ther.* **2017**, *28*, 856–861. [CrossRef] [PubMed]
139. Penaud-Budloo, M.; Francois, A.; Clement, N.; Ayuso, E. Pharmacology of Recombinant Adeno-associated Virus Production. *Mol. Ther. Methods Clin. Dev.* **2018**, *8*, 166–180. [CrossRef] [PubMed]
140. Lebherz, C.; Maguire, A.; Tang, W.; Bennett, J.; Wilson, J.M. Novel AAV serotypes for improved ocular gene transfer. *J. Gene Med.* **2008**, *10*, 375–382. [CrossRef] [PubMed]
141. Naso, M.F.; Tomkowicz, B.; Perry, W.L.; Strohl, W.R. Adeno-Associated Virus (AAV) as a Vector for Gene Therapy. *Biodrugs Clin. Immunother. Biopharm. Gene Ther.* **2017**, *31*, 317–334.
142. Vandenberghe, L.H.; Bell, P.; Maguire, A.M.; Xiao, R.; Hopkins, T.B.; Grant, R.; Bennett, J.; Wilson, J.M. AAV9 targets cone photoreceptors in the nonhuman primate retina. *PLoS ONE* **2013**, *8*, e53463. [CrossRef]
143. Boye, S.E.; Alexander, J.J.; Boye, S.L.; Witherspoon, C.D.; Sandefer, K.J.; Conlon, T.J.; Erger, K.; Sun, J.; Ryals, R.; Chiodo, V.A.; et al. The human rhodopsin kinase promoter in an AAV5 vector confers rod- and cone-specific expression in the primate retina. *Hum. Gene Ther.* **2012**, *23*, 1101–1115. [CrossRef]
144. Virag, T.; Cecchini, S.; Kotin, R.M. Producing recombinant adeno-associated virus in foster cells: Overcoming production limitations using a baculovirus-insect cell expression strategy. *Hum. Gene Ther.* **2009**, *20*, 807–817. [CrossRef]
145. Kotin, R.M.; Snyder, R.O. Manufacturing Clinical Grade Recombinant Adeno-Associated Virus Using Invertebrate Cell Lines. *Hum. Gene Ther.* **2017**, *28*, 350–360. [CrossRef]
146. Kondratov, O.; Marsic, D.; Crosson, S.M.; Mendez-Gomez, H.R.; Moskalenko, O.; Mietzsch, M.; Heilbronn, R.; Allison, J.R.; Green, K.B.; Agbandje-McKenna, M.; et al. Direct Head-to-Head Evaluation of Recombinant Adeno-associated Viral Vectors Manufactured in Human versus Insect Cells. *Mol. Ther. J. Am. Soc. Gene Ther.* **2017**, *25*, 2661–2675. [CrossRef]
147. Robert, M.A.; Chahal, P.S.; Audy, A.; Kamen, A.; Gilbert, R.; Gaillet, B. Manufacturing of recombinant adeno-associated viruses using mammalian expression platforms. *Biotechnol. J.* **2017**, *12*, 1600193. [CrossRef]
148. Graham, F.L.; Smiley, J.; Russell, W.C.; Nairn, R. Characteristics of a human cell line transformed by DNA from human adenovirus type 5. *J. Gen. Virol.* **1977**, *36*, 59–74. [CrossRef]
149. Egan, C.; Bayley, S.T.; Branton, P.E. Binding of the Rb1 protein to E1A products is required for adenovirus transformation. *Oncogene* **1989**, *4*, 383–388. [PubMed]
150. Hacker, D.L.; Bertschinger, M.; Baldi, L.; Wurm, F.M. Reduction of adenovirus E1A mRNA by RNAi results in enhanced recombinant protein expression in transiently transfected HEK293 cells. *Gene* **2004**, *341*, 227–234. [CrossRef] [PubMed]
151. Pear, W.S.; Nolan, G.P.; Scott, M.L.; Baltimore, D. Production of high-titer helper-free retroviruses by transient transfection. *Proc. Natl. Acad. Sci. USA* **1993**, *90*, 8392–8396. [CrossRef] [PubMed]
152. Lin, J.Y.; Simmons, D.T. The ability of large T antigen to complex with p53 is necessary for the increased life span and partial transformation of human cells by simian virus 40. *J. Virol.* **1991**, *65*, 6447–6453. [CrossRef] [PubMed]
153. Emmerling, V.V.; Pegel, A.; Milian, E.G.; Venereo-Sanchez, A.; Kunz, M.; Wegele, J.; Kamen, A.A.; Kochanek, S.; Hoerer, M. Rational plasmid design and bioprocess optimization to enhance recombinant adeno-associated virus (AAV) productivity in mammalian cells. *Biotechnol. J.* **2016**, *11*, 290–297. [CrossRef] [PubMed]
154. World Health Organization. *WHO Guidelines on Tissue Infectivity Distribution in Transmissible Spongiform Encephalopathies*; World Health Organization: Geneva, Switzerland, 2006.
155. Strobel, B.; Miller, F.D.; Rist, W.; Lamla, T. Comparative Analysis of Cesium Chloride- and Iodixanol-Based Purification of Recombinant Adeno-Associated Viral Vectors for Preclinical Applications. *Hum. Gene Ther. Methods* **2015**, *26*, 147–157. [CrossRef]
156. Nass, S.A.; Mattingly, M.A.; Woodcock, D.A.; Burnham, B.L.; Ardinger, J.A.; Osmond, S.E.; Frederick, A.M.; Scaria, A.; Cheng, S.H.; O'Riordan, C.R. Universal Method for the Purification of Recombinant AAV Vectors of Differing Serotypes. *Mol. Ther. Methods Clin. Dev.* **2018**, *9*, 33–46. [CrossRef]
157. Wang, C.; Mulagapati, S.H.R.; Chen, Z.; Du, J.; Zhao, X.; Xi, G.; Chen, L.; Linke, T.; Gao, C.; Schmelzer, A.E.; et al. Developing an Anion Exchange Chromatography Assay for Determining Empty and Full Capsid Contents in AAV6.2. *Mol. Ther. Methods Clin. Dev.* **2019**, *15*, 257–263. [CrossRef]

158. Burnham, B.; Nass, S.; Kong, E.; Mattingly, M.; Woodcock, D.; Song, A.; Wadsworth, S.; Cheng, S.H.; Scaria, A.; O'Riordan, C.R. Analytical Ultracentrifugation as an Approach to Characterize Recombinant Adeno-Associated Viral Vectors. *Hum. Gene Ther. Methods* **2015**, *26*, 228–242. [CrossRef]
159. D'Costa, S.; Blouin, V.; Broucque, F.; Penaud-Budloo, M.; Francois, A.; Perez, I.C.; Le Bec, C.; Moullier, P.; Snyder, R.O.; Ayuso, E. Practical utilization of recombinant AAV vector reference standards: Focus on vector genomes titration by free ITR qPCR. *Mol. Ther. Methods Clin. Dev.* **2016**, *5*, 16019. [CrossRef]
160. Lock, M.; Alvira, M.R.; Chen, S.J.; Wilson, J.M. Absolute determination of single-stranded and self-complementary adeno-associated viral vector genome titers by droplet digital PCR. *Hum. Gene Ther. Methods* **2014**, *25*, 115–125. [CrossRef] [PubMed]
161. Strain, M.C.; Lada, S.M.; Luong, T.; Rought, S.E.; Gianella, S.; Terry, V.H.; Spina, C.A.; Woelk, C.H.; Richman, D.D. Highly precise measurement of HIV DNA by droplet digital PCR. *PLoS ONE* **2013**, *8*, e55943. [CrossRef] [PubMed]
162. Clement, N.; Grieger, J.C. Manufacturing of recombinant adeno-associated viral vectors for clinical trials. *Mol. Ther. Methods Clin. Dev.* **2016**, *3*, 16002. [CrossRef] [PubMed]
163. Lai, Y.; Yue, Y.; Duan, D. Evidence for the failure of adeno-associated virus serotype 5 to package a viral genome > or = 8.2 kb. *Mol. Ther. J. Am. Soc. Gene Ther.* **2010**, *18*, 75–79. [CrossRef] [PubMed]
164. Prusky, G.T.; Alam, N.M.; Beekman, S.; Douglas, R.M. Rapid quantification of adult and developing mouse spatial vision using a virtual optomotor system. *Investig. Ophthalmol. Vis. Sci.* **2004**, *45*, 4611–4616. [CrossRef] [PubMed]
165. Clerin, E.; Wicker, N.; Mohand-Said, S.; Poch, O.; Sahel, J.A.; Leveillard, T. e-conome: An automated tissue counting platform of cone photoreceptors for rodent models of retinitis pigmentosa. *BMC Ophthalmol.* **2011**, *11*, 38. [CrossRef]
166. Cronin, T.; Lyubarsky, A.; Bennett, J. Dark-rearing the rd10 mouse: Implications for therapy. *Adv. Exp. Med. Biol.* **2012**, *723*, 129–136.
167. Barone, I.; Novelli, E.; Piano, I.; Gargini, C.; Strettoi, E. Environmental enrichment extends photoreceptor survival and visual function in a mouse model of retinitis pigmentosa. *PLoS ONE* **2012**, *7*, e50726. [CrossRef]
168. Li, B.; Gografe, S.; Munchow, A.; Lopez-Toledano, M.; Pan, Z.H.; Shen, W. Sex-related differences in the progressive retinal degeneration of the rd10 mouse. *Exp. Eye Res.* **2019**, *187*, 107773. [CrossRef]
169. Narayan, D.S.; Chidlow, G.; Wood, J.P.M.; Casson, R.J. Investigations into Bioenergetic Neuroprotection of Cone Photoreceptors: Relevance to Retinitis Pigmentosa. *Front. Neurosci.* **2019**, *13*, 1234. [CrossRef]
170. The International Council for Harmonisation of Technical Requirements for Pharmaceuticals for Human Use. Guideline ICH. Guidance on nonclinical safety studies for the conduct of human clinical trials and marketing authorization for pharmaceuticals M3 (R2). In *International Conference on Harmonisation of Technical Requirements for Registration of Pharmaceuticals for Human Use*; ICH: Geneva, Switzerland, 2009.
171. European Medicines Agency. *Guideline on the Non-Clinical Studies Required Before First Clinical Use of Gene Therapy Medicinal Products*; EMA: London, UK, 2008.
172. The Food and Drug Administration. *Gene Therapy Guidance Document: Guidance for Industry: Preclinical Assessment of Investigational Cellular and Gene Therapy Products (2013)*; The Food and Drug Administration: White Oak, MD, USA, 2018.
173. Weed, L.; Ammar, M.J.; Zhou, S.; Wei, Z.; Serrano, L.W.; Sun, J.; Lee, V.; Maguire, A.M.; Bennett, J.; Aleman, T.S. Safety of Same-Eye Subretinal Sequential Readministration of AAV2-hRPE65v2 in Non-human Primates. *Mol. Ther. Methods Clin. Dev.* **2019**, *15*, 133–148. [CrossRef] [PubMed]
174. Ding, K.; Shen, J.; Hafiz, Z.; Hackett, S.F.; Silva, R.L.E.; Khan, M.; Lorenc, V.E.; Chen, D.; Chadha, R.; Zhang, M.; et al. AAV8-vectored suprachoroidal gene transfer produces widespread ocular transgene expression. *J. Clin. Investig.* **2019**, *130*, 4901–4911. [CrossRef] [PubMed]
175. Bruewer, A.R.; Mowat, F.M.; Bartoe, J.T.; Boye, S.L.; Hauswirth, W.W.; Petersen-Jones, S.M. Evaluation of lateral spread of transgene expression following subretinal AAV-mediated gene delivery in dogs. *PLoS ONE* **2013**, *8*, e60218. [CrossRef] [PubMed]
176. Singh, H.P.; Wang, S.; Stachelek, K.; Lee, S.; Reid, M.W.; Thornton, M.E.; Craft, C.M.; Grubbs, B.H.; Cobrinik, D. Developmental stage-specific proliferation and retinoblastoma genesis in RB-deficient human but not mouse cone precursors. *Proc. Natl. Acad. Sci. USA* **2018**, *115*, E9391–E9400. [CrossRef] [PubMed]
177. Jauregui, R.; Park, K.S.; Duong, J.K.; Mahajan, V.B.; Tsang, S.H. Quantitative progression of retinitis pigmentosa by optical coherence tomography angiography. *Sci. Rep.* **2018**, *8*, 13130. [CrossRef] [PubMed]

178. Cabral, T.; Sengillo, J.D.; Duong, J.K.; Justus, S.; Boudreault, K.; Schuerch, K.; Belfort, R., Jr.; Mahajan, V.B.; Sparrow, J.R.; Tsang, S.H. Retrospective Analysis of Structural Disease Progression in Retinitis Pigmentosa Utilizing Multimodal Imaging. *Sci. Rep.* **2017**, *7*, 10347. [CrossRef]
179. Yusuf, I.H.; Birtel, J.; Shanks, M.E.; Clouston, P.; Downes, S.M.; Charbel Issa, P.; MacLaren, R.E. Clinical Characterization of Retinitis Pigmentosa Associated With Variants in SNRNP200. *JAMA Ophthalmol.* **2019**, *137*, 1295–1300. [CrossRef]
180. Fujiwara, K.; Ikeda, Y.; Murakami, Y.; Tachibana, T.; Funatsu, J.; Koyanagi, Y.; Nakatake, S.; Yoshida, N.; Nakao, S.; Hisatomi, T.; et al. Assessment of Central Visual Function in Patients with Retinitis Pigmentosa. *Sci. Rep.* **2018**, *8*, 8070. [CrossRef] [PubMed]
181. Comander, J.; Weigel-DiFranco, C.; Sandberg, M.A.; Berson, E.L. Visual Function in Carriers of X-Linked Retinitis Pigmentosa. *Ophthalmology* **2015**, *122*, 1899–1906. [CrossRef] [PubMed]
182. Tee, J.J.L.; Yang, Y.; Kalitzeos, A.; Webster, A.; Bainbridge, J.; Michaelides, M. Natural History Study of Retinal Structure, Progression, and Symmetry Using Ellipzoid Zone Metrics in RPGR-Associated Retinopathy. *Am. J. Ophthalmol.* **2019**, *198*, 111–123. [CrossRef] [PubMed]
183. Cideciyan, A.V.; Charng, J.; Roman, A.J.; Sheplock, R.; Garafalo, A.V.; Heon, E.; Jacobson, S.G. Progression in X-linked Retinitis Pigmentosa Due to ORF15-RPGR Mutations: Assessment of Localized Vision Changes Over 2 Years. *Investig. Ophthalmol. Vis. Sci.* **2018**, *59*, 4558–4566. [CrossRef]
184. Chaumet-Riffaud, A.E.; Chaumet-Riffaud, P.; Cariou, A.; Devisme, C.; Audo, I.; Sahel, J.A.; Mohand-Said, S. Impact of Retinitis Pigmentosa on Quality of Life, Mental Health, and Employment Among Young Adults. *Am. J. Ophthalmol.* **2017**, *177*, 169–174. [CrossRef] [PubMed]
185. Osterberg, G. *Topography of the Layer of Rods and Cones in the Human Retina*; Levin & Munksgaard: Copenhagen, Denmark, 1935.
186. Staurenghi, G.; Sadda, S.; Chakravarthy, U.; Spaide, R.F. International Nomenclature for Optical Coherence Tomography. Proposed lexicon for anatomic landmarks in normal posterior segment spectral-domain optical coherence tomography: The IN*OCT consensus. *Ophthalmology* **2014**, *121*, 1572–1578.
187. Smith, T.B.; Parker, M.A.; Steinkamp, P.N.; Romo, A.; Erker, L.R.; Lujan, B.J.; Smith, N. Reliability of Spectral-Domain OCT Ellipsoid Zone Area and Shape Measurements in Retinitis Pigmentosa. *Transl. Vis. Sci. Technol.* **2019**, *8*, 37. [CrossRef] [PubMed]
188. Nowomiejska, K.; Brzozowska, A.; Koss, M.J.; Weleber, R.G.; Schiefer, U.; Rejdak, K.; Juenemann, A.G.; Maciejewski, R.; Rejdak, R. Quantification of the Visual Field Loss in Retinitis Pigmentosa Using Semi-Automated Kinetic Perimetry. *Curr. Eye Res.* **2016**, *41*, 993–998. [CrossRef] [PubMed]
189. Schuerch, K.; Woods, R.L.; Lee, W.; Duncker, T.; Delori, F.C.; Allikmets, R.; Tsang, S.H.; Sparrow, J.R. Quantifying Fundus Autofluorescence in Patients with Retinitis Pigmentosa. *Investig. Ophthalmol. Vis. Sci.* **2017**, *58*, 1843–1855. [CrossRef] [PubMed]
190. Sandberg, M.A.; Weigel-DiFranco, C.; Dryja, T.P.; Berson, E.L. Clinical expression correlates with location of rhodopsin mutation in dominant retinitis pigmentosa. *Investig. Ophthalmol. Vis. Sci.* **1995**, *36*, 1934–1942.
191. Gerkema, M.P.; Davies, W.I.; Foster, R.G.; Menaker, M.; Hut, R.A. The nocturnal bottleneck and the evolution of activity patterns in mammals. *Proc. Biol. Sci. R. Soc.* **2013**, *280*, 20130508. [CrossRef] [PubMed]
192. Jaillard, C.; Mouret, A.; Niepon, M.L.; Clerin, E.; Yang, Y.; Lee-Rivera, I.; Ait-Ali, N.; Millet-Puel, G.; Cronin, T.; Sedmak, T.; et al. Nxnl2 splicing results in dual functions in neuronal cell survival and maintenance of cell integrity. *Hum. Mol. Genet.* **2012**, *21*, 2298–2311. [CrossRef]

4

Correction of NR2E3 Associated Enhanced S-cone Syndrome Patient-specific iPSCs using CRISPR-Cas9

Laura R. Bohrer, Luke A. Wiley, Erin R. Burnight, Jessica A. Cooke, Joseph C. Giacalone, Kristin R. Anfinson, Jeaneen L. Andorf, Robert F. Mullins, Edwin M. Stone and Budd A. Tucker *

Institute for Vision Research, Department of Ophthalmology and Visual Sciences, University of Iowa, Iowa City, IA 52241, USA; laura-bohrer@uiowa.edu (L.R.B.); luke-wiley@uiowa.edu (L.A.W.); erin-burnight@uiowa.edu (E.R.B.); jessica-cooke@uiowa.edu (J.A.C.); joseph-giacalone@uiowa.edu (J.C.G.); kristin-anfinson@uiowa.edu (K.R.A.); jeaneen-andorf@uiowa.edu (J.L.A.); robert-mullins@uiowa.edu (R.F.M.); edwin-stone@uiowa.edu (E.M.S.)

* Correspondence: budd-tucker@uiowa.edu

Abstract: Enhanced S-cone syndrome (ESCS) is caused by recessive mutations in the photoreceptor cell transcription factor *NR2E3*. Loss of *NR2E3* is characterized by repression of rod photoreceptor cell gene expression, over-expansion of the S-cone photoreceptor cell population, and varying degrees of M- and L-cone photoreceptor cell development. In this study, we developed a CRISPR-based homology-directed repair strategy and corrected two different disease-causing *NR2E3* mutations in patient-derived induced pluripotent stem cells (iPSCs) generated from two affected individuals. In addition, one patient's iPSCs were differentiated into retinal cells and *NR2E3* transcription was evaluated in CRISPR corrected and uncorrected clones. The patient's c.119-2A>C mutation caused the inclusion of a portion of intron 1, the creation of a frame shift, and generation of a premature stop codon. In summary, we used a single set of CRISPR reagents to correct different mutations in iPSCs generated from two individuals with ESCS. In doing so we demonstrate the advantage of using retinal cells derived from affected patients over artificial in vitro model systems when attempting to demonstrate pathophysiologic mechanisms of specific mutations.

Keywords: induced pluripotent stem cell (iPSC); clustered regularly interspaced short palindromic repeats (CRISPR); homology-directed repair (HDR); Enhanced S-Cone Syndrome (ESCS); *NR2E3*

---

1. Introduction

Enhanced S-cone syndrome (ESCS) is an autosomal recessive retinopathy that results from mutations in the photoreceptor cell transcription factor, *NR2E3* (Nuclear Receptor Subfamily 2, Group E, Member 3). *NR2E3*, which is specifically expressed in the outer nuclear layer of the human retina [1], is a direct transcriptional target of NRL, a key regulator of photoreceptor cell genesis. Work in animal models has shown that *NR2E3* acts to repress cone photoreceptor cell gene expression and promote rod photoreceptor cell fate commitment. Specifically, loss of *NR2E3* function hinders rod photoreceptor cell development and drives over-expansion of the S-opsin-positive cone photoreceptor cell population (i.e., blue cones) [2–6], which is normally the least prevalent of the photoreceptor cell subtypes.

Patients with ESCS present with increased sensitivity to blue light (due to overabundance of short wavelength sensitive S-cones), early onset impairment of night vision (due primarily to lack of functional rod development) and varying degrees of sensitivity to green and red light (due to varying abundance of medium wavelength sensitive M-cones and long wavelength sensitive L-cones). Although the disease is progressive in nature, clinically evident retinal degeneration is often highly-variable, ranging from a relatively mild and nearly static disorder in some individuals to a very severe and progressive disease in others [1,7–10].

To date, more than 33 different disease-causing mutations in *NR2E3* have been described [1,11,12]. In addition to ESCS, mutations in NR2E3 can also cause more severe forms of retinal disease, including Goldmann-Farve syndrome (GFS) or autosomal dominant retinitis pigmentosa (adRP). Of these mutations, the majority are in either DNA- (e.g., c.219G>C; p.(Arg73Ser)) or ligand-binding (e.g., c.932G>A; p.(Arg311Gln)) domains of the NR2E3 protein [11,13]. That said, one of the most common *NR2E3* mutations reported in the United States is c.119-2A>C [13], which falls within the canonical splice acceptor site of intron 1. To demonstrate the functional effect of this mutation, Bernal and colleagues transiently transfected COS7 cells with an expression plasmid containing a copy of the *NR2E3* gene harboring the c.119-2A>C variant [14]. Sequence analysis revealed that in addition to the normal transcript, an aberrant transcript that lacked exon 2 and contained a premature stop codon in exon 3 was also present [14].

Understanding how different disease-causing *NR2E3* genotypes alter retinal development and give rise to the observed spectrum of clinical outcomes is of particular interest and relevance to investigators attempting to develop treatments based on photoreceptor cell replacement. Specifically, by understanding exactly how genes such as *NR2E3* function, we may be able to strategically guide developing photoreceptor cells down a more cone-selective path (i.e., alter *NR2E3* function to increase cone genesis without causing widespread photoreceptor cell degeneration). To evaluate the effects of different *NR2E3* variants on photoreceptor cell fate, we have used CRISPR-based genome editing of human patient-derived induced pluripotent stem cells (iPSC). Human iPSCs have several advantages over animal models for this type of work. Unlike animal models, iPSCs can be generated from patients with known disease-causing variants on genetic backgrounds that are demonstrably permissive of the disease. By correcting the patients' mutations one at a time, one can readily evaluate the role of a specific variant on gene expression and phenotypic outcome. Correlating these in vitro findings with the patients' clinical history may provide a better understanding of how variants in each of the different *NR2E3* domains influence photoreceptor cell fate decisions.

To correct retinal disease-causing variants in patient-derived iPSCs, we and others have used CRISPR-based genome editing [15–22]. Unlike the more cumbersome ZFN- and TALEN-based approaches, which require the development of elaborate genomic targeting complexes, the CRISPR method relies on the use of small single guide RNAs (sgRNAs) that can be easily synthesized to direct human codon-optimized Cas9 nuclease to specific genomic targets. Cas9 induces double-strand DNA breaks that can subsequently be repaired via fairly error-prone non-homologous end joining (NHEJ), or via the more precise homology-directed repair (HDR) mechanism [15]. The advantage of the HDR-based strategy, even for mutations within the deep intronic space where NHEJ could be used, is that a single HDR repair template and set of sgRNAs is often sufficient to correct a variety of different mutations that are contained within a limited genomic space (e.g., an HDR template spanning exons 1 through 3 would cover both the above-mentioned c.119-2A>C splice site mutation and the p.(Arg73Ser) variant contained within the *NR2E3*-DNA binding element). By using the same set of reagents to correct a variety of mutations in different cell lines, one can control for differences related to reagent variability while increasing throughput.

In this study, we developed a CRISPR-Cas9-based HDR strategy to correct two different *NR2E3* mutations in iPSCs generated from two patients with clinically-diagnosed and molecularly-confirmed ESCS: Patient 1 harbors homozygous c.119-2A>C mutations, and Patient 2 harbors compound heterozygous p.(Arg73Ser) and p.(Arg311Gln) mutations. The close proximity of c.119-2A>C and p.(Arg73Ser) allowed the same sgRNA and HDR reagents to be used to correct iPSC lines generated from both individuals. Genomic correction of both mutations was confirmed by PCR and Sanger sequencing. To demonstrate the utility of this system for elucidating disease mechanism, iPSCs obtained from Patient 1, both before and after CRISPR correction, were differentiated down a photoreceptor cell lineage. Analysis of the *NR2E3* transcript revealed that, prior to CRISPR correction, patient-derived retinal cells completely lack wild-type messages and instead express a mutant transcript that contains a portion of intron 1, which causes a frameshift and the creation of a premature stop codon. Following monoallelic CRISPR correction, the expression of the wild-type *NR2E3* transcript was restored.

2. Materials and Methods

2.1. Patient-Derived iPSCs

This study was approved by the Institutional Review Board of the University of Iowa (project approval #200202022) and adhered to the tenets set forth in the Declaration of Helsinki. The dermal fibroblast-derived iPSCs used in this study were generated from two patients with molecularly confirmed ESCS. These previously described cell lines were generated using current good manufacturing practices in a clean room environment and validated using scorecard and karyotypic analysis [23]. Consistent with the patients' clinical diagnoses and unlike control individuals, differentiation of these lines gave rise to S-opsin-positive blue cone photoreceptor cell-dominated retinal organoids, which lack rod photoreceptor cells [24].

2.2. Cloning of CRISPR-Cas9 and HDR Donor Constructs

The sgRNAs used in this study were designed to target the region of *NR2E3* that contains the c.119-2A>C (Patient 1) and c.219G>C; p.(Arg73Ser) (Patient 2) mutations using the Benchling platform (www.benchling.com) or the Optimized CRISPR Design Tool (crispr.mit.edu). Guides were cloned into our previously described bicistronic construct expressing a human codon-optimized *Streptococcus pyogenes Cas9* (*spCas9*) nuclease [17,18]. A homology-directed repair (HDR) construct was synthesized by GenScript. As described previously, the HDR plasmid contains 450–750 bp of homologous sequence flanking a floxed puromycin resistance gene followed by the Herpes Simplex Virus type 1 thymidine kinase (vTK) gene [16].

2.3. Screening of NR2E3-specific sgRNAs

sgRNA and CRISPR-Cas9 constructs were transfected into HEK293T cells (ATCC) using Lipofectamine 2000 (Thermo Fisher Scientific) and cleavage was assessed via a T7 endonuclease 1 (T7E1) assay using *NR2E3*-specific primers (Table S1) as described previously [17,18]. Control iPSCs were transfected with 2 µg of plasmid using the Neon transfection system as described previously [16].

2.4. Delivery of sgRNA-Cas9 and the HDR Contruct to NR2E3-Patient-Specific iPSCs

The CRISPR-Cas9 machinery was delivered to iPSCs and analyzed as described previously [16–18]. Briefly, the sg4-spCas9 and HDR plasmids were transfected at a 1:2 molar ratio into patient iPSCs with Lipofectamine Stem (Thermo Fisher Scientific; Patient 1) or Neon electroporation (Thermo Fisher Scientific; Patient 2). Puromycin (0.5 µg/mL) selection was performed as previously described [16], and surviving colonies were PCR screened for HDR incorporation and sequenced to confirm correction. The puroR-vTK cassette was removed by Lipofectamine Stem transfection of Cre recombinase, and cells were treated with 40–400 nM Ganciclovir to select for those with vTK removal. The top off-target sites (Table S2) were determined using the Benchling platform (https://benchling.com/) and analyzed using the T7E1 assays as described above.

2.5. Retinal Differentiation

Undifferentiated iPSCs cultured on Laminin-521 coated culture dishes in Essential 8 medium (Thermo Fisher Scientific) were transitioned to Matrigel (Corning) coated culture dishes in mTESR1 medium (StemCell Technologies). Transitioned cells were passaged every 4–5 days using 1mg/ml dispase (Thermo Fisher Scientific). Differentiation was initiated through embryoid body (EB) formation as previously described [25]. Briefly, EBs were generated on ultra-low adhesion plates and transitioned from mTESR1 to neural induction medium (NIM - DMEM/F12 (1:1), 1% N2 supplement, 1% non-essential amino acids, 1% Glutamax (Thermo Fisher Scientific), 2 μg/ml heparin (Sigma) and 0.2% Primocin (Invivogen)) over a three day time period. EBs were maintained free-floating in NIM until day 7, at which time they were induced to adhere to tissue culture-treated plates overnight in NIM supplemented with 25% fetal bovine serum (FBS). Media was replaced with NIM minus FBS on day 8 and the adherent EBs were fed with NIM every other day until day 16. On day 16, the entire EB outgrowth was mechanically lifted using a cell scraper and transferred to retinal differentiation medium (RDM - DMEM/F12 (3:1), 2% B27 supplement, 1% non-essential amino acids, 1% Glutamax and 0.2% Primocin). Three-dimensional aggregates maintained in RDM give rise to both retinal organoids and non-retinal neurospheres that can be isolated based on their morphological appearances. Retinal organoids were isolated and dissociated at 5–6 weeks using Accutase (StemCell Technologies) and cells were subsequently plated onto laminin (Sigma) coated tissue culture plates. Cells were maintained in RDM and collected at a series of time points for RNA analysis.

2.6. Reverse Transcription PCR

Total RNA was extracted from cells using either the NucleoSpin RNA extraction kit (Machery-Nagel) or TRIzol (Thermo Fisher Scientific) following the manufacturer's protocol. cDNA was generated with the High Capacity cDNA Reverse Transcription Kit (Applied Biosystems) using 200 ng of RNA template. *NR2E3* transcript was amplified using BIOLASE DNA polymerase (Bioline) and *NR2E3* specific primers (Table S1). PCR products were separated on an agarose gel and bands were excised, purified using the QIAquick Gel Extraction Kit (Qiagen) and subcloned using the PCR2.1 TOPO TA cloning kit (Invitrogen). Colonies were subsequently picked and Sanger sequenced using M13(-20)F or M13R primers.

3. Results

3.1. Testing CRISPR-Cas9 Guide Cleavage in HEK293T Cells and iPSCs

The goal of this study was to develop a CRISPR-Cas9 homology-directed repair strategy suitable for the correction of disease-causing mutations in iPSCs generated from two independent patients with molecularly confirmed *NR2E3*-associated enhanced S-cone syndrome (Figure 1A,B). As enhanced S-cone syndrome has a recessive mode of inheritance (such that correction of only one allele would be expected to mitigate the disease phenotype) and the p.(Arg73Ser) mutation on the paternal allele of Patient 2 is within 100 bps of the c.119-2A>C mutations in Patient 1, we hypothesized that a single CRISPR-Cas9 HDR cassette would be sufficient for the correction of iPSCs generated from both individuals. We began by designing and testing 5 different sgRNAs that utilized the spCas9 PAM sites. To determine the efficiency of cleavage, we evaluated nonhomologous end joining (NHEJ) using T7E1 assays in HEK293T cells transfected with each sgRNA and spCas9. While no cleavage was detected in controls (i.e., untransfected cells), all 5 guides induced cleavage and indel formation with similar efficiencies in the transfected cells (Figure 1C). The ability of all 5 guides to direct specific DNA cleavage was subsequently evaluated in iPSCs generated from a normal non-diseased individual. As with HEK293T cells, all 5 guides induced DNA cleavage and indel formation; however, more robust cleavage was detected in cells that received sg2 and sg4 (Figure 1D). As the PAM sequence used by sg4 could be readily modified with a synonymous mutation in the HDR cassette that would prevent re-cleavage events without altering the predicted amino acid sequence, this guide was chosen for all subsequent patient-specific genome repair experiments.

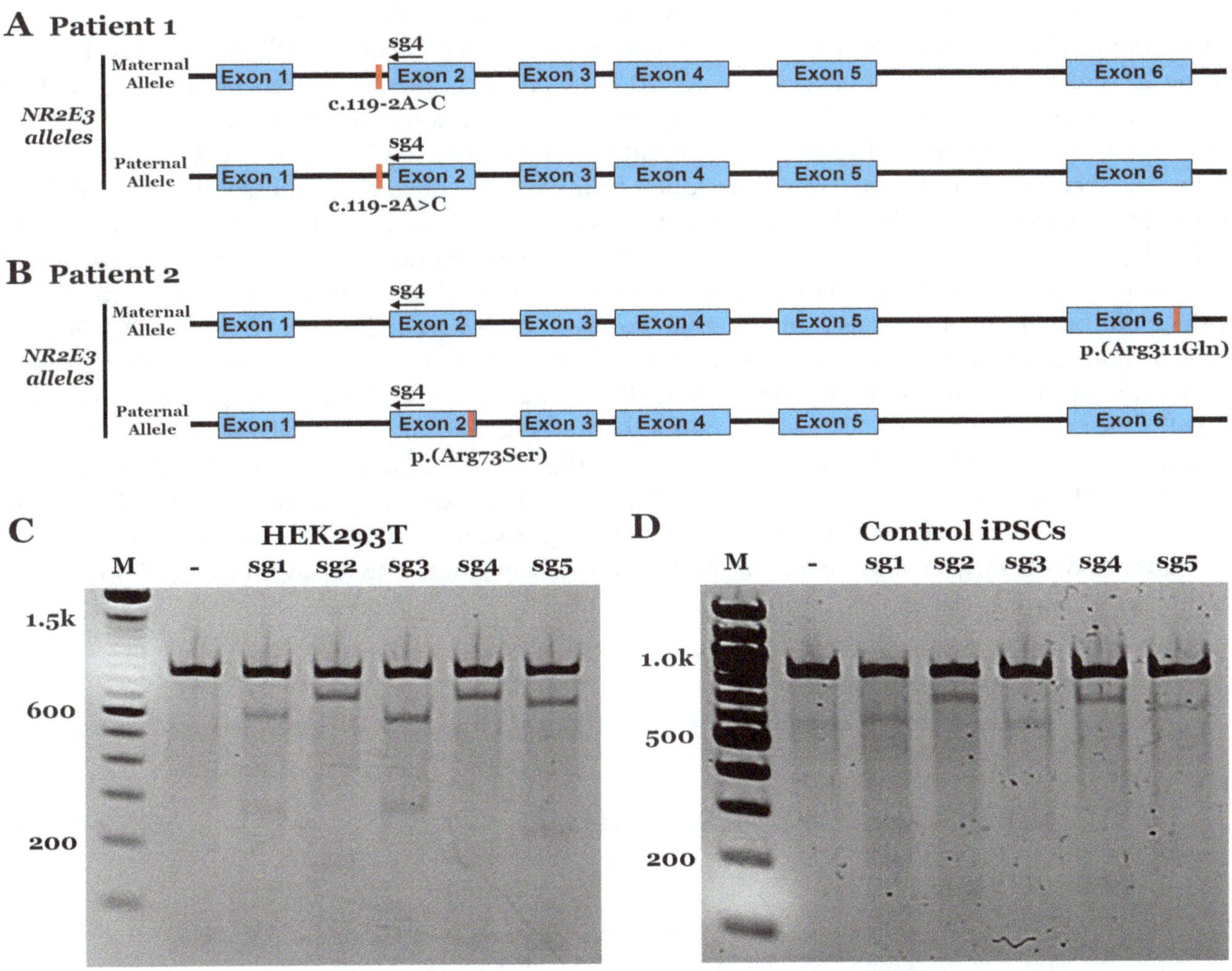

Figure 1. Analysis of CRISPR-Cas9 sgRNA mediated cleavage efficiency. **A,B:** Schematics depicting genomic disease-causing mutations in Patient 1—homozygous c.119-2A>C mutations (**A**) and Patient 2—compound heterozygous p.(Arg73Ser) and p.(Arg311Gln) mutations (**B**). **C,D:** Representative gel images of T7E1 assays in HEK293T (**C**) and control induced pluripotent stem cells (iPSCs) (**D**) for 5 different sgRNAs. No transfection control: (-).

3.2. CRISPR Correction of the NR2E3 c.119-2A>C mutation in Patient-Specific iPSCs using Homology-Directed Repair (HDR)

To correct the c.119-2A>C and p.(Arg73Ser) variants in iPSCs generated from the patients described in Figure 1, we designed an HDR donor cassette with ~500 bps of homologous sequence upstream and downstream of the sg4 cleavage site (Figure 2A). As indicated above, to prevent re-cleavage events, we included a synonymous variant in the sg4 PAM site (CGG>CGA). To select for cells that incorporated the HDR sequence, a puromycin resistance cassette under the control of the mPGK promoter was added to intron 1 as previously described [16,18]. In addition, the stop codon in the puromycin resistance sequence was replaced with a porcine 2A peptide (P2A) coding sequence, followed by the Herpes Simplex Virus type 1 thymidine kinase (vTK) gene (thymidine kinase phosphorylates ganciclovir, a nucleoside analog, which disrupts DNA synthesis and induces cell death) and a downstream polyadenylation sequence (PA) [16]. The entire cassette, mPGK-PuroR-vTK-PA, was flanked by loxP sites that enabled removal of the cassette via Cre recombinase [16]. Following Cre recombinase transfection, treatment of cells with ganciclovir allowed for the selection of cells that had lost the cassette [16]. Patient 1 iPSCs were transfected with sg4NR2E3-spCas9 and the HDR construct via lipofection. Puromycin selection was subsequently performed as described in the methods section. Following selection, cells were clonally expanded and screened for incorporation of the HDR sequence via PCR using a forward primer in the PA sequence (Figure 2A,F1) and a reverse primer outside the HDR cassette (Figure 2A,R1). Eighteen of the 25 screened clones amplified the expected PCR product, indicating incorporation of the HDR cassette (Figure S1). We chose 2 clones, clone 16 and clone 17, to confirm genomic correction. PCR was performed using primers that spanned the mutation (Figure 2A,F2,R2) and the PCR product was TA cloned. Sequencing demonstrated that all products from clone 17 still had the disease-causing c.119-2A>C mutation. However, 5 of the 12 clones from the clone 16 PCR product showed a normal sequence, indicating a monoallelic correction of the c.119-2A>C variant (Figure S2). Clone 16 was subsequently transfected with Cre recombinase to remove the floxed PuroR-vTK cassette. After a second transfection with Cre recombinase, some cells containing the PuroR-vTK cassette still remained (Figure 2C). To select for cells that lacked the PuroR-vTK cassette, cultures were treated with ganciclovir, which resulted in the removal of the PuroR-vTK containing cells (Figure 2C). PCR products using primers outside the PuroR-vTK cassette (Figure 2D,F2) and homology arm (Figure 2D,R2) demonstrated equal amounts of genomic DNA. To evaluate off-target cutting events, the top 10 off-target sites and 2 additional exonic loci selected from the top 24 off-target sites, each predicted via Benchling, were analyzed. T7E1 assays were performed with genomic DNA from unmodified control and CRISPR-corrected cells. We observed no evidence of off-target events at any of the genomic loci evaluated; that is, we observed no cleavage products that were specific to the corrected cells (Figure S3).

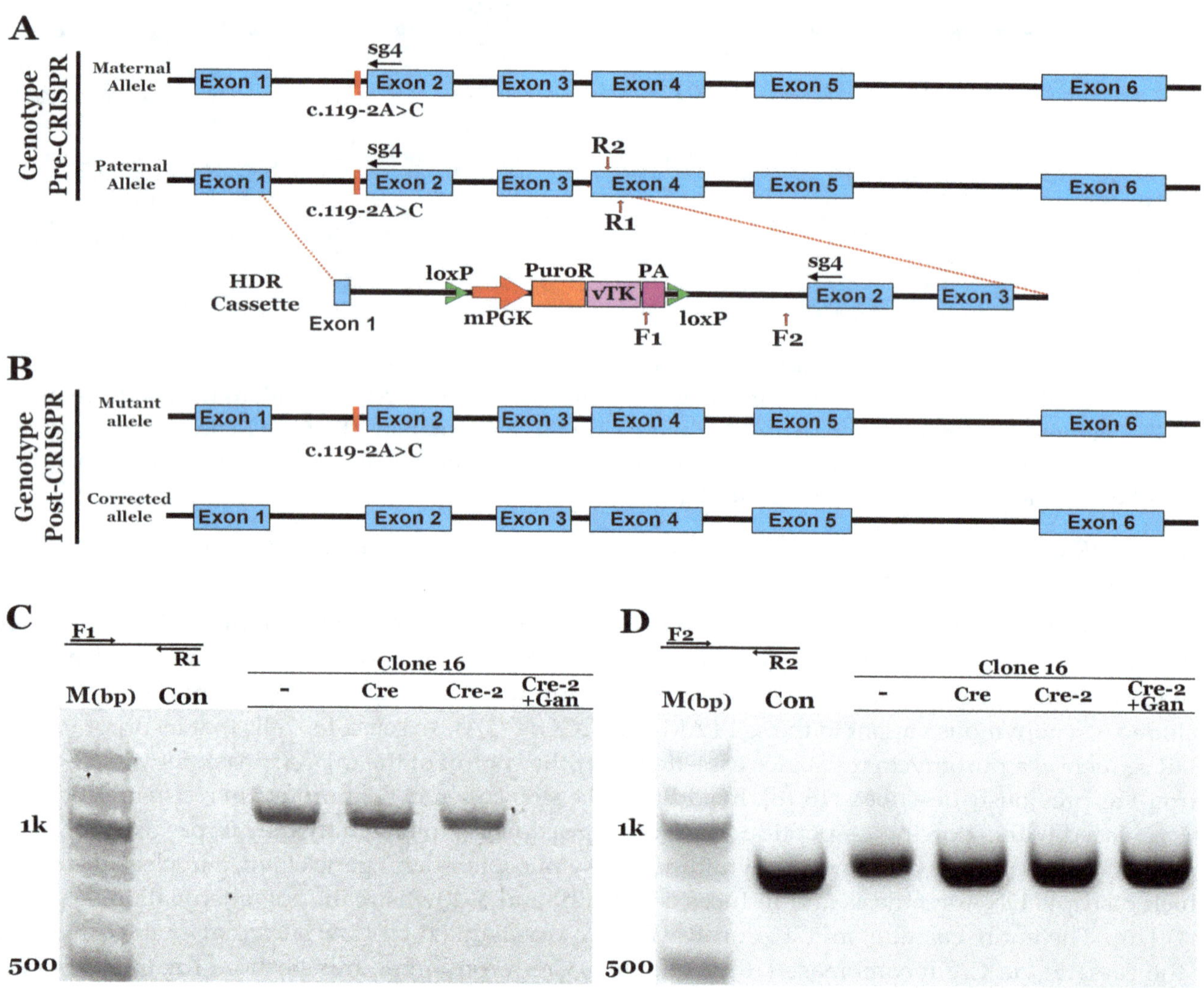

Figure 2. CRISPR-based homology-directed repair of the c.119-2A>C mutation in patient-derived iPSCs. (**A**): Schematic diagram depicting the genotype pre-CRISPR correction and the homology-directed repair (HDR) cassette designed to repair the c.119-2A>C mutation: Homologous sequence upstream

and downstream of the loxP flanked puromycin resistance (PuroR), viral thymidine kinase (vTK), and SV40 polyadenylation (PA). (**B**): Schematic depicting the genotype following CRISPR-based repair: Monoallelic correction results in a cell line that contains one corrected allele and one mutant allele. (**C**): Representative gel image of the genomic PCR confirming incorporation of HDR cassette in clone 16 and cassette removal following transfection of Cre recombinase and selection with ganciclovir (Cre-2, +Gan). (**D**): Representative gel image of genomic PCR from the same samples presented in panel C to demonstrate similar amounts of DNA. PCR products were also used for sequencing to confirm the correction of clone 16.

3.3. *CRISPR Correction of the NR2E3 p.(Arg73Ser) Mutation in Patient-Specific iPSCs using HDR*

As indicated above, the p.(Arg73Ser) mutation in Patient 2 is located 100 bps away from the c.119-2A>C mutations in Patient 1. We therefore wanted to determine if the same HDR cassette and genome editing strategy used to correct Patient 1's iPSCs could be used to correct iPSCs generated from this individual (Figure 3A). The same plasmids were delivered; however, instead of Lipofectamine Stem, electroporation was used to determine if a different delivery method could also be used to achieve robust correction. We observed a similar efficiency with electroporation; specifically, 20 of 24 clones screened had a PCR product that indicated incorporation of the HDR cassette (Figure S4,F1,R1 primers). Patient 2 is a compound heterozygote, and only the p.(Arg73Ser) mutation was targeted using this HDR cassette. As a result, extra screening was needed to identify clones that had the HDR sequence specifically incorporated into the p.(Arg73Ser)-containing paternal allele as opposed to the maternal allele, which is wild-type at this location (Figure 3A). To identify patient-derived iPSCs that had the paternal p.(Arg73Ser) allele corrected, PCR products obtained from 6 clonally expanded iPSC lines were sequenced using the F2/R2 primer pair. Following this analysis, clone 6 was found to be corrected. None of the 18 sequencing reactions performed on DNA obtained from clone 6 contained the p.(Arg73Ser) variant (Figure S5). Not surprisingly, the p.(Arg311Gln) mutation in exon 6, which lies outside of the region of homology covered by the HDR cassette, was still present (Figure S5). A single transfection with Cre recombinase and subsequent selection with ganciclovir resulted in the removal of cells containing the PuroR-vTK cassette (Figure 3C, Cre+Gan). PCR products using both sequencing primer sets F2/R2 and F3/R3 revealed equal amounts of genomic DNA (Figure 3D,E). Using the same strategy described for Patient 1 above, Patient 2 iPSCs were evaluated for off-target cleavage events. As shown in Figure S6, indel formation was identified in OT7. However, as OT7 is located within the middle of an intronic region of a non-retinal gene, it would not be predicted to affect retinal cell development, health, and/or function. Collectively, the above-described findings indicate that a single HDR cassette can be used to successfully correct iPSCs obtained from two independent patients with separate disease-causing mutations in the gene *NR2E3*.

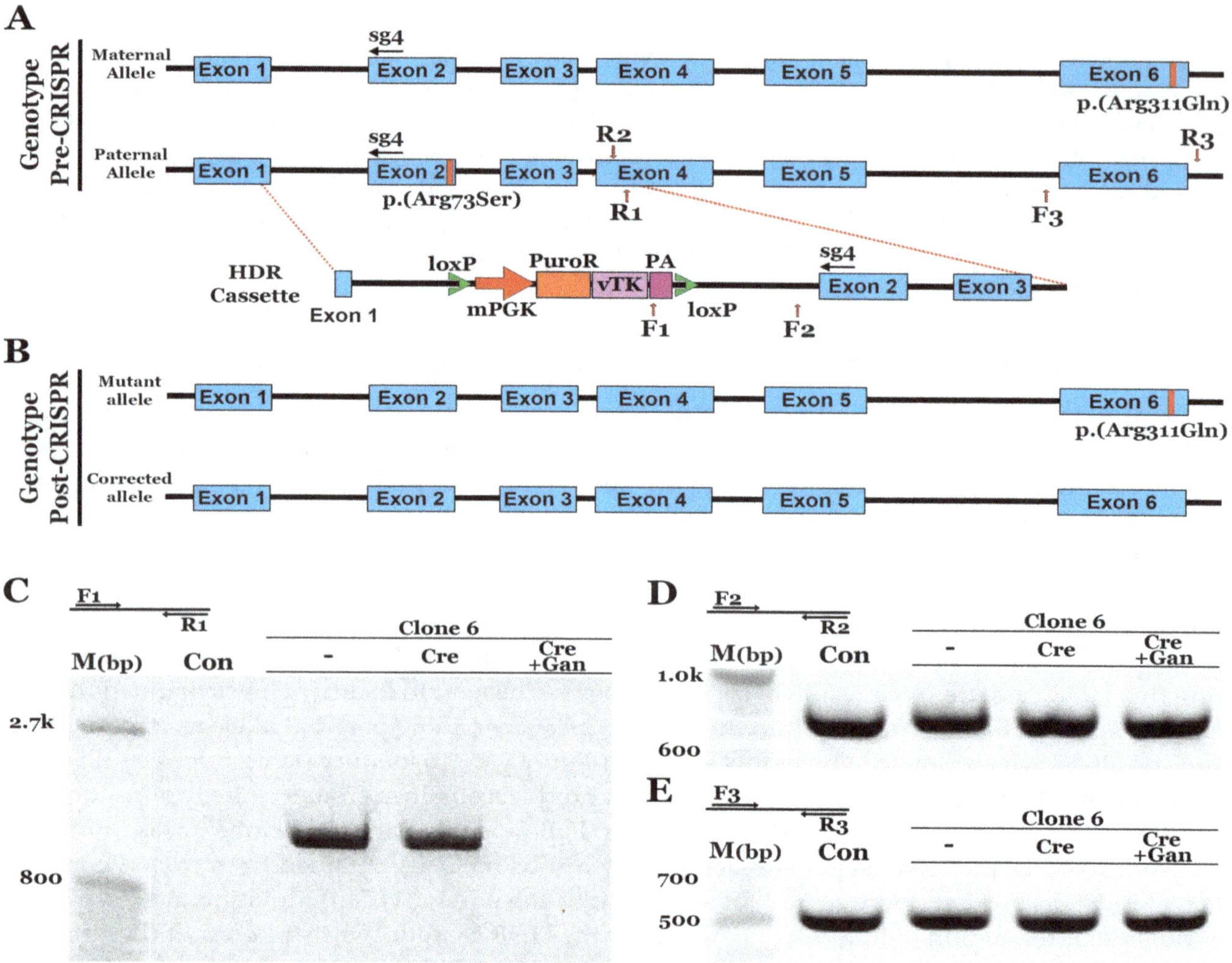

Figure 3. CRISPR-based homology-directed repair of the p.(Arg73Ser) mutation in patient-derived iPSCs. (**A**): Schematic diagram depicting the genotype pre-CRISPR correction and the HDR cassette used to repair the p.(Arg73Ser) mutation: Homologous sequence upstream and downstream of the loxP flanked puromycin resistance (PuroR), viral thymidine kinase (vTK), and SV40 polyadenylation (PA). (**B**): Schematic depicting the genotype following CRISPR-based repair: One corrected allele and one mutant allele harboring the p.(Arg311Gln) mutation. (**C**): Representative gel image of the genomic PCR confirming incorporation of the HDR cassette in clone 6 and cassette removal following transfection of Cre recombinase and selection with ganciclovir (Cre, +Gan). **D**,**E**: Representative gel images of the genomic PCR using the same samples in panel C to demonstrate similar amounts of DNA. PCR products were also used for sequencing to confirm the correction of clone 6 in one allele (**D**) and the presence of the p.(Arg311Gln) mutation in the other allele (**E**).

3.4. CRISPR-based Restoration of the NR2E3 Transcript in Patient-derived Retinal Cells

NR2E3 is a nuclear transcription factor that is required for rod photoreceptor cell genesis; thus, to confirm that CRISPR-based genomic correction restores expression of *NR2E3* transcript, iPSCs (Figure 4A–C) were differentiated toward a retinal cell fate. The iPSCs generated from Patient 1, who is homozygous for the c.119-2A>C splice site mutation, were predicted to have the most overt molecular phenotype. Thus, Patient 1's cells were chosen for the transcriptional analysis. As shown in Figure 4, at 5–6 weeks post-differentiation, three-dimensional optic vesicles generated from control (D), affected patient (E), and CRISPR-corrected (F) iPSCs appear to develop normally. To evaluate the normal kinetics of *NR2E3* expression, control iPSC-derived retinal cells were harvested at 6–20 weeks following initiation of differentiation. *NR2E3* expression is first detected after approximately 10 weeks of differentiation and is strongly expressed between weeks 13–20 (Figure 4G). After 9 weeks of differentiation, the wild-type *NR2E3* transcript was detectable in CRISPR-corrected as opposed to non-corrected iPSC-derived retinal progenitor cells (Figure 4G). By week 14, the robust expression of wild-type *NR2E3* transcript could be detected in CRISPR-corrected retinal cells (Figure 4G). Interestingly, at this timepoint, a second larger transcript could also be detected in both corrected and uncorrected cells (Figure 4G). Following gel purification and sequencing, we found that the upper band actually contained two novel transcripts that differ by only 32 bps (which explains why they appear as a single product on a 2% agarose gel). The larger transcript included 143 bps of intron 1 followed by exon 2, and the smaller contained 111 bps of intron 1 followed by exon 2. In both cases, the inclusion of this intronic sequence resulted in a frame shift and the creation of a premature stop codon just 47 bps downstream of the canonical exon 1 boundary (Figure S7). In summary, monoallelic genomic correction of the c.119-2A>C variant in patient-derived iPSCs restores the cells ability to make wild-type *NR2E3* transcript during retinal cell differentiation.

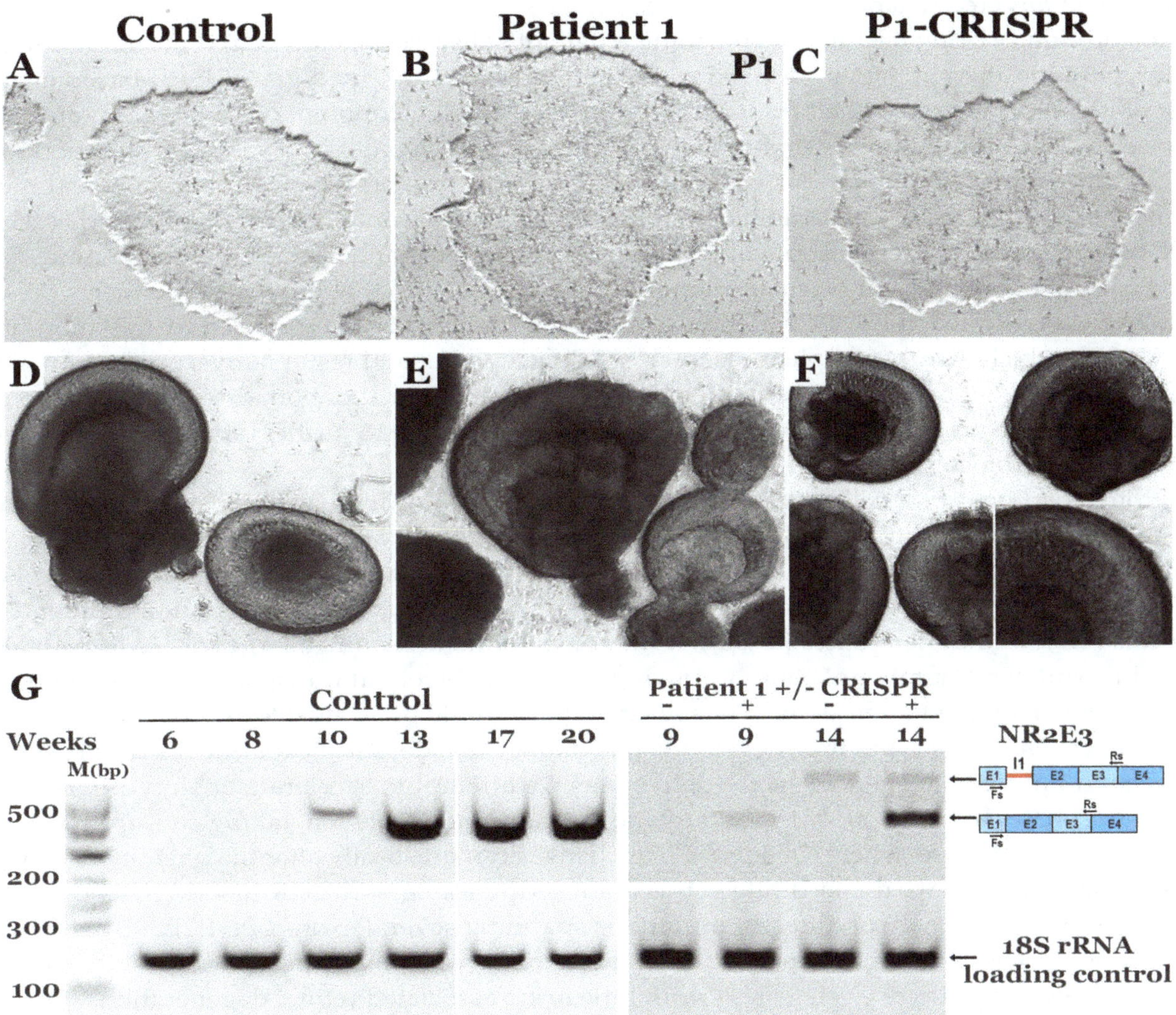

Figure 4. Correction of c.119-2A>C restores expression of normal *NR2E3* transcript in patient-derived retinal cells. **A–C**: Bright-field images of control (**A**), Patient 1 (**B**) and CRISPR-corrected Patient 1 (**C**) iPSCs. **D–F**: Bright-field images of control (**D**), Patient 1 (**E**) and CRISPR-corrected Patient 1 (**F**) optic vesicles at 5 weeks following initiation of differentiation. **G**: *NR2E3* transcript analysis by semi-quantitative PCR in control and Patient 1 iPSC derived retinal cells before (-) and after (+) CRISPR correction at various time points following the initiation of differentiation; 18S rRNA was amplified as a loading control.

4. Discussion

The discovery of iPSCs, the creation of protocols for successful tissue-specific differentiation, and the development of CRISPR-based genome editing have collectively enabled scientists to study pathophysiology in human tissues like the retina that are usually inaccessible in living individuals. For example, our ability to generate photoreceptor cells from patients with molecularly-undiagnosed retinitis pigmentosa allowed us to demonstrate how a newly identified mutation in the gene male germ cell associated kinase (MAK) causes photoreceptor cell-specific disease [26]. Similarly, by generating retinal pigmented epithelial cells from a patient with suspected RPE65 associated Leber congenital amaurosis (LCA), we were able to demonstrate that a novel intronic variant in a child of Haitian ancestry, which could have easily been a non-disease causing ethnic polymorphism, altered splicing and normal transcript production [27]. In the burgeoning field of retinal gene therapy, where molecular confirmation of a patient's disease-causing genotype is required for enrollment in a clinical gene augmentation trial, the ability to use these approaches to demonstrate that a patient truly has the disease being targeted will be invaluable.

In addition to being useful for confirming a patient's disease-causing genotype, disease-specific phenotypes identified in patient-derived cells (which can be confirmed via CRISPR-based genomic correction) are proving to be helpful for the evaluation and development of novel therapeutics. For instance, we recently demonstrated how AAV-based replacement of *CLN3* and mitigation of the molecular phenotype in patient-derived photoreceptor cells was preferable for the demonstration of treatment efficacy to the use of an animal model that does not accurately recapitulate the disease [28]. In the current study, we demonstrate how patient-derived iPSCs and CRISPR-based genome editing can be used to evaluate the molecular phenotype associated with the rare disease, enhanced S-cone syndrome. As indicated in the introduction, enhanced S-cone syndrome is caused by mutations in the gene *NR2E3*, which disrupt rod photoreceptor cell development and result in overproduction of blue cones. By identifying how genetic alterations in *NR2E3* expression alter both disease progression and the percentage of cone and rod photoreceptor cells, we may be able to further refine our current retinal differentiation protocols.

From a photoreceptor cell replacement perspective, to restore high-acuity vision, transplantation of high-density cone photoreceptor cells will be required. There are a few promising strategies for isolating cones from retinal organoids, which depending on cell line and differentiation protocol used can have different percentages of rods vs. cones that result from using current retinal differentiation protocols (reviewed in References [29,30]); however, all of them require a large scale culture in order to obtain a sufficient number of cones following selection for retinal transplantation. A method for directing retinal differentiation along a cone selective path would be a valuable improvement. Typically, we and others have taken cues from developmental biology and designed experiments to vary the type, dosage, and timing of exogenous factor delivery as we attempt to accelerate or shift differentiation in one direction or another [31–35]. Although not a traditional approach, taking cues from naturally occurring genetic disease, where single base pair changes can drastically alter the phenotypic outcome, may also be useful. As we demonstrate in this manuscript, a single CRISPR-based HDR strategy can be used to correct a variety of different mutations spanning several exons of NR2E3. By comparing these changes to both in vitro phenotype and patient history, it may be possible to identify variants that selectively promote cone cell genesis with little or no associated retinal degeneration.

Although unexpected, one of the more interesting findings that we report in this study pertains to the molecular mechanism of the c.119-2A>C variant and is in opposition to a previous publication on this subject [14]. It is important to note that the previous study was performed prior to the widespread use of iPSCs and the development of CRISPR-based genome editing, and as a result, the authors elected to test the function of this variant by transiently transfecting COS7 cells (transformed green monkey kidney cells) with an expression plasmid that contained the *NR2E3* gene harboring the c.119-2A>C mutation. Transcriptional analysis in their system indicated that this mutation resulted in skipping of exon 2, which caused a frameshift and creation of a premature stop codon in exon 3 [14]. In our study, by focusing on endogenously expressed *NR2E3* in human patient-derived photoreceptor cells, we found that the c.119-2A>C mutation in fact generates an abnormal transcript that includes a segment of intron 1 followed by exon 2, which also causes a frameshift and the creation of a premature stop codon. Interestingly, analysis of the wild-type and mutant alleles using the ESEFinder 3.0 program (rulai.cshl.edu) revealed a difference in predicted splicing factor binding sites. An SRSF1 site was found to be present in the wild-type but absent in the mutant, and an SRSF6 site that is absent in wild-type was found to be present in the mutant. We suspect that the change in splice factor binding activated a cryptic splice acceptor site in intron 1 in the iPSC-derived retinal cells rather than a skipping of exon 2 as observed in the previous COS7 study. The reason that the cryptic splice site was not used in the COS7 system could simply be due to species and cell type-specific differences in the splicing machinery. That is, it is possible that the splicing machinery used by monkey kidney cells is somewhat different from that used by human photoreceptor cells. Regardless, this finding illustrates the importance of using the appropriate cell type, obtained from the species of interest, when making inferences about the function of different genetic variants. This will be especially true when attempting to determine the pathogenicity of newly identified genetic variants in the age of clinical molecular medicine.

Author Contributions: Study conceptualization, L.R.B., L.A.W., R.F.M., E.M.S. and B.A.T.; methodology, L.R.B., L.A.W., E.R.B., J.A.C., J.C.G., K.R.A. and J.L.A.; data curation, L.R.B., L.A.W., E.R.B., J.A.C., J.C.G., K.R.A. and J.L.A.; writing—original draft preparation, L.R.B., R.F.M., E.M.S. and B.A.T.; writing—review and editing, L.R.B., L.A.W., E.R.B., J.A.C., J.L.A., R.F.M., E.M.S. and B.A.T.; supervision, R.F.M., E.M.S. and B.A.T.; funding acquisition, R.F.M., E.M.S. and B.A.T.

Acknowledgments: We would like to thank the patients for donating skin biopsies from which the iPSCs used in this study were generated. We would like to thank the Carver Non-Profit Genetic Testing Laboratory for providing sequencing support and molecular confirmation of the patients' disease-causing genotype.

References

1. Haider, N.B.; Jacobson, S.G.; Cideciyan, A.V.; Swiderski, R.; Streb, L.M.; Searby, C.; Beck, G.; Hockey, R.; Hanna, D.B.; Gorman, S.; et al. Mutation of a nuclear receptor gene, NR2E3, causes enhanced S cone syndrome, a disorder of retinal cell fate. *Nat. Genet.* **2000**, *24*, 127–131. [CrossRef] [PubMed]
2. Haider, N.B.; Naggert, J.K.; Nishina, P.M. Excess cone cell proliferation due to lack of a functional NR2E3 causes retinal dysplasia and degeneration in rd7/rd7 mice. *Hum. Mol. Genet.* **2001**, *10*, 1619–1626. [CrossRef] [PubMed]
3. Haider, N.B.; Demarco, P.; Nystuen, A.M.; Huang, X.; Smith, R.S.; McCall, M.A.; Naggert, J.K.; Nishina, P.M. The transcription factor Nr2e3 functions in retinal progenitors to suppress cone cell generation. *Vis. Neurosci.* **2006**, *23*, 917–929. [CrossRef] [PubMed]
4. Haider, N.B.; Mollema, N.; Gaule, M.; Yuan, Y.; Sachs, A.J.; Nystuen, A.M.; Naggert, J.K.; Nishina, P.M. Nr2e3-directed transcriptional regulation of genes involved in photoreceptor development and cell-type specific phototransduction. *Exp. Eye Res.* **2009**, *89*, 365–372. [CrossRef] [PubMed]
5. Cheng, H.; Khan, N.W.; Roger, J.E.; Swaroop, A. Excess cones in the retinal degeneration rd7 mouse, caused by the loss of function of orphan nuclear receptor Nr2e3, originate from early-born photoreceptor precursors. *Hum. Mol. Genet.* **2011**, *20*, 4102–4115. [CrossRef] [PubMed]
6. Chen, J.; Rattner, A.; Nathans, J. The rod photoreceptor-specific nuclear receptor Nr2e3 represses transcription of multiple cone-specific genes. *J. Neurosci.* **2005**, *25*, 118–129. [CrossRef]
7. Marmor, M.F.; Jacobson, S.G.; Foerster, M.H.; Kellner, U.; Weleber, R.G. Diagnostic clinical findings of a new syndrome with night blindness, maculopathy, and enhanced S cone sensitivity. *Am. J. Ophthalmol.* **1990**, *110*, 124–134. [CrossRef]
8. Fishman, G.A.; Jampol, L.M.; Goldberg, M.F. Diagnostic features of the Favre-Goldmann syndrome. *Br. J. Ophthalmol* **1976**, *60*, 345–353. [CrossRef]
9. Garafalo, A.V.; Calzetti, G.; Cideciyan, A.V.; Roman, A.J.; Saxena, S.; Sumaroka, A.; Choi, W.; Wright, A.F.;

Jacobson, S.G. Cone Vision Changes in the Enhanced S-Cone Syndrome Caused by NR2E3 Gene Mutations. *Invest. Ophthalmol. Vis. Sci.* **2018**, *59*, 3209–3219. [CrossRef]

10. Yzer, S.; Barbazetto, I.; Allikmets, R.; van Schooneveld, M.J.; Bergen, A.; Tsang, S.H.; Jacobson, S.G.; Yannuzzi, L.A. Expanded clinical spectrum of enhanced S-cone syndrome. *JAMA Ophthalmol* **2013**, *131*, 1324–1330. [CrossRef] [PubMed]
11. Schorderet, D.F.; Escher, P. NR2E3 mutations in enhanced S-cone sensitivity syndrome (ESCS), Goldmann-Favre syndrome (GFS), clumped pigmentary retinal degeneration (CPRD), and retinitis pigmentosa (RP). *Hum. Mutat.* **2009**, *30*, 1475–1485. [CrossRef] [PubMed]
12. Escher, P.; Gouras, P.; Roduit, R.; Tiab, L.; Bolay, S.; Delarive, T.; Chen, S.; Tsai, C.-C.; Hayashi, M.; Zernant, J.; et al. Mutations in NR2E3 can cause dominant or recessive retinal degenerations in the same family. *Hum. Mutat.* **2009**, *30*, 342–351. [CrossRef] [PubMed]
13. Stone, E.M.; Andorf, J.L.; Whitmore, S.S.; DeLuca, A.P.; Giacalone, J.C.; Streb, L.M.; Braun, T.A.; Mullins, R.F.; Scheetz, T.E.; Sheffield, V.C.; et al. Clinically Focused Molecular Investigation of 1000 Consecutive Families with Inherited Retinal Disease. *Ophthalmology* **2017**, *124*, 1314–1331. [CrossRef] [PubMed]
14. Bernal, S.; Solans, T.; Gamundi, M.J.; Hernan, I.; de Jorge, L.; Carballo, M.; Navarro, R.; Tizzano, E.; Ayuso, C.; Baiget, M. Analysis of the involvement of the NR2E3 gene in autosomal recessive retinal dystrophies. *Clin. Genet.* **2008**, *73*, 360–366. [CrossRef]
15. Burnight, E.R.; Giacalone, J.C.; Cooke, J.A.; Thompson, J.R.; Bohrer, L.R.; Chirco, K.R.; Drack, A.V.; Fingert, J.H.; Worthington, K.S.; Wiley, L.A.; et al. CRISPR-Cas9 genome engineering: Treating inherited retinal degeneration. *Prog Retin Eye Res.* **2018**, *65*, 28–49. [CrossRef] [PubMed]
16. Giacalone, J.C.; Sharma, T.P.; Burnight, E.R.; Fingert, J.F.; Mullins, R.F.; Stone, E.M.; Tucker, B.A. CRISPR-Cas9-Based Genome Editing of Human Induced Pluripotent Stem Cells. *Curr Protoc Stem Cell Biol* **2018**, *44*, 5B.7.1–5B.7.22. [PubMed]
17. Burnight, E.R.; Gupta, M.; Wiley, L.A.; Anfinson, K.R.; Tran, A.; Triboulet, R.; Hoffmann, J.M.; Klaahsen, D.L.; Andorf, J.L.; Jiao, C.; et al. Using CRISPR-Cas9 to Generate Gene-Corrected Autologous iPSCs for the Treatment of Inherited Retinal Degeneration. *Mol. Ther.* **2017**, *25*, 1999–2013. [CrossRef]
18. Burnight, E.R.; Bohrer, L.R.; Giacalone, J.C.; Klaahsen, D.L.; Daggett, H.T.; East, J.S.; Madumba, R.A.; Worthington, K.S.; Mullins, R.F.; Stone, E.M.; et al. CRISPR-Cas9-Mediated Correction of the 1.02 kb Common Deletion in CLN3 in Induced Pluripotent Stem Cells from Patients with Batten Disease. *The CRISPR Journal* **2018**, *1*, 75–87. [CrossRef]
19. Buskin, A.; Zhu, L.; Chichagova, V.; Basu, B.; Mozaffari-Jovin, S.; Dolan, D.; Droop, A.; Collin, J.; Bronstein, R.; Mehrotra, S.; et al. Disrupted alternative splicing for genes implicated in splicing and ciliogenesis causes PRPF31 retinitis pigmentosa. *Nat. Commun* **2018**, *9*, 4234. [CrossRef]
20. Steyer, B.; Bu, Q.; Cory, E.; Jiang, K.; Duong, S.; Sinha, D.; Steltzer, S.; Gamm, D.; Chang, Q.; Saha, K. Scarless Genome Editing of Human Pluripotent Stem Cells via Transient Puromycin Selection. *Stem Cell Reports* **2018**, *10*, 642–654. [CrossRef]
21. Deng, W.-L.; Gao, M.-L.; Lei, X.-L.; Lv, J.-N.; Zhao, H.; He, K.-W.; Xia, X.-X.; Li, L.-Y.; Chen, Y.-C.; Li, Y.-P.; et al. Gene Correction Reverses Ciliopathy and Photoreceptor Loss in iPSC-Derived Retinal Organoids from Retinitis Pigmentosa Patients. *Stem Cell Reports* **2018**, *10*, 1267–1281. [CrossRef]
22. Maeder, M.L.; Stefanidakis, M.; Wilson, C.J.; Baral, R.; Barrera, L.A.; Bounoutas, G.S.; Bumcrot, D.; Chao, H.; Ciulla, D.M.; DaSilva, J.A.; et al. Development of a gene-editing approach to restore vision loss in Leber congenital amaurosis type 10. *Nat. Med.* **2019**, *25*, 229–233. [CrossRef] [PubMed]
23. Wiley, L.A.; Anfinson, K.R.; Cranston, C.M.; Kaalberg, E.E.; Collins, M.M.; Mullins, R.F.; Stone, E.M.; Tucker, B.A. Generation of Xeno-Free, cGMP-Compliant Patient-Specific iPSCs from Skin Biopsy. *Curr Protoc Stem Cell Biol* **2017**, *42*, 4A.12.1–4A.12.14. [PubMed]
24. Wiley, L.A.; Burnight, E.R.; DeLuca, A.P.; Anfinson, K.R.; Cranston, C.M.; Kaalberg, E.E.; Penticoff, J.A.; Affatigato, L.M.; Mullins, R.F.; Stone, E.M.; et al. cGMP production of patient-specific iPSCs and photoreceptor precursor cells to treat retinal degenerative blindness. *Sci Rep.* **2016**, *6*, 30742. [CrossRef] [PubMed]
25. Ohlemacher, S.K.; Iglesias, C.L.; Sridhar, A.; Gamm, D.M.; Meyer, J.S. Generation of highly enriched populations of optic vesicle-like retinal cells from human pluripotent stem cells. *Curr Protoc Stem Cell Biol.* **2015**, *32*, 1H.8.1–1H.8.20. [PubMed]

26. Tucker, B.A.; Scheetz, T.E.; Mullins, R.F.; DeLuca, A.P.; Hoffmann, J.M.; Johnston, R.M.; Jacobson, S.G.; Sheffield, V.C.; Stone, E.M. Exome sequencing and analysis of induced pluripotent stem cells identify the cilia-related gene male germ cell-associated kinase (MAK) as a cause of retinitis pigmentosa. *Proc. Natl. Acad. Sci. USA* **2011**, *108*, E569–E576. [CrossRef] [PubMed]
27. Tucker, B.A.; Cranston, C.M.; Anfinson, K.A.; Shrestha, S.; Streb, L.M.; Leon, A.; Mullins, R.F.; Stone, E.M. Using patient-specific induced pluripotent stem cells to interrogate the pathogenicity of a novel retinal pigment epithelium-specific 65 kDa cryptic splice site mutation and confirm eligibility for enrollment into a clinical gene augmentation trial. *Transl Res.* **2015**, *166*, 740–749.e1. [CrossRef] [PubMed]
28. Wiley, L.A.; Burnight, E.R.; Drack, A.V.; Banach, B.B.; Ochoa, D.; Cranston, C.M.; Madumba, R.A.; East, J.S.; Mullins, R.F.; Stone, E.M.; et al. Using Patient-Specific Induced Pluripotent Stem Cells and Wild-Type Mice to Develop a Gene Augmentation-Based Strategy to Treat CLN3-Associated Retinal Degeneration. *Hum. Gene Ther.* **2016**, *27*, 835–846. [CrossRef] [PubMed]
29. Llonch, S.; Carido, M.; Ader, M. Organoid technology for retinal repair. *Dev. Biol.* **2018**, *433*, 132–143. [CrossRef]
30. Achberger, K.; Haderspeck, J.C.; Kleger, A.; Liebau, S. Stem cell-based retina models. *Adv. Drug Deliv. Rev.* **2018**. [CrossRef]
31. Tucker, B.A.; Park, I.-H.; Qi, S.D.; Klassen, H.J.; Jiang, C.; Yao, J.; Redenti, S.; Daley, G.Q.; Young, M.J. Transplantation of adult mouse iPS cell-derived photoreceptor precursors restores retinal structure and function in degenerative mice. *PLoS ONE* **2011**, *6*, e18992. [CrossRef] [PubMed]
32. Ueda, K.; Onishi, A.; Ito, S.-I.; Nakamura, M.; Takahashi, M. Generation of three-dimensional retinal organoids expressing rhodopsin and S- and M-cone opsins from mouse stem cells. *Biochem. Biophys. Res. Commun.* **2018**, *495*, 2595–2601. [CrossRef] [PubMed]
33. Riazifar, H.; Jia, Y.; Chen, J.; Lynch, G.; Huang, T. Chemically induced specification of retinal ganglion cells from human embryonic and induced pluripotent stem cells. *Stem Cells Transl Med.* **2014**, *3*, 424–432. [CrossRef] [PubMed]
34. Tucker, B.A.; Anfinson, K.R.; Mullins, R.F.; Stone, E.M.; Young, M.J. Use of a synthetic xeno-free culture substrate for induced pluripotent stem cell induction and retinal differentiation. *Stem Cells Transl Med.* **2013**, *2*, 16–24. [CrossRef] [PubMed]
35. Nelson, B.R.; Hartman, B.H.; Georgi, S.A.; Lan, M.S.; Reh, T.A. Transient inactivation of Notch signaling synchronizes differentiation of neural progenitor cells. *Dev. Biol.* **2007**, *304*, 479–498. [CrossRef] [PubMed]

5

Phosphoinositides in Retinal Function and Disease

Theodore G. Wensel

Verna and Marrs McLean Department of Biochemistry and Molecular Biology, Baylor College of Medicine, Houston, TX 77030, USA; twensel@bcm.edu

Abstract: Phosphatidylinositol and its phosphorylated derivatives, the phosphoinositides, play many important roles in all eukaryotic cells. These include modulation of physical properties of membranes, activation or inhibition of membrane-associated proteins, recruitment of peripheral membrane proteins that act as effectors, and control of membrane trafficking. They also serve as precursors for important second messengers, inositol (1,4,5) trisphosphate and diacylglycerol. Animal models and human diseases involving defects in phosphoinositide regulatory pathways have revealed their importance for function in the mammalian retina and retinal pigmented epithelium. New technologies for localizing, measuring and genetically manipulating them are revealing new information about their importance for the function and health of the vertebrate retina.

Keywords: phosphoinositides; retinal lipids; membrane trafficking

---

1. Introduction

Phosphoinositides are membrane phospholipids with the six-member cyclic polyol *myo*-inositol, $(CHOH)_6$, or O-phosphorylated forms of inositol, as their headgroup (Figure 1). The phosphorylated forms are of low abundance in eukaryotic cells of all types, generally comprising 1% or less of total phospholipid. Nevertheless, they play critical roles in cellular regulation, and defects in their synthesis and regulation lead to devastating diseases [1–6]. The retina is clearly no exception to this generality, but surprisingly few details have been worked out in what is arguably one of the most extensively studied tissues in our bodies, about the regulation and regulatory roles of retinal phosphoinositides. Recent technological advances make it possible to make substantial advances in this field in the next few years.

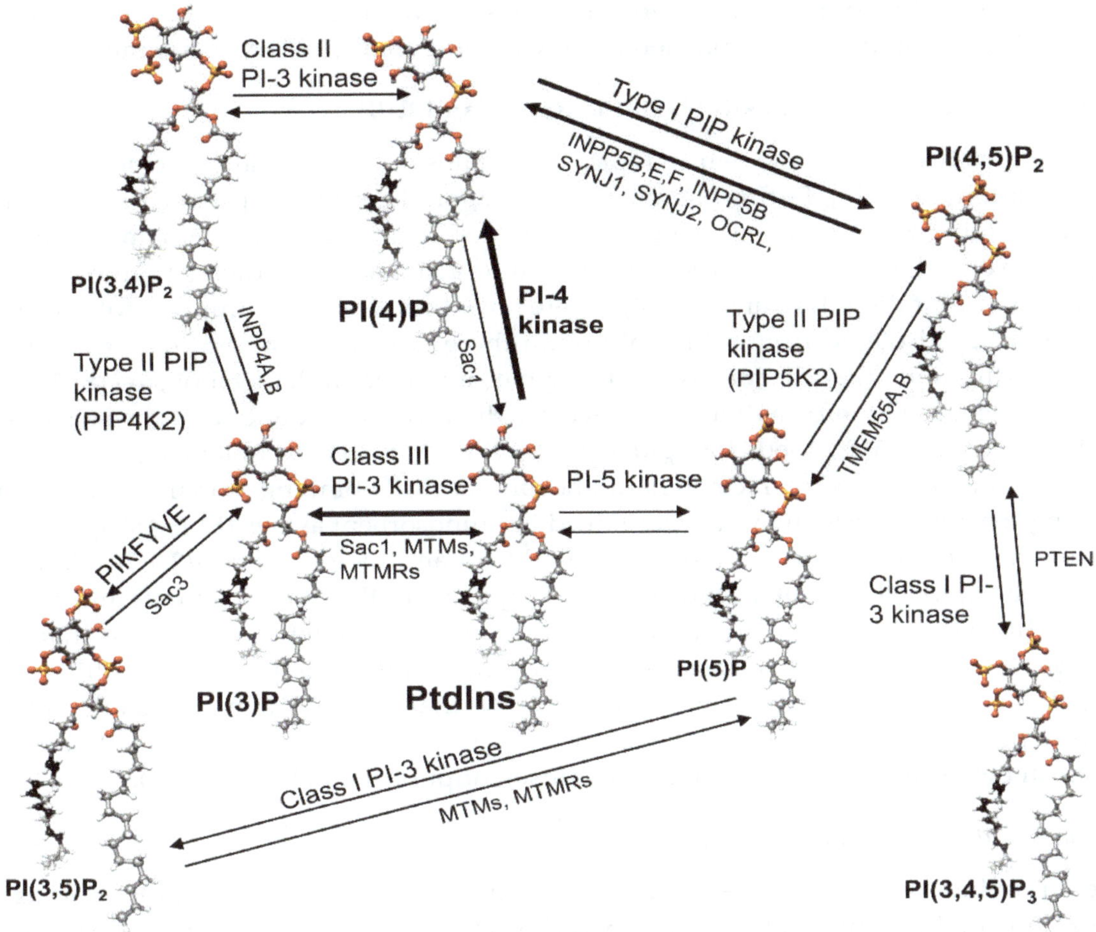

Figure 1. Structures of the cellular phosphoinositides and enzymes responsible for their synthesis and interconversion. Phosphoinositides (PI) species are shown with the acyl chains most commonly found on phosphatidylinositol, which is the starting point for all the others, arachidonic acid (20:4) and stearic acid (C18). Relative font sizes correlate with relative abundance.

2. Chemical Structures of Phosphoinositides

Phosphoinositides (abbreviated here as "PI") include phosphatidylinositol (PtdIns), in which the 1′-position of the inositol ring is attached via a phosphodiester bond to the *sn*-3 position of (1, 2) diacyl glycerol, and derivatives of PtdIns with one, two, or three phosphates attached in various combinations to the 4′, 5′ or 3′ hydroxyls of PtdIns. Including PtdIns, a total of eight different PI head groups are commonly found in eukaryotic cells (Figure 1) [4,5].

3. Phosphatidylinositol Content in the Retina and RPE

PtdIns is a relatively substantial component of the membranes of most cells in metazoans, with mole fractions ranging from ~4%–20% of total phospholipid [4]. Early reports stated that retina phospholipids contained 4.4%–6.4% PtdIns across six different mammalian species [7–9]. Interestingly, rod outer segment (ROS) membranes were found to have much lower levels, 1.5% to 2.5% in bovine and 2.1% in frog [10–13]. Retinal pigment epithelial cells (RPE), in contrast, have higher levels of PtdIns, at 6.5% of total phospholipid [14], while ER membranes isolated from bovine retinas contain 9.6% PtdIns [10]. The general picture that emerges is that total PtdIns content in total retinal membranes outside of outer segments and that of RPE are more or less "normal" as compared to other tissues and cell types, consistent with the notion that widespread roles of PI are likely to be conserved in many retinal cell types. In contrast, ROS have an unusually low PtdIns content, suggesting different roles for this lipid class in that organelle. This idea is consistent with findings discussed below, indicating different lipid compositions in plasma membranes as compared to ciliary membranes.

4. Content of Minor Phosphoinositides in the Retina and RPE

As a negatively charged lipid, which typically contains one polyunsaturated side chain fatty acid, such as arachidonic acid [8], PtdIns has a major impact on the physical properties of the membrane domains containing it. In contrast, the phosphorylated forms are much less abundant, and exert their influence on cell physiology largely through interactions with proteins with high-affinity and high-specificity PI-binding domains [15–17]. There have been few measurements of phosphorylated PI in retina or cells isolated from retina, although there have been several papers addressing the turnover of PtdIns and other PI, or activity of enzymes involved in PI metabolism [18–21]. The likely reason for the absence of information on PI levels is their low abundance and the lack of sensitivity provided by conventional methods for lipid analysis. More sensitive techniques have been developed recently, including one based on recombinant phosphoinositide-binding domains fused to an epitope tag, allowing sensitive detection by enzyme-linked immunosorbent assays (ELISAs) and measurement of chemiluminescence [22]. This technique was used to quantify PI(3)P and PI(3,4,5)P_3 in preparations of rod cells that contain both outer segments and fragments of the inner segments and demonstrated levels of PI(3)P at 0.0035 mol% of total phospholipid under illumination conditions that yielded the highest levels of that lipid, and at least 10-fold lower (i.e., undetectable) levels of PI(3,4,5)P_3. PI(4)P and PI(4,5)P_2 are, in general, found at much higher levels than the 3-phosphorylated PI, but even those appear to be present in rods at very low levels, which are only about 10-fold higher than the levels of PI(3)P, i.e., on the order of 0.04 mol% (He and Wensel, unpublished observations).

Comparison to Other Tissues and Cell Types

These numbers are comparable to those found in other eukaryotic cells, reported as PtdIns3P, 0.002% of phospholipid mass; PtdIns4P, 0.05%; PtdIns5P, 0.002%; PtdIns(4,5)P, 0.05%; PtdIns(3,4)P, 0.0001%; PtdIns(3,5)P, 0.0001% [17], see also references in [23]. A more recent mass spectrometry study reported PI(3,4,5)3 levels as 50-fold or more lower than those of the more common PIs in mammalian U87MG cells [24]. An interesting observation derived from measurements of PI levels in cultured cells is that, generally, they do not change greatly upon activation with extracellular stimuli; for the more common forms, PtdIns, PI(4)P, PI(4,5)P_2 and PI(3)P, the change is generally less than 30% [17]. The implication, for PI(4,5)P_2, which is rapidly degraded to form $InsP_3$ and diacylglycerol upon activation of phospholipase C isozymes by G-protein-coupled receptors or growth factor receptors [25,26], is that homeostatic mechanisms are in place to regenerate rapidly the pools of both PI(4,5)P_2 and its precursor PI(4)P upon PLC activation. In contrast, PI(3,4,5)P_3 level changes due to receptor stimulation are generally too low to have a major impact on levels of its precursor, PI(4,5)P_2.

5. Importance of PI Generally

Despite their low abundance, phosphoinositides play major roles in regulation of cell signaling and membrane dynamics, and are essential for control of a wide range of processes including development, proliferation and differentiation, membrane excitability, exocytosis, phagocytosis, cell motility, and detection of extracellular signals [4]. These functional roles are primarily mediated by a plethora of enzymes, scaffold proteins and complex-nucleating proteins containing phosphoinositide-binding domains of high affinity and high specificity. Genetic defects in the enzymes responsible for their regulation are, in most cases, lethal at the embryo stage, except for some cases of redundancy (i.e., more than one gene encoding enzymes or PI-binding proteins with similar activities). Cell-type specific deletion of these enzymes leads to more specific pathologies, e.g., neurodegeneration in the case of the type III PI-3 kinase, Vps34 (also known as PIK3C3) [27,28]. Some of these enzymes, such as type I PI-3 kinases, can act as oncogenes when mutations disrupt their regulation, and are considered prime targets for cancer chemotherapy, whereas others, such as the phosphoinositide phosphatase, PTEN, are considered tumor suppressor genes [29]; these therapeutic targets are present in the retina, where their roles in retinal function, and any effects of drugs targeting them are unknown.

Importance of Phosphoinositides for Dynamics and Functions of Membranes in Retina and RPE

Among the most important roles of phosphoinositides and their protein effectors are those mediating intracellular membrane traffic, by directing membrane proteins and lipids from one compartment to another in response to cellular needs and changing environments. For example, PI(3)P is found in early and recycling endosomes, and is important for recruiting key proteins that regulate trafficking to these compartments [30]. It is also important for autophagy, a survival-promoting pathway leading to the lysosomal degradation of organelles [31]. PI(4)P is enriched in the Golgi apparatus, and is thought to be important for membrane trafficking through the Golgi compartments and from the Golgi to the plasma membrane and other subcellular compartments [32], likely including disk membranes. PI(4,5)P_2 plays a key role in clathrin-mediated endocytosis, and serves to direct many effector proteins to the plasma membrane where it is primarily found [33].

PI(4,5)P_2 and other phosphoinositides directly regulate the activity of ion channels, transporters and enzymes in membranes [34,35]. In addition, PI(4,5)P_2 serves as the substrate for phosphoinositide-specific phospholipase C, leading to production of the important second messengers, inositol (1,4,5) trisphosphate (InsP_3) and diacylglycerol [25,26,36,37]. Phosphoinositides are also critically important for regulating interactions between membranes and cytoskeletal elements [38,39]. Changes in these interactions are critical for cell growth and mobility, and for remodeling of intracellular structures. They may well play a role in cytoskeleton-dependent disk morphogenesis in rods.

6. Membrane Trafficking in Retina and RPE

Every aspect of retinal biology depends heavily on the correct organization and composition of highly specialized membranes, from the unique disc membranes of the photoreceptor sensory cilia, to the ribbon synapses of rods, cones, and bipolar cells, to the apical processes of RPE (retinal pigmented epithelium) cells, uniquely tuned to the detection and engulfment of shed outer segment fragments. The formation, maintenance, and functions of these membranes rely heavily on the phosphorylated phosphoinositides [2–4,40]. Despite the intense interest in phosphoinositide research in recent decades, surprisingly little is known about their regulation and functional roles in the retina, although it is known that disruption of phosphoinositide regulation can lead to blindness in human patients and animal models [41–48]. The membranes and pathways they regulate are known to be essential for the function and health of the retina as well as for disease processes and cellular responses to disease states.

One of the reasons for the dearth of knowledge has been a lack of tools for studying these very low-abundance lipids within the multiple cell types of the retina and the adjacent retinal pigment epithelium. Recently, tools developed by the broader PI field have begun to be applied to the unique challenges and opportunities posed by the retina [22,49]. Doing so will have enormous impact on our understanding of the cell biology of the retina and its disruption in disease. This can help to inform the design and optimization of therapies aimed at treating and preventing retinal dysfunction and degeneration.

7. Features of the Retina that Make It Ideal for Studies of Phosphoinositide Regulation In Vivo

The field of phosphoinositide regulation has long been dominated by studies in cultured immortalized cell lines, giving rise to a critical need for elucidation of their physiological regulation in terminally differentiated neurons. For this reason, in vivo studies have broad significance for this field. There are several features of the retina that make it particularly amenable to studies of phosphoinositide regulation in vivo. These include the ability to assay both structure and function non-invasively, the ease of making cell-type-specific knockouts, the ability to isolate rod cells for either biochemical analysis or ultrastructure determination, an extensive understanding of biochemistry and cell biology, especially of rods, which exceeds that of any of other vertebrate neurons, and a wealth of knowledge of RPE cell biology.

8. Importance of Phosphoinositides for Membrane Trafficking in Retina

Despite years of study, no convincing evidence has accumulated for an important role for phosphoinositides in the phototransduction cascade. In contrast, a steady stream of evidence supports a central role for these lipids in membrane trafficking and sorting in all mammalian cell types, just as a critical role in photoreceptors for membrane sorting and trafficking has long been established [3,50,51]. A review article in 2011 covered advances in understanding the roles of phosphoinositides in photoreceptors [6]. It is highly likely that events such as endocytosis and exocytosis, endosomal sorting, membrane budding, post-Golgi vesicle trafficking, and disk morphogenesis all depend on phosphoinositide dynamics, and published reports support a role for PI(3)P and PI(4,5)P_2 in rhodopsin trafficking [52,53]. For example, PI(4,5)P_2-binding proteins, ezrin and moesin, were reported to colocalize with Rac1 and Rab8 on rhodopsin transport carrier vesicles at the site of their fusion with the plasma membrane. A recent report suggesting the involvement of actin-nucleating proteins Arp2/Arp3 in basal disc extension [54] potentially implicates local pools or PI(4,5)P_2, which are known to be critical for their function [55,56].

In cone photoreceptors, ablation of a type I PI-3 kinase leads to enhanced sensitivity to light damage [57]. Mutations in the phosphoinositide phosphatase, synaptojanin 1 lead to defects in synaptic vesicle trafficking in cone cells [44].

9. Retinal Cilia and Phosphoinositides

Phosphoinositides, and especially PI(4,5)P_2 and PI(4)P, have been proposed to play important roles in assembly, disassembly, and regulation of primary cilia [52,58–62]. The lipid content of cilia is different from that of the plasma membrane, and a membrane diffusion barrier surrounding the cilium has been demonstrated (see [63] for a review). Two PI-5-phosphatases, INPP5E and OCRL, essential for cilium function have been reported to be localized to the cilium [41,64–66]

Phosphoinositides and the BBSome

The BBSome, a heterooctameric protein complex involved in ciliary trafficking, whose defects lead to the blinding ciliopathy, Bardet–Biedl syndrome, binds to membranes, and shows a preference for acidic lipids, including phosphoinositides [67,68], and isolated BBS5 which contains pleckstrin homology domains, binds to phosphoinositides, especially PI(3)P [68]. More recently, it was shown that a core BBSome complex containing BBS 1, 4, 5, 8, 9 and 18 and a smaller sub-complex lacking BBS1 and BBS5 bind phosphoinositides with similar specificities. A caveat for these studies is that the commercial "PIP strips" used have local surface densities of phosphoinositides that far exceed anything found under physiological conditions, so further investigation of phosphoinositide-binding of the BBSome and its sub-complexes is warranted.

10. Autophagy and other Stress Responses Involving Redirection of Membrane Traffic and Phosphoinositides

It has been reported that light exposure induces elements of the autophagy pathway in rods and that autophagy plays an important role in photoreceptor homeostasis [69–73]. This pathway has been suggested to be a neuroprotective one that forestalls apoptosis under conditions of stress [69,74]. This process may be part of a more general neuroprotective response involving re-direction of membrane traffic and phosphoinositides. As discussed below, Synaptojanin-1 has been implicated in autophagy in zebrafish cones [75].

11. Evidence for Effects of Light on Phosphoinositide Metabolism

A number of early reports in the 1980s suggested that light had measurable impacts on PI metabolism in photoreceptors or the retina generally. Based on measurement of ^{32}Pi incorporated into PtdIns by metabolic labeling, it was reported that exposure of isolated frog retina to light decreased levels of PIP_2 by 14% after 5 s and 37% after 15 s, while levels of PI(4)P, PtdIns and other acidic lipids remained essentially constant [76]. Subsequent publications from the same group reported increased levels of ^{3}H inositol and ^{32}P into phosphoinositides upon illumination [77]. They also reported PI(4,5)P_2-specific phospholipase C (PLC) activity in frog photoreceptors, and PLC immunoreactivity in bovine rod outer segments [78,79], as well as PI-kinase and PIP-kinase activities in frog ROS [19]. Another group found that exposure of rat retinas to light led to decreased staining of rod outer segments with anti-PI(4,5)P_2 antibodies [80,81]. The caveats of those experiments are that it is known that physical properties of outer segment membranes and their protein composition are altered by bright light exposure, and that it is difficult to establish the specificity of such antibody staining. In addition to light, reports on regulation of photoreceptor PLC by Ca^{2+} [82] or by subunits of the phototransduction G protein, transducin [83], were published, also suggesting a possible influence of light exposure, which is known to control levels of Ca^{2+} and active and inactive forms of transducin subunits.

In contrast, another group [84] reported that bovine rod outer segments have very little PIP kinase activity as compared to the rest of the retina (consistent with the previously reported low level of PI(4,5)P_2 in outer segment membranes), and that light adaptation had no measurable effect on phosphoinositide metabolism as compared to in vivo dark adaptation. Yet another group, using metabolic labeling with [^{3}H]inositol, reported that light led to decreases in PIP_2 levels without generation of $InsP_3$, suggesting light-dependent activity of a phosphatase rather than of phospholipase C [85]. In vitro studies demonstrated that the presence of PI(4,5)P_2 in membranes could affect the activity of components of the phototransduction cascade [86,87], including the cGMP-gated cation channel and the cGMP phosphodiesterase-transducin complex. The physiological relevance of effects of PI(4,5)P_2 on phototransduction or of effects of light on PI(4,5)P_2 metabolism remains untested, and it seems to be possible to explain the entire time-course of rod light responses without invoking any participation by phosphoinositide metabolism [88]. Antibodies specific for isoforms of phospholipase C or $G_{\alpha q/11}$ PLC-coupled subunits revealed the presence of PLCβ4 and $G_{\alpha q/11}$ in rod outer segments, and $G_{\alpha q}$ and other PKC isoforms elsewhere in the retina [89]. The functional roles of these proteins in outer segments are not known. There have been suggestions that slower effects of prolonged light exposure, such as arrestin translocation from the inner to outer segments of rod cells, may be mediated by a phospholipase C cascade [90].

Light Regulation of PI-3 Kinase

Interest has turned toward Type I PI-3 kinase and PI(3,4,5)P_3, with reports of effects of light on the activity of this enzyme in bovine rod outer segments [91,92], which were reported to be mediated by light-stimulated activation and tyrosine phosphorylation of the insulin receptor [93–95]. Deletion of the p85α regulatory subunit of Type I PI-3 kinase in cone cells resulted in progressive degeneration of cones, without observable effects on rod survival [57]. Likewise, cone-specific inactivation of the gene encoding the p110α catalytic subunit also resulted in defects in cone survival [96].

In contrast, Type I PI-3 kinase and its product, PI(3,4,5)P_3, seem to be much less important for rod function. Rod-specific ablation of the p85α gene using two different rod-specific Cre transgenes yielded no obvious defects in retinal morphology or rod cell survival [22,97], although modest effects on kinetics of light response recovery and arrestin translocation were reported in one case [97]. Quantitative analysis of PI(3,4,5)P_3 levels in rods isolated from dark-adapted or light-adapted retinas revealed levels of this phosphoinositide of more than one order magnitude lower than those found for PI(3)P in the light, or at least two orders of magnitude lower than light-stimulated levels of PI(4,5)P_2 [22].

12. $PI(4,5)P_2$ and Phospholipase C in Intrinsically Photosensitive Ganglion Cells

In addition to image-forming light detection mediated by rods and cones, the vertebrate retina also contains intrinsically photosensitive retinal ganglion cells. These contain phototransduction cascades reminiscent of that found in invertebrate rhabdomeric photoreceptors [98–104]. Light activates melanopsin, encoded by the *Opn4* gene, a visual pigment which is more closely related to invertebrate opsins than to vertebrate opsin [105]. In M1-type ganglion cells, melanopsin photoisomerization leads to activation of a $G_{\alpha q/11/14}$ class G-protein, which activates the phosphoinositide-specific phospholipase C isoform, PLCβ4; the phospholipase presumably acts on $PI(4,5)P_2$ as in other cell types, including *Drosophila* photoreceptors, which contain a homologous phospholipase, to produce diacylglycerol and $InsP_3$. $PI(4,5)P_2$ hydrolysis, in turn, leads to the activation of the cation channels TRPC6 and TRPC7 [104]. In M4 ganglion cells, a different phototransduction cascade involving cyclic nucleotides and cyclic nucleotide-regulated HCN channels, whereas in M2 ganglion cells, both of these cascades operate [102].

13. Studies of PI Metabolism in the RPE

A variety of extracellular stimuli acting on tyrosine kinase-associated receptors or G protein-coupled-receptors have been reported to stimulate release of inositol phosphates in cultured RPE cells, presumably derived from PLC action of $PI(4,5)P_2$, on a timescale of tens of minutes; effective stimuli included fetal bovine serum, agonists for muscarinic, histamine, and serotonin, peptides, including bradykinin, arginine vasopressin, bombesin and oxytocin, [106–109]. The physiological relevance of these observations was not explored, but an in vivo study using frogs demonstrated dramatic acceleration of inositol phosphate release, especially of $InsP_3$, following stimulation by light [21]. Acutely isolated rat RPE cells were reported to release $InsP_3$ in response to induction of phagocytosis by addition of isolated rod outer segments [110]; this $InsP_3$ release was not observed in cells from Royal College of Surgeon (RCS) rats, which have a defect in OS phagocytosis due to a deficiency in the receptor tyrosine kinase, MERTK [111]. As in many other cell types, insulin has been reported to stimulate activity of Type I PI-3 kinase to produce $PI(3,4,5)P_3$ [95,112,113]. Responses to hypoxia [112,114,115] and elevated glucose [116,117] are also reported to involve this pathway in RPE.

A number of important processes in RPE are known to rely on phosphoinositides, but how they are regulated in these cells is not well understood. Phagocytosis, autophagy, endocytosis and endosome processing, establishment of epithelial cell polarity and extension of microvilli membranes are all known to critically depend on phosphoinositides. For example, both autophagy and phagocytosis involve the recruitment of the ubiquitin-like protein, LC3 [118–120], whose recruitment to membranes depends on PI(3)P. Phagocytosis is also thought to require $PI(4,5)P_2$ and lysosomal fusion may involve other phosphoinositides such as $PI(3,5)P_2$ and PI(5)P [22,121–125].

14. Phosphoinositide Kinases and Phosphatase

In mammals, there are 47 genes encoding 19 PI-kinase and PIP-kinases and 28 PIP phosphatases [126].

14.1. Kinases

The kinase isoforms are divided into three major families: PI 4-kinases (PI4Ks), the PI 3-kinases (PI3Ks), and PIP (PIP) kinases (PIPKs) [127]. The nomenclature for these is a bit confusing, as some enzymes termed "PI-kinases" actually act primarily as PIP kinases. For example, Type I PI-3 kinases primarily use $PI(4,5)P_2$ as their substrate to produce $PI(3,4,5)P_3$, and there is little evidence for a substantial portion of cellular PI(3)P being formed by these enzymes. When the Type III PI-3 kinase, Vps34, was knocked out in mouse rod cells and phosphoinositide levels measured, the results suggested complete ablation of PI(3)P despite the presence of the Type I enzyme [22]. Several of these have been reported to be expressed in retina or RPE at the level of protein, mRNA or enzyme activity and most, if not all, are likely present at some level; however, as far as their functions, only the Type I and Type III PI-3 kinase have been studied using gene knockouts in the retina and RPE [22,49,57,128]. Global knockouts have been produced for the α, β, and γ isoforms of Type I PIP-kinases, which are the major source of PI(4,5)P_2 in most cells [16]. Of these, the γ isoform seems to have the highest expression in the retina [129] and in other neurons [130,131] and leads to severe neuronal phenotypes and early postnatal mortality when knocked out [132]. Type II PIP-kinases have been observed in retina and are reported to be regulated by tyrosine phosphorylation [133]. The proteins encoded by the mouse genes, Pip4k2a, Pip4k2b, Pip4k2c, Pip5k1a, and Pip5k1c were all observed in a proteomic study of mouse retina [134].

14.2. Phosphatases

The phosphoinositide phosphatases encoded by Inpp1, Inpp4a, Inpp4b, Inpp5e, Mtmr2 and Synj1 (synaptojanin-1) have also been detected in retina by proteomics [134]. As noted below, defects in synaptojanin-1 and INPP5E are associated with retinal defects, as is the phosphoinositide 5-phosphatase, OCRL (oculocerebrorenal syndrome of Lowe) [135,136]. Among the other enzymes detected, almost none were enriched in the rod outer segment fraction as compared to the rest of the retina, consistent with the relatively low PI content of that organelle. One exception was Pip4k2c, the PI(5)P-4-kinase Type II γ isoform. Inactivation of the mouse *Pip4kc2* gene was found to lead to hyperactivation of the immune system, but the retinal phenotype was not examined [137].

15. Retinal Phenotypes of Genetic Defects in Genes Related to Phosphoinositide Metabolism and Signaling

Rods and cones have a very high rate of metabolism and biosynthesis of membrane components, due to the energetic demands of the phototransduction cascade and the daily shedding of ~10% of the disk membranes (based on observation of a rate of 9%–13% in the rhesus monkey [138], which have to be engulfed and recycled by the RPE. As highly polarized cells, their function and health depend critically on efficient and accurate transport of the correct proteins and lipids to the correct compartments. A host of human blinding diseases have been linked to defects in membrane transport and sorting [139,140]. In RPE cells, massive amounts of membrane traffic are associated with their role as professional phagophores. Defects in RPE phagocytosis, as in MERTK deficiency [111,141] and Bestrophin deficiency [142–145], cause retinal degeneration in humans and animal models and have been proposed to play a role in age-related macular degeneration [146].

15.1. Phosphatases and Inherited Retinopathies

Inherited defects in the phosphoinositide phosphatase, INPP5E, are associated with the multi-syndromic ciliopathies, Joubert syndrome and Bardet–Biedl syndrome [147–150], and with retinal degeneration. The substrates for this phosphatase are PI(4,5)P_2 and PI(3,4,5)P_3, and its critical role in the cilia suggests that regulating levels of PI(4,5)P_2 may be important in ciliogenesis and cilium stability.

Synaptojanins are phosphoinositide phosphatases associated with synaptic function [151–153], including vesicle uncoating and endocytosis. Synaptojanin-1 deficiency causes severe cone defects in zebrafish and has been implicated in the regulation of autophagy in cones [45,46,75].

Defects in another phosphoinositide phosphatase, OCRL, are associated with a severe ciliopathy, oculocerebrorenal syndrome of Lowe [136]. Symptoms of this disease include glaucoma, a disease of the retina.

15.2. PI3NM3

The phosphatidyl inositol transfer protein PIT3NM3 (aka CCL118) is the mammalian homologue of the *Drosophila* retinal degeneration gene, *rdgB*, and defects in it are associated with autosomal dominant cone-rod dystrophy CORD5 [154–159]. The protein has also been implicated in cancer metastasis [160]. In zebrafish, the Class I phosphatidylinositol transfer protein β isoform, Pitpnb, is essential for biogenesis and maintenance of double cones [161].

15.3. PI Binding Proteins

Proteins with phosphoinositide-binding domains have also been associated with retinal disease. These include the product of the *tub/TUB* gene [162,163] and a related protein, TULP1 [47,164–166]. Tub was discovered as the protein encoded by a gene whose mutation in *tubby* mice causes obesity, deafness and blindness. The widely expressed members of the tubby family, including TULP1-TULP4, have a characteristic carboxyl-terminal tubby domain consisting of an alpha helix surrounded by a beta barrel which has been shown to bind to specific phosphoinositides [167]. Both Tub and Tulp1 are expressed in the retina, and TULP1 mutations cause retinitis pigmentosa [47,168].

16. Conclusions

While the overall field of phosphoinositide regulation and signaling has made dramatic advances in recent years, our understanding of specific regulatory pathways in specific cell types of the retina remains limited. The emergence of new technologies for cell-type-specific gene manipulation, along with imaging techniques for subcellular localization of phosphoinositides, their regulatory enzymes and their effector proteins, and the development of more sensitive methods for measuring PI levels, bodes well for rapid progress in understanding the roles of retinal phosphoinositides in the coming years.

References

1. Phan, T.K.; Williams, S.A.; Bindra, G.K.; Lay, F.T.; Poon, I.K.H.; Hulett, M.D. Phosphoinositides: Multipurpose cellular lipids with emerging roles in cell death. *Cell Death Differ.* **2019**, *26*, 781–793. [CrossRef] [PubMed]
2. Dickson, E.J.; Hille, B. Understanding phosphoinositides: Rare, dynamic, and essential membrane phospholipids. *Biochem. J.* **2019**, *476*, 1–23. [CrossRef] [PubMed]
3. Schink, K.O.; Tan, K.W.; Stenmark, H. Phosphoinositides in Control of Membrane Dynamics. *Annu. Rev. Cell Dev. Biol.* **2016**, *32*, 143–171. [CrossRef] [PubMed]
4. Balla, T. Phosphoinositides: Tiny lipids with giant impact on cell regulation. *Physiol. Rev.* **2013**, *93*, 1019–1137. [CrossRef]
5. Maffucci, T. An introduction to phosphoinositides. *Curr. Top. Microbiol. Immunol.* **2012**, *362*, 1–42. [CrossRef]
6. Brockerhoff, S.E. Phosphoinositides and photoreceptors. *Mol. Neurobiol.* **2011**, *44*, 420–425. [CrossRef]
7. Broekhuyse, R.M. Phospholipids in tissues of the eye. I. Isolation, characterization and quantitative analysis by two-dimensional thin-layer chromatography of diacyl and vinyl-ether phospholipids. *Biochim. Biophys. Acta* **1968**, *152*, 307–315. [CrossRef]
8. Anderson, R.E.; Feldman, L.S.; Feldman, G.L. Lipids of ocular tissues. II. The phospholipids of mature bovine and rabbit whole retina. *Biochim. Biophys. Acta* **1970**, *202*, 367–373. [CrossRef]
9. Anderson, R.E. Lipids of ocular tissues. IV. A comparison of the phospholipids from the retina of six mammalian species. *Exp. Eye Res.* **1970**, *10*, 339–344. [CrossRef]
10. Anderson, R.E.; Maude, M.B.; Zimmerman, W. Lipids of ocular tissues–X. Lipid composition of subcellular fractions of bovine retina. *Vision Res.* **1975**, *15*, 1087–1090. [CrossRef]
11. Anderson, R.E.; Maude, M.B. Phospholipids of bovine outer segments. *Biochemistry* **1970**, *9*, 3624–3628. [CrossRef] [PubMed]
12. Nielsen, N.C.; Fleischer, S.; McConnell, D.G. Lipid composition of bovine retinal outer segment fragments. *Biochim. Biophys. Acta* **1970**, *211*, 10–19. [CrossRef]
13. Anderson, R.E.; Risk, M. Lipids of ocular tissues. IX. The phospholipids of frog photoreceptor membranes. *Vision Res.* **1974**, *14*, 129–131. [CrossRef]

14. Anderson, R.E.; Lissandrello, P.M.; Maude, M.B.; Matthes, M.T. Lipids of bovine retinal pigment epithelium. *Exp. Eye Res.* **1976**, *23*, 149–157. [CrossRef]
15. Balla, T. Inositol-lipid binding motifs: Signal integrators through protein-lipid and protein-protein interactions. *J. Cell Sci.* **2005**, *118*, 2093–2104. [CrossRef] [PubMed]
16. Choi, S.; Thapa, N.; Tan, X.; Hedman, A.C.; Anderson, R.A. PIP kinases define PI4,5P(2)signaling specificity by association with effectors. *Biochim. Biophys. Acta* **2015**, *1851*, 711–723. [CrossRef]
17. Lemmon, M.A. Membrane recognition by phospholipid-binding domains. *Nat. Rev. Mol. Cell Biol.* **2008**, *9*, 99–111. [CrossRef]
18. Anderson, R.E.; Maude, M.B.; Kelleher, P.A. Metabolism of phosphatidylinositol in the frog retina. *Biochim. Biophys. Acta* **1980**, *620*, 236–246. [CrossRef]
19. Choe, H.G.; Ghalayini, A.J.; Anderson, R.E. Phosphoinositide metabolism in frog rod outer segments. *Exp. Eye Res.* **1990**, *51*, 167–176. [CrossRef]
20. Gehm, B.D.; Mc Connell, D.G. Phosphoinositide synthesis in bovine rod outer segments. *Biochemistry* **1990**, *29*, 5442–5446. [CrossRef]
21. Rodriguez de Turco, E.B.; Gordon, W.C.; Bazan, N.G. Light stimulates in vivo inositol lipid turnover in frog retinal pigment epithelial cells at the onset of shedding and phagocytosis of photoreceptor membranes. *Exp. Eye Res.* **1992**, *55*, 719–725. [CrossRef]
22. He, F.; Agosto, M.A.; Anastassov, I.A.; Tse, D.Y.; Wu, S.M.; Wensel, T.G. Phosphatidylinositol-3-phosphate is light-regulated and essential for survival in retinal rods. *Sci. Rep.* **2016**, *6*, 26978. [CrossRef]
23. Stephens, L.R.; Jackson, T.R.; Hawkins, P.T. Agonist-stimulated synthesis of phosphatidylinositol(3,4,5)-trisphosphate: A new intracellular signalling system? *Biochim. Biophys. Acta* **1993**, *1179*, 27–75. [CrossRef]
24. Bui, H.H.; Sanders, P.E.; Bodenmiller, D.; Kuo, M.S.; Donoho, G.P.; Fischl, A.S. Direct analysis of PI(3,4,5)P3 using liquid chromatography electrospray ionization tandem mass spectrometry. *Anal. Biochem.* **2018**, *547*, 66–76. [CrossRef]
25. Kadamur, G.; Ross, E.M. Mammalian phospholipase C. *Annu. Rev. Physiol.* **2013**, *75*, 127–154. [CrossRef]
26. Trebak, M.; Lemonnier, L.; Smyth, J.T.; Vazquez, G.; Putney, J.W., Jr. Phospholipase C-coupled receptors and activation of TRPC channels. *Handb Exp. Pharmacol.* **2007**, 593–614.
27. Wang, L.; Budolfson, K.; Wang, F. Pik3c3 deletion in pyramidal neurons results in loss of synapses, extensive gliosis and progressive neurodegeneration. *Neuroscience* **2011**, *172*, 427–442. [CrossRef]
28. Zhou, X.; Wang, L.; Hasegawa, H.; Amin, P.; Han, B.X.; Kaneko, S.; He, Y.; Wang, F. Deletion of PIK3C3/Vps34 in sensory neurons causes rapid neurodegeneration by disrupting the endosomal but not the autophagic pathway. *Proc. Natl. Acad. Sci. USA* **2010**, *107*, 9424–9429. [CrossRef]
29. Carnero, A.; Blanco-Aparicio, C.; Renner, O.; Link, W.; Leal, J.F. The PTEN/PI3K/AKT signalling pathway in cancer, therapeutic implications. *Curr. Cancer Drug Targets* **2008**, *8*, 187–198. [CrossRef]
30. Carpentier, S.; N'Kuli, F.; Grieco, G.; Van Der Smissen, P.; Janssens, V.; Emonard, H.; Bilanges, B.; Vanhaesebroeck, B.; Gaide Chevronnay, H.P.; Pierreux, C.E.; et al. Class III phosphoinositide 3-kinase/VPS34 and dynamin are critical for apical endocytic recycling. *Traffic* **2013**, *14*, 933–948. [CrossRef]
31. Dall'Armi, C.; Devereaux, K.A.; Di Paolo, G. The role of lipids in the control of autophagy. *Curr. Biol.* **2013**, *23*, R33–R45. [CrossRef]
32. Lenoir, M.; Overduin, M. PtdIns(4)P signalling and recognition systems. *Adv. Exp. Med. Biol.* **2013**, *991*, 59–83. [CrossRef]
33. McLaughlin, S.; Wang, J.; Gambhir, A.; Murray, D. PIP(2) and proteins: Interactions, organization, and information flow. *Annu. Rev. Biophys. Biomol. Struct.* **2002**, *31*, 151–175. [CrossRef]
34. Falkenburger, B.H.; Jensen, J.B.; Dickson, E.J.; Suh, B.C.; Hille, B. Phosphoinositides: Lipid regulators of membrane proteins. *J. Physiol.* **2010**, *588*, 3179–3185. [CrossRef]
35. Hilgemann, D.W.; Feng, S.; Nasuhoglu, C. The complex and intriguing lives of PIP2 with ion channels and transporters. *Sci. STKE* **2001**, *2001*, re19. [CrossRef]
36. Fukami, K.; Inanobe, S.; Kanemaru, K.; Nakamura, Y. Phospholipase C is a key enzyme regulating intracellular calcium and modulating the phosphoinositide balance. *Prog. Lipid Res.* **2010**, *49*, 429–437. [CrossRef]
37. Vines, C.M. Phospholipase C. *Adv. Exp. Med. Biol.* **2012**, *740*, 235–254. [CrossRef]
38. Shewan, A.; Eastburn, D.J.; Mostov, K. Phosphoinositides in cell architecture. *Cold Spring Harb. Perspect. Biol.* **2011**, *3*, a004796. [CrossRef]

39. Yin, H.L.; Janmey, P.A. Phosphoinositide regulation of the actin cytoskeleton. *Annu. Rev. Physiol.* **2003**, *65*, 761–789. [CrossRef]
40. Hille, B.; Dickson, E.J.; Kruse, M.; Vivas, O.; Suh, B.C. Phosphoinositides regulate ion channels. *Biochim. Biophys. Acta* **2015**, *1851*, 844–856. [CrossRef]
41. Bielas, S.L.; Silhavy, J.L.; Brancati, F.; Kisseleva, M.V.; Al-Gazali, L.; Sztriha, L.; Bayoumi, R.A.; Zaki, M.S.; Abdel-Aleem, A.; Rosti, R.O.; et al. Mutations in INPP5E, encoding inositol polyphosphate-5-phosphatase E, link phosphatidyl inositol signaling to the ciliopathies. *Nat. Genet.* **2009**, *41*, 1032–1036. [CrossRef]
42. Jacoby, M.; Cox, J.J.; Gayral, S.; Hampshire, D.J.; Ayub, M.; Blockmans, M.; Pernot, E.; Kisseleva, M.V.; Compere, P.; Schiffmann, S.N.; et al. INPP5E mutations cause primary cilium signaling defects, ciliary instability and ciliopathies in human and mouse. *Nat. Genet.* **2009**, *41*, 1027–1031. [CrossRef]
43. Saar, K.; Al-Gazali, L.; Sztriha, L.; Rueschendorf, F.; Nur, E.K.M.; Reis, A.; Bayoumi, R. Homozygosity mapping in families with Joubert syndrome identifies a locus on chromosome 9q34.3 and evidence for genetic heterogeneity. *Am. J. Hum. Genet.* **1999**, *65*, 1666–1671. [CrossRef] [PubMed]
44. George, A.A.; Hayden, S.; Holzhausen, L.C.; Ma, E.Y.; Suzuki, S.C.; Brockerhoff, S.E. Synaptojanin 1 is required for endolysosomal trafficking of synaptic proteins in cone photoreceptor inner segments. *PLoS ONE* **2014**, *9*, e84394. [CrossRef] [PubMed]
45. Holzhausen, L.C.; Lewis, A.A.; Cheong, K.K.; Brockerhoff, S.E. Differential role for synaptojanin 1 in rod and cone photoreceptors. *J. Comp. Neurol.* **2009**, *517*, 633–644. [CrossRef]
46. Van Epps, H.A.; Hayashi, M.; Lucast, L.; Stearns, G.W.; Hurley, J.B.; De Camilli, P.; Brockerhoff, S.E. The zebrafish nrc mutant reveals a role for the polyphosphoinositide phosphatase synaptojanin 1 in cone photoreceptor ribbon anchoring. *J. Neurosci.* **2004**, *24*, 8641–8650. [CrossRef]
47. Hagstrom, S.A.; North, M.A.; Nishina, P.L.; Berson, E.L.; Dryja, T.P. Recessive mutations in the gene encoding the tubby-like protein TULP1 in patients with retinitis pigmentosa. *Nat. Genet.* **1998**, *18*, 174–176. [CrossRef]
48. Jacobson, S.G.; Cideciyan, A.V.; Huang, W.C.; Sumaroka, A.; Roman, A.J.; Schwartz, S.B.; Luo, X.; Sheplock, R.; Dauber, J.M.; Swider, M.; et al. TULP1 mutations causing early-onset retinal degeneration: Preserved but insensitive macular cones. *Invest. Ophthalmol. Vis. Sci.* **2014**, *55*, 5354–5364. [CrossRef]
49. He, F.; Nichols, R.M.; Kailasam, L.; Wensel, T.G.; Agosto, M.A. Critical Role for Phosphatidylinositol-3 Kinase Vps34/PIK3C3 in ON-Bipolar Cells. *Invest. Ophthalmol. Vis. Sci.* **2019**, *60*, 2861–2874. [CrossRef]
50. Hammond, G.R.; Hong, Y. Phosphoinositides and Membrane Targeting in Cell Polarity. *Cold Spring Harb. Perspect. Biol.* **2018**, *10*. [CrossRef]
51. Mayinger, P. Phosphoinositides and vesicular membrane traffic. *Biochim. Biophys. Acta* **2012**, *1821*, 1104–1113. [CrossRef] [PubMed]
52. Chuang, J.Z.; Zhao, Y.; Sung, C.H. SARA-regulated vesicular targeting underlies formation of the light-sensing organelle in mammalian rods. *Cell* **2007**, *130*, 535–547. [CrossRef] [PubMed]
53. Deretic, D.; Traverso, V.; Parkins, N.; Jackson, F.; Rodriguez de Turco, E.B.; Ransom, N. Phosphoinositides, ezrin/moesin, and rac1 regulate fusion of rhodopsin transport carriers in retinal photoreceptors. *Mol. Biol. Cell* **2004**, *15*, 359–370. [CrossRef] [PubMed]
54. Spencer, W.J.; Lewis, T.R.; Phan, S.; Cady, M.A.; Serebrovskaya, E.O.; Schneider, N.F.; Kim, K.Y.; Cameron, L.A.; Skiba, N.P.; Ellisman, M.H.; et al. Photoreceptor disc membranes are formed through an Arp2/3-dependent lamellipodium-like mechanism. *Proc. Natl. Acad. Sci. USA* **2019**. [CrossRef]
55. Bucki, R.; Wang, Y.H.; Yang, C.; Kandy, S.K.; Fatunmbi, O.; Bradley, R.; Pogoda, K.; Svitkina, T.; Radhakrishnan, R.; Janmey, P.A. Lateral distribution of phosphatidylinositol 4,5-bisphosphate in membranes regulates formin- and ARP2/3-mediated actin nucleation. *J. Biol. Chem.* **2019**, *294*, 4704–4722. [CrossRef]
56. Daste, F.; Walrant, A.; Holst, M.R.; Gadsby, J.R.; Mason, J.; Lee, J.E.; Brook, D.; Mettlen, M.; Larsson, E.; Lee, S.F.; et al. Control of actin polymerization via the coincidence of phosphoinositides and high membrane curvature. *J. Cell Biol.* **2017**, *216*, 3745–3765. [CrossRef]
57. Ivanovic, I.; Anderson, R.E.; Le, Y.Z.; Fliesler, S.J.; Sherry, D.M.; Rajala, R.V. Deletion of the p85alpha regulatory subunit of phosphoinositide 3-kinase in cone photoreceptor cells results in cone photoreceptor degeneration. *Invest. Ophthalmol. Vis. Sci.* **2011**, *52*, 3775–3783. [CrossRef]
58. Xu, W.; Jin, M.; Huang, W.; Wang, H.; Hu, R.; Li, J.; Cao, Y. Apical PtdIns(4,5)P2 is required for ciliogenesis and suppression of polycystic kidney disease. *FASEB J.* **2019**, *33*, 2848–2857. [CrossRef]
59. Phua, S.C.; Nihongaki, Y.; Inoue, T. Autonomy declared by primary cilia through compartmentalization of membrane phosphoinositides. *Curr. Opin. Cell Biol.* **2018**, *50*, 72–78. [CrossRef]

60. Park, J.; Lee, N.; Kavoussi, A.; Seo, J.T.; Kim, C.H.; Moon, S.J. Ciliary Phosphoinositide Regulates Ciliary Protein Trafficking in Drosophila. *Cell Rep.* **2015**, *13*, 2808–2816. [CrossRef]
61. Garcia-Gonzalo, F.R.; Phua, S.C.; Roberson, E.C.; Garcia, G., 3rd; Abedin, M.; Schurmans, S.; Inoue, T.; Reiter, J.F. Phosphoinositides Regulate Ciliary Protein Trafficking to Modulate Hedgehog Signaling. *Dev. Cell* **2015**, *34*, 400–409. [CrossRef] [PubMed]
62. Vieira, O.V.; Gaus, K.; Verkade, P.; Fullekrug, J.; Vaz, W.L.; Simons, K. FAPP2, cilium formation, and compartmentalization of the apical membrane in polarized Madin-Darby canine kidney (MDCK) cells. *Proc. Natl. Acad. Sci. USA* **2006**, *103*, 18556–18561. [CrossRef] [PubMed]
63. Nachury, M.V.; Seeley, E.S.; Jin, H. Trafficking to the ciliary membrane: How to get across the periciliary diffusion barrier? *Annu. Rev. Cell Dev. Biol.* **2010**, *26*, 59–87. [CrossRef] [PubMed]
64. Luo, N.; West, C.C.; Murga-Zamalloa, C.A.; Sun, L.; Anderson, R.M.; Wells, C.D.; Weinreb, R.N.; Travers, J.B.; Khanna, H.; Sun, Y. OCRL localizes to the primary cilium: A new role for cilia in Lowe syndrome. *Hum. Mol. Genet.* **2012**, *21*, 3333–3344. [CrossRef] [PubMed]
65. Coon, B.G.; Hernandez, V.; Madhivanan, K.; Mukherjee, D.; Hanna, C.B.; Barinaga-Rementeria Ramirez, I.; Lowe, M.; Beales, P.L.; Aguilar, R.C. The Lowe syndrome protein OCRL1 is involved in primary cilia assembly. *Hum. Mol. Genet.* **2012**, *21*, 1835–1847. [CrossRef] [PubMed]
66. Humbert, M.C.; Weihbrecht, K.; Searby, C.C.; Li, Y.; Pope, R.M.; Sheffield, V.C.; Seo, S. ARL13B, PDE6D, and CEP164 form a functional network for INPP5E ciliary targeting. *Proc. Natl. Acad. Sci. USA* **2012**, *109*, 19691–19696. [CrossRef] [PubMed]
67. Jin, H.; White, S.R.; Shida, T.; Schulz, S.; Aguiar, M.; Gygi, S.P.; Bazan, J.F.; Nachury, M.V. The conserved Bardet-Biedl syndrome proteins assemble a coat that traffics membrane proteins to cilia. *Cell* **2010**, *141*, 1208–1219. [CrossRef]
68. Nachury, M.V.; Loktev, A.V.; Zhang, Q.; Westlake, C.J.; Peranen, J.; Merdes, A.; Slusarski, D.C.; Scheller, R.H.; Bazan, J.F.; Sheffield, V.C.; et al. A core complex of BBS proteins cooperates with the GTPase Rab8 to promote ciliary membrane biogenesis. *Cell* **2007**, *129*, 1201–1213. [CrossRef]
69. Chinskey, N.D.; Zheng, Q.D.; Zacks, D.N. Control of Photoreceptor Autophagy after Retinal Detachment: The Switch from Survival to Death. *Invest. Ophthalmol. Vis. Sci.* **2014**, *55*, 688–695. [CrossRef]
70. Reme, C.; Drinker, C.K.; Aeberhard, B. Modification of autophagic degradation by medium- and illumination conditions in frog visual cells in vitro. *Doc. Ophthalmol.* **1984**, *56*, 377–383. [CrossRef]
71. Reme, C. Autophagy in rods and cones of the vertebrate retina. *Dev. Ophthalmol.* **1981**, *4*, 101–148.
72. Reme, C.E.; Sulser, M. Diurnal variation of autophagy in rod visual cells in the rat. *Albrecht Von Graefes Arch. Klin. Exp. Ophthalmol.* **1977**, *203*, 261–270. [CrossRef]
73. Chen, Y.; Sawada, O.; Kohno, H.; Le, Y.Z.; Subauste, C.; Maeda, T.; Maeda, A. Autophagy protects the retina from light-induced degeneration. *J. Biol. Chem.* **2013**, *288*, 7506–7518. [CrossRef] [PubMed]
74. Besirli, C.G.; Chinskey, N.D.; Zheng, Q.D.; Zacks, D.N. Autophagy activation in the injured photoreceptor inhibits fas-mediated apoptosis. *Invest. Ophthalmol. Vis. Sci.* **2011**, *52*, 4193–4199. [CrossRef] [PubMed]
75. George, A.A.; Hayden, S.; Stanton, G.R.; Brockerhoff, S.E. Arf6 and the 5′phosphatase of synaptojanin 1 regulate autophagy in cone photoreceptors. *Bioessays* **2016**, *38* (Suppl. 1), S119–S135. [CrossRef]
76. Ghalayini, A.; Anderson, R.E. Phosphatidylinositol 4,5-bisphosphate: Light-mediated breakdown in the vertebrate retina. *Biochem. Biophys. Res. Commun.* **1984**, *124*, 503–506. [CrossRef]
77. Anderson, R.E.; Maude, M.B.; Pu, G.A.; Hollyfield, J.G. Effect of light on the metabolism of lipids in the rat retina. *J. Neurochem.* **1985**, *44*, 773–778. [CrossRef] [PubMed]
78. Tarver, A.P.; Anderson, R.E. Phospholipase C activity and substrate specificity in frog photoreceptors. *Exp. Eye Res.* **1988**, *46*, 29–35. [CrossRef]
79. Ghalayini, A.J.; Tarver, A.P.; Mackin, W.M.; Koutz, C.A.; Anderson, R.E. Identification and immunolocalization of phospholipase C in bovine rod outer segments. *J. Neurochem.* **1991**, *57*, 1405–1412. [CrossRef]
80. Das, N.D.; Yoshioka, T.; Samuelson, D.; Shichi, H. Immunocytochemical localization of phosphatidylinositol-4,5-bisphosphate in dark- and light-adapted rat retinas. *Cell Struct. Funct.* **1986**, *11*, 53–63. [CrossRef]
81. Das, N.D.; Yoshioka, T.; Samuelson, D.; Cohen, R.J.; Shichi, H. Immunochemical evidence for the light-regulated modulation of phosphatidylinositol-4,5-bisphosphate in rat photoreceptor cells. *Cell Struct. Funct.* **1987**, *12*, 471–481. [CrossRef] [PubMed]

82. Panfoli, I.; Morelli, A.; Pepe, I. Calcium ion-regulated phospholipase C activity in bovine rod outer segments. *Biochem. Biophys. Res. Commun.* **1990**, *173*, 283–288. [CrossRef]
83. Grigorjev, I.V.; Grits, A.I.; Artamonov, I.D.; Baranova, L.A.; Volotovski, I.D. betagamma-Transducin stimulates hydrolysis and synthesis of phosphatidylinositol 4,5-bisphosphate in bovine rod outer segment membranes. *Biochim. Biophys. Acta* **1996**, *1310*, 131–136. [CrossRef]
84. Van Rooijen, L.A.; Bazan, N.G. The inositide cycle in bovine photoreceptor membranes. *Life Sci.* **1986**, *38*, 1685–1693. [CrossRef]
85. Millar, F.A.; Fisher, S.C.; Muir, C.A.; Edwards, E.; Hawthorne, J.N. Polyphosphoinositide hydrolysis in response to light stimulation of rat and chick retina and retinal rod outer segments. *Biochim. Biophys. Acta* **1988**, *970*, 205–211. [CrossRef]
86. He, F.; Mao, M.; Wensel, T.G. Enhancement of phototransduction g protein-effector interactions by phosphoinositides. *J. Biol. Chem.* **2004**, *279*, 8986–8990. [CrossRef]
87. Womack, K.B.; Gordon, S.E.; He, F.; Wensel, T.G.; Lu, C.C.; Hilgemann, D.W. Do phosphatidylinositides modulate vertebrate phototransduction? *J. Neurosci.* **2000**, *20*, 2792–2799. [CrossRef]
88. Gross, O.P.; Pugh, E.N., Jr.; Burns, M.E. Spatiotemporal cGMP dynamics in living mouse rods. *Biophys J.* **2012**, *102*, 1775–1784. [CrossRef]
89. Peng, Y.W.; Rhee, S.G.; Yu, W.P.; Ho, Y.K.; Schoen, T.; Chader, G.J.; Yau, K.W. Identification of components of a phosphoinositide signaling pathway in retinal rod outer segments. *Proc. Natl. Acad. Sci. USA* **1997**, *94*, 1995–2000. [CrossRef]
90. Orisme, W.; Li, J.; Goldmann, T.; Bolch, S.; Wolfrum, U.; Smith, W.C. Light-dependent translocation of arrestin in rod photoreceptors is signaled through a phospholipase C cascade and requires ATP. *Cell Signal.* **2010**, *22*, 447–456. [CrossRef]
91. Guo, X.; Ghalayini, A.J.; Chen, H.; Anderson, R.E. Phosphatidylinositol 3-kinase in bovine photoreceptor rod outer segments. *Invest. Ophthalmol. Vis. Sci.* **1997**, *38*, 1873–1882. [PubMed]
92. Guo, X.X.; Huang, Z.; Bell, M.W.; Chen, H.; Anderson, R.E. Tyrosine phosphorylation is involved in phosphatidylinositol 3-kinase activation in bovine rod outer segments. *Mol. Vis.* **2000**, *6*, 216–221. [PubMed]
93. Rajala, R.V.; McClellan, M.E.; Chan, M.D.; Tsiokas, L.; Anderson, R.E. Interaction of the retinal insulin receptor beta-subunit with the p85 subunit of phosphoinositide 3-kinase. *Biochemistry* **2004**, *43*, 5637–5650. [CrossRef] [PubMed]
94. Rajala, R.V.; Anderson, R.E. Light regulation of the insulin receptor in the retina. *Mol. Neurobiol.* **2003**, *28*, 123–138. [CrossRef]
95. Rajala, R.V.; McClellan, M.E.; Ash, J.D.; Anderson, R.E. In vivo regulation of phosphoinositide 3-kinase in retina through light-induced tyrosine phosphorylation of the insulin receptor beta-subunit. *J. Biol. Chem.* **2002**, *277*, 43319–43326. [CrossRef] [PubMed]
96. Rajala, R.V.; Ranjo-Bishop, M.; Wang, Y.; Rajala, A.; Anderson, R.E. The p110alpha isoform of phosphoinositide 3-kinase is essential for cone photoreceptor survival. *Biochimie* **2015**, *112*, 35–40. [CrossRef] [PubMed]
97. Ivanovic, I.; Allen, D.T.; Dighe, R.; Le, Y.Z.; Anderson, R.E.; Rajala, R.V. Phosphoinositide 3-kinase signaling in retinal rod photoreceptors. *Invest. Ophthalmol. Vis. Sci.* **2011**, *52*, 6355–6362. [CrossRef]
98. Detwiler, P.B. Phototransduction in Retinal Ganglion Cells. *Yale J. Biol. Med.* **2018**, *91*, 49–52.
99. Graham, D.M.; Wong, K.Y.; Shapiro, P.; Frederick, C.; Pattabiraman, K.; Berson, D.M. Melanopsin ganglion cells use a membrane-associated rhabdomeric phototransduction cascade. *J. Neurophysiol.* **2008**, *99*, 2522–2532. [CrossRef]
100. Hardie, R.C. Photosensitive TRPs. *Handb. Exp. Pharmacol.* **2014**, *223*, 795–826. [CrossRef]
101. Isoldi, M.C.; Rollag, M.D.; Castrucci, A.M.; Provencio, I. Rhabdomeric phototransduction initiated by the vertebrate photopigment melanopsin. *Proc. Natl. Acad. Sci. USA* **2005**, *102*, 1217–1221. [CrossRef] [PubMed]
102. Jiang, Z.; Yue, W.W.S.; Chen, L.; Sheng, Y.; Yau, K.W. Cyclic-Nucleotide- and HCN-Channel-Mediated Phototransduction in Intrinsically Photosensitive Retinal Ganglion Cells. *Cell* **2018**, *175*, 652–664 e612. [CrossRef]
103. Montell, C. Drosophila visual transduction. *Trends Neurosci.* **2012**, *35*, 356–363. [CrossRef] [PubMed]
104. Xue, T.; Do, M.T.; Riccio, A.; Jiang, Z.; Hsieh, J.; Wang, H.C.; Merbs, S.L.; Welsbie, D.S.; Yoshioka, T.; Weissgerber, P.; et al. Melanopsin signalling in mammalian iris and retina. *Nature* **2011**, *479*, 67–73. [CrossRef] [PubMed]
105. Arendt, D. Evolution of eyes and photoreceptor cell types. *Int. J. Dev. Biol.* **2003**, *47*, 563–571. [PubMed]

106. Kuriyama, S.; Ohuchi, T.; Yoshimura, N.; Honda, Y. Growth factor-induced cytosolic calcium ion transients in cultured human retinal pigment epithelial cells. *Invest. Ophthalmol. Vis. Sci.* **1991**, *32*, 2882–2890.
107. Osborne, N.N.; FitzGibbon, F.; Schwartz, G. Muscarinic acetylcholine receptor-mediated phosphoinositide turnover in cultured human retinal pigment epithelium cells. *Vision Res.* **1991**, *31*, 1119–1127. [CrossRef]
108. Feldman, E.L.; Randolph, A.E.; Johnston, G.C.; DelMonte, M.A.; Greene, D.A. Receptor-coupled phosphoinositide hydrolysis in human retinal pigment epithelium. *J. Neurochem.* **1991**, *56*, 2094–2100. [CrossRef]
109. York, N.; Halbach, P.; Chiu, M.A.; Bird, I.M.; Pillers, D.M.; Pattnaik, B.R. Oxytocin (OXT)-stimulated inhibition of Kir7.1 activity is through PIP2-dependent Ca(2+) response of the oxytocin receptor in the retinal pigment epithelium in vitro. *Cell Signal.* **2017**, *37*, 93–102. [CrossRef]
110. Heth, C.A.; Marescalchi, P.A. Inositol triphosphate generation in cultured rat retinal pigment epithelium. *Invest. Ophthalmol. Vis. Sci.* **1994**, *35*, 409–416.
111. D'Cruz, P.M.; Yasumura, D.; Weir, J.; Matthes, M.T.; Abderrahim, H.; LaVail, M.M.; Vollrath, D. Mutation of the receptor tyrosine kinase gene Mertk in the retinal dystrophic RCS rat. *Hum. Mol. Genet.* **2000**, *9*, 645–651. [CrossRef] [PubMed]
112. Treins, C.; Giorgetti-Peraldi, S.; Murdaca, J.; Semenza, G.L.; Van Obberghen, E. Insulin stimulates hypoxia-inducible factor 1 through a phosphatidylinositol 3-kinase/target of rapamycin-dependent signaling pathway. *J. Biol. Chem.* **2002**, *277*, 27975–27981. [CrossRef] [PubMed]
113. Geraldes, P.; Yagi, K.; Ohshiro, Y.; He, Z.; Maeno, Y.; Yamamoto-Hiraoka, J.; Rask-Madsen, C.; Chung, S.W.; Perrella, M.A.; King, G.L. Selective regulation of heme oxygenase-1 expression and function by insulin through IRS1/phosphoinositide 3-kinase/Akt-2 pathway. *J. Biol. Chem.* **2008**, *283*, 34327–34336. [CrossRef]
114. Mwaikambo, B.R.; Yang, C.; Chemtob, S.; Hardy, P. Hypoxia up-regulates CD36 expression and function via hypoxia-inducible factor-1- and phosphatidylinositol 3-kinase-dependent mechanisms. *J. Biol. Chem.* **2009**, *284*, 26695–26707. [CrossRef]
115. Yang, X.M.; Wang, Y.S.; Zhang, J.; Li, Y.; Xu, J.F.; Zhu, J.; Zhao, W.; Chu, D.K.; Wiedemann, P. Role of PI3K/Akt and MEK/ERK in mediating hypoxia-induced expression of HIF-1alpha and VEGF in laser-induced rat choroidal neovascularization. *Invest. Ophthalmol. Vis. Sci.* **2009**, *50*, 1873–1879. [CrossRef]
116. Kim, D.I.; Lim, S.K.; Park, M.J.; Han, H.J.; Kim, G.Y.; Park, S.H. The involvement of phosphatidylinositol 3-kinase/Akt signaling in high glucose-induced downregulation of GLUT-1 expression in ARPE cells. *Life Sci.* **2007**, *80*, 626–632. [CrossRef]
117. Qin, D.; Zhang, G.M.; Xu, X.; Wang, L.Y. The PI3K/Akt signaling pathway mediates the high glucose-induced expression of extracellular matrix molecules in human retinal pigment epithelial cells. *J. Diabetes Res.* **2015**, *2015*, 920280. [CrossRef]
118. Ferguson, T.A.; Green, D.R. Autophagy and phagocytosis converge for better vision. *Autophagy* **2014**, *10*, 165–167. [CrossRef]
119. Kim, J.Y.; Zhao, H.; Martinez, J.; Doggett, T.A.; Kolesnikov, A.V.; Tang, P.H.; Ablonczy, Z.; Chan, C.C.; Zhou, Z.; Green, D.R.; et al. Noncanonical autophagy promotes the visual cycle. *Cell* **2013**, *154*, 365–376. [CrossRef]
120. Muniz-Feliciano, L.; Doggett, T.A.; Zhou, Z.; Ferguson, T.A. RUBCN/rubicon and EGFR regulate lysosomal degradative processes in the retinal pigment epithelium (RPE) of the eye. *Autophagy* **2017**, *13*, 2072–2085. [CrossRef]
121. Shaw, J.D.; Hama, H.; Sohrabi, F.; DeWald, D.B.; Wendland, B. PtdIns(3,5)P2 is required for delivery of endocytic cargo into the multivesicular body. *Traffic* **2003**, *4*, 479–490. [CrossRef]
122. Ketel, K.; Krauss, M.; Nicot, A.S.; Puchkov, D.; Wieffer, M.; Muller, R.; Subramanian, D.; Schultz, C.; Laporte, J.; Haucke, V. A phosphoinositide conversion mechanism for exit from endosomes. *Nature* **2016**, *529*, 408–412. [CrossRef]
123. Isobe, Y.; Nigorikawa, K.; Tsurumi, G.; Takemasu, S.; Takasuga, S.; Kofuji, S.; Hazeki, K. PIKfyve accelerates phagosome acidification through activation of TRPML1 while arrests aberrant vacuolation independent of the Ca2+ channel. *J. Biochem.* **2019**, *165*, 75–84. [CrossRef]
124. Ikonomov, O.C.; Sbrissa, D.; Shisheva, A. Localized PtdIns 3,5-P2 synthesis to regulate early endosome dynamics and fusion. *Am. J. Physiol. Cell Physiol.* **2006**, *291*, C393–C404. [CrossRef]

125. Dong, X.P.; Shen, D.; Wang, X.; Dawson, T.; Li, X.; Zhang, Q.; Cheng, X.; Zhang, Y.; Weisman, L.S.; Delling, M.; et al. PI(3,5)P(2) controls membrane trafficking by direct activation of mucolipin Ca(2+) release channels in the endolysosome. *Nat. Commun.* **2010**, *1*, 38. [CrossRef]
126. Sasaki, T.; Takasuga, S.; Sasaki, J.; Kofuji, S.; Eguchi, S.; Yamazaki, M.; Suzuki, A. Mammalian phosphoinositide kinases and phosphatases. *Prog. Lipid Res.* **2009**, *48*, 307–343. [CrossRef]
127. Brown, J.R.; Auger, K.R. Phylogenomics of phosphoinositide lipid kinases: Perspectives on the evolution of second messenger signaling and drug discovery. *BMC Evol. Biol.* **2011**, *11*, 4. [CrossRef]
128. Azadi, S.; Brush, R.S.; Anderson, R.E.; Rajala, R.V. Class I Phosphoinositide 3-Kinase Exerts a Differential Role on Cell Survival and Cell Trafficking in Retina. *Adv. Exp. Med. Biol.* **2016**, *854*, 363–369. [CrossRef]
129. Sakagami, H.; Katsumata, O.; Hara, Y.; Tamaki, H.; Fukaya, M. Preferential localization of type I phosphatidylinositol 4-phosphate 5-kinase gamma at the periactive zone of mouse photoreceptor ribbon synapses. *Brain Res.* **2014**, *1586*, 23–33. [CrossRef]
130. Wenk, M.R.; Pellegrini, L.; Klenchin, V.A.; Di Paolo, G.; Chang, S.; Daniell, L.; Arioka, M.; Martin, T.F.; De Camilli, P. PIP kinase Igamma is the major PI(4,5)P(2) synthesizing enzyme at the synapse. *Neuron* **2001**, *32*, 79–88. [CrossRef]
131. Wright, B.D.; Loo, L.; Street, S.E.; Ma, A.; Taylor-Blake, B.; Stashko, M.A.; Jin, J.; Janzen, W.P.; Frye, S.V.; Zylka, M.J. The lipid kinase PIP5K1C regulates pain signaling and sensitization. *Neuron* **2014**, *82*, 836–847. [CrossRef]
132. Di Paolo, G.; Moskowitz, H.S.; Gipson, K.; Wenk, M.R.; Voronov, S.; Obayashi, M.; Flavell, R.; Fitzsimonds, R.M.; Ryan, T.A.; De Camilli, P. Impaired PtdIns(4,5)P2 synthesis in nerve terminals produces defects in synaptic vesicle trafficking. *Nature* **2004**, *431*, 415–422. [CrossRef]
133. Huang, Z.; Guo, X.X.; Chen, S.X.; Alvarez, K.M.; Bell, M.W.; Anderson, R.E. Regulation of type II phosphatidylinositol phosphate kinase by tyrosine phosphorylation in bovine rod outer segments. *Biochemistry* **2001**, *40*, 4550–4559. [CrossRef]
134. Zhao, L.; Chen, Y.; Bajaj, A.O.; Eblimit, A.; Xu, M.; Soens, Z.T.; Wang, F.; Ge, Z.; Jung, S.Y.; He, F.; et al. Integrative subcellular proteomic analysis allows accurate prediction of human disease-causing genes. *Genome Res.* **2016**, *26*, 660–669. [CrossRef]
135. Prosseda, P.P.; Luo, N.; Wang, B.; Alvarado, J.A.; Hu, Y.; Sun, Y. Loss of OCRL increases ciliary PI(4,5)P2 in Lowe oculocerebrorenal syndrome. *J. Cell Sci.* **2017**, *130*, 3447–3454. [CrossRef]
136. Attree, O.; Olivos, I.M.; Okabe, I.; Bailey, L.C.; Nelson, D.L.; Lewis, R.A.; McInnes, R.R.; Nussbaum, R.L. The Lowe's oculocerebrorenal syndrome gene encodes a protein highly homologous to inositol polyphosphate-5-phosphatase. *Nature* **1992**, *358*, 239–242. [CrossRef]
137. Shim, H.; Wu, C.; Ramsamooj, S.; Bosch, K.N.; Chen, Z.; Emerling, B.M.; Yun, J.; Liu, H.; Choo-Wing, R.; Yang, Z.; et al. Deletion of the gene Pip4k2c, a novel phosphatidylinositol kinase, results in hyperactivation of the immune system. *Proc. Natl. Acad. Sci. USA* **2016**, *113*, 7596–7601. [CrossRef]
138. Young, R.W. The renewal of rod and cone outer segments in the rhesus monkey. *J. Cell Biol.* **1971**, *49*, 303–318. [CrossRef]
139. Adams, N.A.; Awadein, A.; Toma, H.S. The retinal ciliopathies. *Ophthalmic Genet.* **2007**, *28*, 113–125. [CrossRef]
140. Wheway, G.; Parry, D.A.; Johnson, C.A. The role of primary cilia in the development and disease of the retina. *Organogenesis* **2013**, *10*, 69–85. [CrossRef]
141. Gal, A.; Li, Y.; Thompson, D.A.; Weir, J.; Orth, U.; Jacobson, S.G.; Apfelstedt-Sylla, E.; Vollrath, D. Mutations in MERTK, the human orthologue of the RCS rat retinal dystrophy gene, cause retinitis pigmentosa. *Nat. Genet.* **2000**, *26*, 270–271. [CrossRef]
142. Marmorstein, A.D.; Johnson, A.A.; Bachman, L.A.; Andrews-Pfannkoch, C.; Knudsen, T.; Gilles, B.J.; Hill, M.; Gandhi, J.K.; Marmorstein, L.Y.; Pulido, J.S. Mutant Best1 Expression and Impaired Phagocytosis in an iPSC Model of Autosomal Recessive Bestrophinopathy. *Sci Rep.* **2018**, *8*, 4487. [CrossRef]
143. Strauss, O.; Reichhart, N.; Gomez, N.M.; Muller, C. Contribution of Ion Channels in Calcium Signaling Regulating Phagocytosis: MaxiK, Cav1.3 and Bestrophin-1. *Adv. Exp. Med. Biol.* **2016**, *854*, 739–744. [CrossRef]
144. Muller, C.; Mas Gomez, N.; Ruth, P.; Strauss, O. CaV1.3 L-type channels, maxiK Ca(2+)-dependent K(+) channels and bestrophin-1 regulate rhythmic photoreceptor outer segment phagocytosis by retinal pigment epithelial cells. *Cell Signal.* **2014**, *26*, 968–978. [CrossRef]

145. Xiao, Q.; Hartzell, H.C.; Yu, K. Bestrophins and retinopathies. *Pflugers Arch.* **2010**, *460*, 559–569. [CrossRef]
146. Strauss, O. The retinal pigment epithelium in visual function. *Physiol. Rev.* **2005**, *85*, 845–881. [CrossRef]
147. Luo, N.; Lu, J.; Sun, Y. Evidence of a role of inositol polyphosphate 5-phosphatase INPP5E in cilia formation in zebrafish. *Vision Res.* **2012**, *75*, 98–107. [CrossRef]
148. Travaglini, L.; Brancati, F.; Silhavy, J.; Iannicelli, M.; Nickerson, E.; Elkhartoufi, N.; Scott, E.; Spencer, E.; Gabriel, S.; Thomas, S.; et al. Phenotypic spectrum and prevalence of INPP5E mutations in Joubert syndrome and related disorders. *Eur. J. Hum. Genet.* **2013**, *21*, 1074–1078. [CrossRef]
149. Plotnikova, O.V.; Seo, S.; Cottle, D.L.; Conduit, S.; Hakim, S.; Dyson, J.M.; Mitchell, C.A.; Smyth, I.M. INPP5E interacts with AURKA, linking phosphoinositide signaling to primary cilium stability. *J. Cell Sci.* **2015**, *128*, 364–372. [CrossRef]
150. Xu, W.; Jin, M.; Hu, R.; Wang, H.; Zhang, F.; Yuan, S.; Cao, Y. The Joubert Syndrome Protein Inpp5e Controls Ciliogenesis by Regulating Phosphoinositides at the Apical Membrane. *J. Am. Soc. Nephrol.* **2017**, *28*, 118–129. [CrossRef]
151. Verstreken, P.; Koh, T.W.; Schulze, K.L.; Zhai, R.G.; Hiesinger, P.R.; Zhou, Y.; Mehta, S.Q.; Cao, Y.; Roos, J.; Bellen, H.J. Synaptojanin is recruited by endophilin to promote synaptic vesicle uncoating. *Neuron* **2003**, *40*, 733–748. [CrossRef]
152. Chi, Y.; Zhou, B.; Wang, W.Q.; Chung, S.K.; Kwon, Y.U.; Ahn, Y.H.; Chang, Y.T.; Tsujishita, Y.; Hurley, J.H.; Zhang, Z.Y. Comparative mechanistic and substrate specificity study of inositol polyphosphate 5-phosphatase Schizosaccharomyces pombe Synaptojanin and SHIP2. *J. Biol. Chem.* **2004**, *279*, 44987–44995. [CrossRef]
153. Chang-Ileto, B.; Frere, S.G.; Chan, R.B.; Voronov, S.V.; Roux, A.; Di Paolo, G. Synaptojanin 1-mediated PI(4,5)P2 hydrolysis is modulated by membrane curvature and facilitates membrane fission. *Dev. Cell* **2011**, *20*, 206–218. [CrossRef] [PubMed]
154. Lev, S.; Hernandez, J.; Martinez, R.; Chen, A.; Plowman, G.; Schlessinger, J. Identification of a novel family of targets of PYK2 related to Drosophila retinal degeneration B (rdgB) protein. *Mol. Cell Biol.* **1999**, *19*, 2278–2288. [CrossRef]
155. Tian, D.; Lev, S. Cellular and developmental distribution of human homologues of the Drosophilia rdgB protein in the rat retina. *Invest. Ophthalmol. Vis. Sci.* **2002**, *43*, 1946–1953.
156. Kohn, L.; Kadzhaev, K.; Burstedt, M.S.I.; Haraldsson, S.; Hallberg, B.; Sandgren, O.; Golovleva, I. Mutation in the PYK2-binding domain of PITPNM3 causes autosomal dominant cone dystrophy (CORD5) in two Swedish families. *Eur. J. Hum. Genet.* **2007**, *15*, 664–671. [CrossRef]
157. Kohn, L.; Kadzhaev, K.; Burstedt, M.S.I.; Haraldsson, S.; Sandgren, O.; Golovleva, I. Mutation in the PYK2-binding domain of PITPNM3 causes autosomal dominant cone dystrophy (CORD5) in two Swedish families. *Rencent Adv. Exp. Med. Biol.* **2008**, *613*, 229–234. [CrossRef]
158. Kohn, L.; Kohl, S.; Bowne, S.J.; Sullivan, L.S.; Kellner, U.; Daiger, S.P.; Sandgren, O.; Golovleva, I. PITPNM3 is an uncommon cause of cone and cone-rod dystrophies. *Ophthalmic Genet.* **2010**, *31*, 139–140. [CrossRef]
159. Bakhoum, M.F.; Sengillo, J.D.; Cui, X.; Tsang, S.H. Autoimmune retinopathy in a patient with a missense mutation in PITPNM3. *Retin Cases Brief. Rep.* **2018**, *12* (Suppl. 1), S72–S75. [CrossRef]
160. Lin, Z.; Li, W.; Zhang, H.; Wu, W.; Peng, Y.; Zeng, Y.; Wan, Y.; Wang, J.; Ouyang, N. CCL18/PITPNM3 enhances migration, invasion, and EMT through the NF-kappaB signaling pathway in hepatocellular carcinoma. *Tumour Biol.* **2016**, *37*, 3461–3468. [CrossRef]
161. Ile, K.E.; Kassen, S.; Cao, C.; Vihtehlic, T.; Shah, S.D.; Mousley, C.J.; Alb, J.G., Jr.; Huijbregts, R.P.; Stearns, G.W.; Brockerhoff, S.E.; et al. Zebrafish class 1 phosphatidylinositol transfer proteins: PITPbeta and double cone cell outer segment integrity in retina. *Traffic* **2010**, *11*, 1151–1167. [CrossRef] [PubMed]
162. Chang, B.; Hawes, N.L.; Hurd, R.E.; Davisson, M.T.; Nusinowitz, S.; Heckenlively, J.R. Retinal degeneration mutants in the mouse. *Vision Res.* **2002**, *42*, 517–525. [CrossRef]
163. Borman, A.D.; Pearce, L.R.; Mackay, D.S.; Nagel-Wolfrum, K.; Davidson, A.E.; Henderson, R.; Garg, S.; Waseem, N.H.; Webster, A.R.; Plagnol, V.; et al. A homozygous mutation in the TUB gene associated with retinal dystrophy and obesity. *Hum. Mutat.* **2014**, *35*, 289–293. [CrossRef] [PubMed]
164. Hagstrom, S.A.; Watson, R.F.; Pauer, G.J.; Grossman, G.H. Tulp1 is involved in specific photoreceptor protein transport pathways. *Adv. Exp. Med. Biol.* **2012**, *723*, 783–789. [CrossRef] [PubMed]
165. Xi, Q.; Pauer, G.J.; Traboulsi, E.I.; Hagstrom, S.A. Mutation screen of the TUB gene in patients with retinitis pigmentosa and Leber congenital amaurosis. *Exp. Eye Res.* **2006**, *83*, 569–573. [CrossRef] [PubMed]

166. Xi, Q.; Pauer, G.J.; West, K.A.; Crabb, J.W.; Hagstrom, S.A. Retinal degeneration caused by mutations in TULP1. *Adv. Exp. Med. Biol.* **2003**, *533*, 303–308. [CrossRef]
167. Mukhopadhyay, S.; Jackson, P.K. The tubby family proteins. *Genome Biol.* **2011**, *12*, 225. [CrossRef]
168. Hagstrom, S.A.; Duyao, M.; North, M.A.; Li, T. Retinal degeneration in tulp1-/- mice: Vesicular accumulation in the interphotoreceptor matrix. *Invest. Ophthalmol. Vis. Sci.* **1999**, *40*, 2795–2802.

6

Retinal miRNA Functions in Health and Disease

Marta Zuzic [1], Jesus Eduardo Rojo Arias [1], Stefanie Gabriele Wohl [2] and Volker Busskamp [1,*]

1 Center for Regenerative Therapies Dresden (CRTD), Technische Universität Dresden, 01307 Dresden, Germany; marta.zuzic@tu-dresden.de (M.Z.); Jesus_Eduardo.Rojo_Arias@tu-dresden.de (J.E.R.A.)

2 Department of Biological and Vision Sciences, The State University of New York, College of Optometry, New York, NY 10036, USA; swohl@sunyopt.edu

* Correspondence: volker.busskamp@tu-dresden.de

Abstract: The health and function of our visual system relies on accurate gene expression. While many genetic mutations are associated with visual impairment and blindness, we are just beginning to understand the complex interplay between gene regulation and retinal pathologies. MicroRNAs (miRNAs), a class of non-coding RNAs, are important regulators of gene expression that exert their function through post-transcriptional silencing of complementary mRNA targets. According to recent transcriptomic analyses, certain miRNA species are expressed in all retinal cell types, while others are cell type-specific. As miRNAs play important roles in homeostasis, cellular function, and survival of differentiated retinal cell types, their dysregulation is associated with retinal degenerative diseases. Thus, advancing our understanding of the genetic networks modulated by miRNAs is central to harnessing their potential as therapeutic agents to overcome visual impairment. In this review, we summarize the role of distinct miRNAs in specific retinal cell types, the current knowledge on their implication in inherited retinal disorders, and their potential as therapeutic agents.

Keywords: microRNA; retina; photoreceptors; rods; cones; bipolar cells; Müller glia; retinal inherited disorders; retinitis pigmentosa; retinal degeneration

---

1. miRNA Biogenesis and Function

MicroRNAs (miRNAs) are a class of highly conserved ~22 nucleotide (nt)-long non-coding RNAs that have a repressive impact on gene expression in a sequence-specific manner (Figure 1). These miRNAs are derived from partially complementary primary RNA transcripts (pri-miRNA) produced mainly by RNA polymerase II, but also by RNA polymerase III. Pri-miRNAs self-anneal to form hairpin or stem–loop structures, which are subsequently cleaved 11 base pairs (bp) from the base of the hairpin stem by the miRNA-processing complex, a protein ensemble that contains the Drosha ribonuclease and the DiGeorge Critical Region 8 (Dgcr8) protein [1]. The resulting 70 nt-long sequence is known as precursor miRNA (pre-miRNA) and is characterized by a 5′ phosphate and a 2-nt overhang at the 3′ end [2]. Alternatively, miRNAs also result from splicing events independently of Drosha and Dgcr8 [3]. Pre-miRNAs are subsequently exported out of the nucleus for the next processing step in which the Dicer endoribonuclease creates a cut ~22 nt away from the cleaving site of the miRNA-processing complex. Thereby, an additional 5′ phosphate and a new 2-nt 3′ overhang are generated at the opposite end of the double-stranded RNA [4]. The final miRNA structure is thus a duplex formed by partially complementary 22 nt-long RNA sequences with 5′ phosphates and 2-nt 3′ overhangs at both ends. In the last processing step, these duplexes are incorporated into the Argonaute protein, which is a member of the RNA-induced silencing complex (RISC), where one of the strands is removed. The strand that remains bound to Argonaute coordinates the search of, and pairing to, partially complementary target mRNA transcripts [1,5]. Upon binding their mRNA targets, miRNAs either induce their degradation, promote their deadenylation, or reduce their translational efficacy [6]. As individual miRNAs can have thousands of mRNA targets, they represent potent regulators of gene expression at the systems level [7,8]. To date, there are 1917 annotated human miRNA sequences (miRbase v22, access date 2019-05-13) [9].

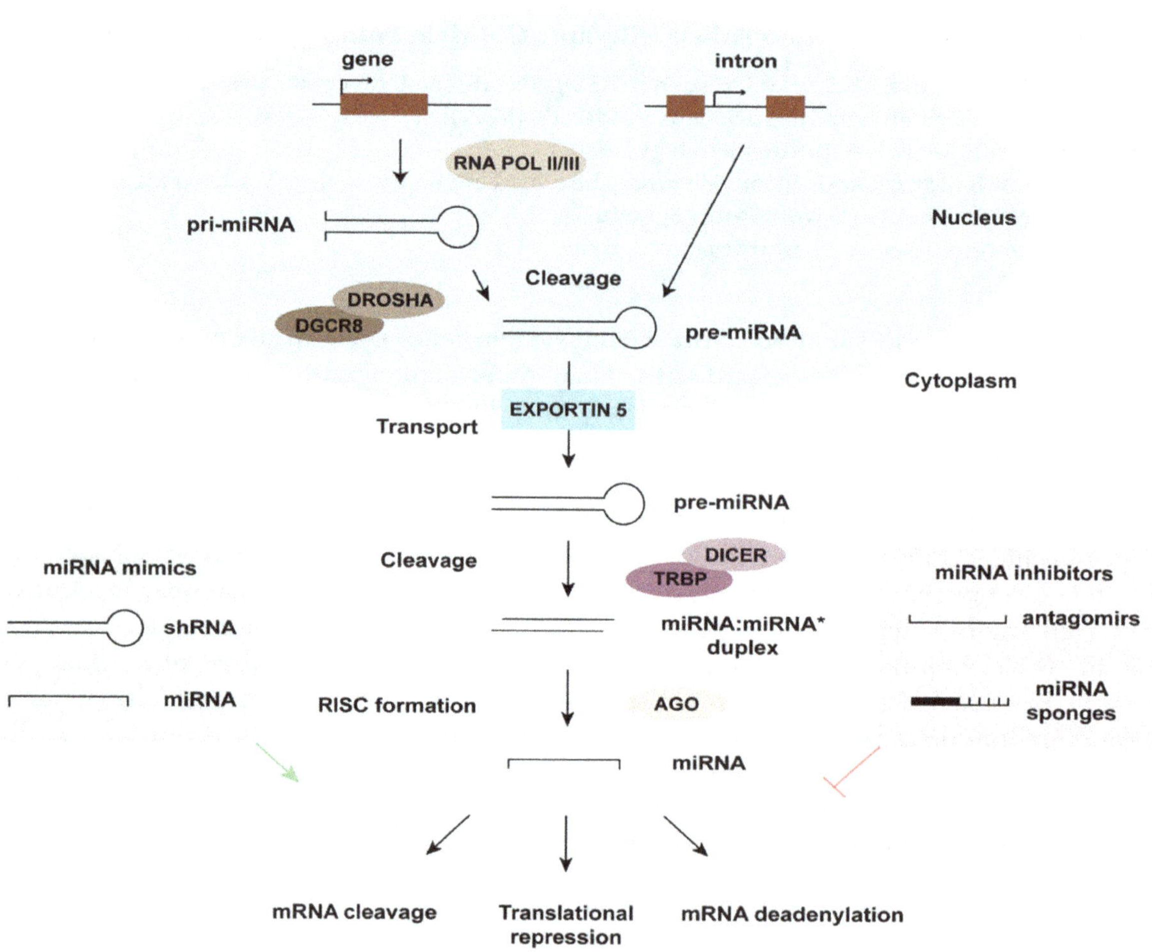

Figure 1. MicroRNA (miRNA) pathway. miRNA biogenesis starts in the nucleus where partially self-complementary RNA polymerase II or III transcripts from a miRNA gene or from an intronic region assemble into a hairpin-like structure known as primary (pri)-miRNA. Pri-miRNAs are cleaved by the DiGeorge Critical Region 8 (Dgcr8)/Drosha complex and transported to the cytoplasm via Exportin 5. In the cytoplasm, pre-miRNAs are cleaved by the Dicer/HIV-1 TAR RNA binding protein (TRBP) nuclease complex, thereby giving rise to a miRNA duplex. This duplex is then loaded onto the Argonaute (AGO) protein, a component of the RNA-induced silencing complex (RISC), where one of the two strands is discarded while the other serves to search complementary transcripts. Targets bound by miRNAs exhibit reduced translational efficiency, mainly as a consequence of mRNA cleavage or deadenylation. The miRNA pathway can be modulated by introducing miRNA mimics (green) or miRNA inhibitors (red). shRNA is small hairpin RNA.

Dysregulated miRNA expression during development can lead to severe defects and is connected to many pathological conditions such as cancer, neurodegenerative diseases, heart failure, diabetes, and inherited genetic disorders [10]. In mature organs and tissues, miRNAs support the robustness of gene networks and buffer against the fluctuations in gene expression often resulting from stochastic modulation and environmental stress [11]. As their metabolic activity is considerably high and they are often exposed to high levels of external stress, photoreceptors are highly vulnerable to cell death in retinal degenerative diseases. In this context, miRNAs play an important role in photoreceptor survival and function [12]. Moreover, as not all retinal disease phenotypes have been linked to specific genes, altered miRNA expression may underlie the emergence and progression of certain retinal disorders. Thus, exploring the function and gene regulatory networks of these and other non-coding RNAs is of the utmost importance. A dominant mutation in miR-204, for instance, is the genetic cause of retinal degeneration associated with ocular coloboma, a genetic developmental disorder characterized by keyhole-shaped defects in various eye structures [13]. It is thus tempting to speculate that miR-204 is not the sole case of a miRNA giving rise to an ocular disease, and that altered expression of non-coding RNAs might lead to other retinal disorders. Here, we discuss some of the known functions of miRNAs in the adult retina.

2. Controlling Cellular miRNA Expression

The deliberate modulation of gene expression through the use of non-coding RNAs, commonly referred to as RNA interference [14], has been extensively utilized in basic and biomedical research. Small hairpin RNAs (shRNAs), for instance, are artificial RNA molecules with a hairpin region processed by the same machinery as miRNAs and effectively acting as miRNA mimics [15,16]. Normally, shRNAs are designed to match the sequence of specific RNA molecules, which they target and downregulate upon delivery. The production of such shRNA molecules is driven by regular promoter elements within a plasmid or a viral vector. Standard gene delivery techniques can be applied to express the shRNA of interest in target cells. This system can also be used to overexpress specific miRNAs [17]. Alternatively, the consequences of miRNA overexpression can be studied by inserting them within artificial intron systems. In general, shRNA vectors are particularly interesting for silencing dominant disease-causing transcripts and their use in retinal cell types was established already over a decade ago [18].

Vice versa, for downregulating or silencing miRNAs, commonly used techniques include "antagomirs" [19] and so-called miRNA "sponges" [20]. Whereas antagomirs are chemically engineered oligonucleotides, miRNA sponges are RNAs with artificial tandem binding site arrays for specific miRNAs. Hence, these sponge sequences compete with physiological targets for miRNA binding, which ultimately leads to reduced silencing of primary mRNA targets. Sponge cassettes can be delivered to retinal cell types by adeno-associated viruses (AAV) [21], which are powerful clinically approved vectors for ocular gene transfer [22,23]. Thus, the therapeutic use of non-coding RNAs is presently growing at an accelerated pace due to increased knowledge of miRNA functions and the wide adoption of technologies that facilitate control of their expression levels in distinct retinal cell types.

3. Photoreceptor–miRNAs as Cell Maintenance and Survival Regulators

Rod photoreceptors are sensory neurons essential to night vision. To investigate the impact of miRNA deficiency in these cells, rod photoreceptor-specific Dicer conditional knock-out (cKO) mice have been generated. As mentioned above, Dicer is the endoribonuclease responsible for the second cleavage step in the canonical miRNA biosynthesis pathway. These mice were generated by crossing a *Dicer1*$^{fl/fl}$ line with mice expressing Cre recombinase exclusively in mature rods. Loss of *Dicer1* at postnatal day 28 (P28), a time-point at which rods are mature and postmitotic, was reported to lead to outer segment disorganization in eight-week-old mice, followed by robust retinal degeneration and loss of visual function by 14 weeks. Notably, cKO mice did not exhibit significant defects in either phototransduction or the visual cycle before the onset of retinal degeneration, suggesting that the main role of miRNAs in rods is to support photoreceptor survival [24].

Additional studies have aimed at revealing the functions of miRNAs in cone photoreceptors, which are essential for high-acuity and daylight vision. Cone photoreceptor-specific miRNA-deficient mice have been generated by crossing *Dgcr8*$^{fl/fl}$ animals with mice expressing Cre recombinase solely in differentiated cones. In these mice, the Dgcr8 protein was only gradually depleted over time as a consequence of its prolonged half-life. Thus, loss of miRNA processing was first detected at P30 and was complete only by P60. The lack of miRNAs in these animals resulted in the progressive loss of cone outer segments, and therefore in low sensitivity to high light levels. However, cones without outer segments did not degenerate in spite of their severely altered gene expression profiles. The latter suggests a crucial role for miRNAs in regulating genetic pathways essential to cone outer segment maintenance and function, but not to cone survival [17]. On the other hand, a recent study reported that the conditional knockout of Dicer in cones results not only in outer segment loss but also in a more severe phenotype with enhanced cone cell death [25]. For proper phenotype interpretation, the targeted miRNA biogenesis proteins, Dgcr8 versus Dicer, are of importance as Dgcr8 knockouts may have residual miRNA expression from splicing products. Although these reports also differed in the cone-specific Cre driver lines used and in the onset of miRNA loss, together they provide strong evidence for the importance of miRNAs on photoreceptor homeostasis, function, and survival.

4. The Impact of the miR-183/96/182 Cluster on Photoreceptors

The miRNAs of the miR-183/96/182 cluster play important functional roles in multiple sensory tissues, as evidenced by their expression not only in the retina [26,27], but also in the inner ear [28], the olfactory and gustatory epithelium [27], and in dorsal root ganglia mechanosensory neurons [29]. miR-183, -96, and -182 are expressed as a single polycistronic transcript and exhibit significant sequence similarity in their seed regions. Thereby, they possess shared targets and can partially substitute each other's function. This overlap in function explains why targeted deletion of only one of these three miRNAs, i.e., miR-182, results in no visible alterations in retinal development [30]. More importantly, although these three miRNAs possess distinct targets, the majority of such targets are involved in identical pathways [31]. In the retina, the miR-183/96/182 cluster is enriched in rod and cone photoreceptors with transcript levels reduced in dark and increased in light conditions (Figure 2). Such dynamic changes in expression levels are the consequences of rapid miRNA decay and of increased transcription, respectively. The latter suggests that miRNA metabolism, in general, is higher in neurons than in other cell types, possibly due to neuronal activity [21].

The function of the miR-183/96/182 cluster was examined in a transgenic mouse line expressing a miRNA sponge for all three cluster miRNAs exclusively in mature rods [32]. Retinae from these mice displayed no detectable morphological or functional changes, likely because the sponge activity was insufficient to capture all mature miRNA molecules of such a highly expressed cluster. Nonetheless, after 30 min exposure to high light intensities (10,000 lux), transgenic mice but not wild type animals showed severe retinal degeneration, indicating that reduced levels of cluster miRNAs have an impact on rod function and survival. More severe retinal defects and retinal degeneration were observed in a miR-183/96/182 cluster knockout mouse model [33], although the miRNAs of the cluster were also missing during photoreceptor development, when cluster expression is tightly controlled [34]. Hence, in this case it is impossible to distinguish the functions of the miR-183/96/182 cluster in development from those in adulthood. Nevertheless, together these knockdown and knockout studies suggest that this cluster plays a neuroprotective role in the retina. Remarkably, re-introducing miR-182 and -183 in Dgcr8 cKO cones, i.e., cones depleted of all other miRNAs, has been reported to prevent the loss of cone outer segments [17]. Considering that miR-182 and -183 constitutes around 70% of all cone miRNA content, it is likely that these play major roles in cone functionality, including in the modulation of outer segment maintenance. Furthermore, overexpression of the miR-183/96/182 cluster in embryonic stem cell-derived retinal organoids induces the formation of light-responsive short outer segments [17], while in human RPE cells in vitro it triggers their reprogramming to neurons [35]. In this sense, a number of the cluster's targets have been validated, including pro-apoptotic genes, like *Casp2* [32], genes important for survival such as *Rac1* coding for the small GTP-binding protein [36], and neurotransmitter transporters like the voltage-dependent glutamate transporter *Slc1a1* [21] as well as the sodium- and chloride-dependent glycine transporter *Slc6a9* [36]. The latter, together with the neurogenic effects of overexpressing the miRNAs within this cluster in different cell types, suggests that the miR-183/96/182 cluster is central to photoreceptor homeostasis and serves as a pro-survival factor in stress conditions.

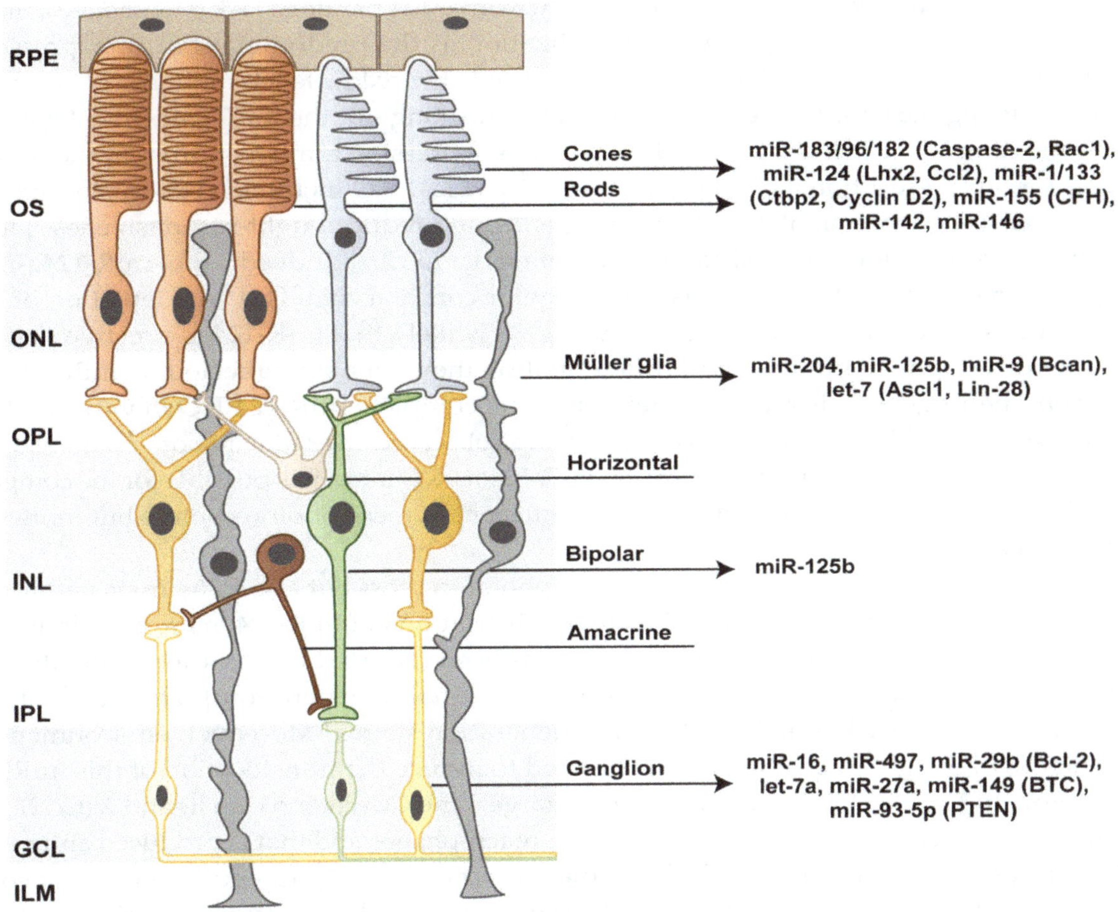

Figure 2. MiRNAs acting as modulators of retinal cell behavior. In the vertebrate eye, the retinal pigment epithelium (RPE) separates the retina from the subretinal space. Within the outermost layer of the retina, rod and cone photoreceptors sense light with their outer segments (OS). Photoreceptor bodies reside within the outer nuclear layer (ONL), and their axons protrude into the outer plexiform layer (OPL), where they synapse with excitatory bipolar cells and inhibitory horizontal cells. The bodies of these cells, as well as of amacrine cells, which create inhibitory synapses with the axons of bipolar cells, reside in turn within the inner nuclear layer (INL). The electrochemical signal produced by photoreceptors during phototransduction is transmitted through bipolar cells to ganglion cells via synaptic connections in the inner plexiform layer (IPL). In a final step, ganglion cells send this information to higher brain areas through their axons, which bundle up to form the optic nerve. An additional cell type within the retina is Müller glia. These cells play key roles in the support of neuronal functions and in mediating the reaction to a number of physiological signals, including immune responses. Müller glia feet form the outer limiting membrane (OLM), which separates photoreceptor OS from their somata. Within the retina, miRNAs play central roles in health and disease. Recognized miRNA species associated to the functionality of specific retinal cell types are shown with validated targets between parentheses. GCL, ganglion cell layer; ILM, inner limiting membrane.

5. miR-124 Protects Photoreceptors from Apoptosis

MiR-124 is enriched in neurons of the central nervous system [37,38] including the retina [39], and is one of the most well studied miRNA species. In the retina, miR-124 is expressed in all neuronal cell layers, but most prominently in photoreceptor outer (OS) and inner segments (IS). As both humans and mice possess three miR-124 loci, the generation of a complete miR-124 knockout model has been challenging. Recently, a full miR-124 KO (i.e., all six genomic copies) was achieved in a human induced pluripotent stem cell model of neurogenesis [8]. Neurons generated from KO cells displayed altered morphological and functional features and decreased long-term viability, pointing to the importance of miR-124 in neuronal survival. Of note, among the three miR-124 paralogs (a-1, a-2, and a-3), miR-124a-1 has been previously identified by in situ hybridization as the predominant form expressed in the developing mouse retina, with miR-124a-2 being detected at very low levels and miR-124a-3 expression being almost negligible [40]. In agreement with this, knocking out the miR-124a-1 host gene, i.e., the retinal non-coding RNA 3 (*Rncr3*), abolishes miR-124 expression almost entirely in the mouse cone photoreceptor layer. Additional consequences of miR-124a-1 KO included cone mislocalization and apoptosis, decreased expression of cone-specific genes, and reduced light-responsiveness [40].

A validated target of miR-124a in the retina is *Lhx2*. Indeed, the miR-124a-mediated downregulation of *Lhx2* mRNA levels is necessary for cone survival [40]. As depletion of Dgcr8 in adult cones does not cause cone degeneration, it is very likely that miR-124 is effective in these cells early during development but that after differentiation they remain unaffected by miR-124 deletion. In agreement, neurogenesis is hindered neither in the complete miR-124 KO in vitro model nor in miR-124a-1 KO mice, although increased apoptosis was observed over time in both cases. Moreover, as cones but no other retinal neurons degenerate in miR-124a-1 KO mice, it is possible for the compensatory effects of the other two miR-124 paralogs to be insufficient in these photoreceptors but more potent in other retinal cell types.

In the retina, miR-124 is expressed not only in photoreceptors but also in neurons within the inner nuclear layer and the ganglion cell layer. An altered distribution of miR-124 expression from primarily the outer nuclear layer to the inner nuclear layer has been reported to occur in age-related macular degeneration (AMD) patients and mouse models of retinal degeneration [41], with such changes being followed by miR-124 depletion at later degeneration stages. Moreover, environmental stress factors, such as high light intensities, are speculated to induce the translocation of this miRNA from photoreceptors to Müller glia (MG) cells, where it targets the CC-chemokine ligand 2 (*Ccl2*). Ccl2 is a pro-inflammatory chemokine that attracts microglia/macrophages and that is produced and released by MG cells in response to retinal damage [42]. Further, this chemokine is upregulated in both neovascular and atrophic forms of AMD [43] and in retinitis pigmentosa [44]. By downregulating *Ccl2*, miR-124 translocation would thus dampen the inflammatory cascade and promote photoreceptor survival. After prolonged stress, on the other hand, miR-124 depletion results in highly pro-inflammatory environments and thereby in subsequent photoreceptor degeneration. Supporting these observations, *Ccl2* downregulation has been shown to reduce photoreceptor cell death in animal models of retinal degeneration [44–46]. Notably, intravitreal administration of miR-124 mimics decreases retinal inflammation and photoreceptor cell death, while preserving retinal function [41]. The latter might be a consequence, at least partially, of increased *Ccl2* targeting.

6. miRNA Functions in Inner Retinal Neurons

For the maintenance and survival of retinal cell types other than photoreceptors, miRNAs are also remarkably important. For example, miR-125b has been described as a regulator of neuritogenesis during remodeling in rod bipolar cells after retinal degeneration [47]. Similarly, in retinal ganglion cells (RGCs), miRNA expression profiles and functions have been investigated. RGCs are responsible for sending the visual information collected by photoreceptors to higher brain areas via the optic nerve, and their damage is a hallmark of glaucoma. In retinae of a glaucoma mouse model, nine miRNAs (out of 17 tested) were identified as differentially expressed relative to controls. Among those nine miRNAs, the pro-apoptotic miR-16, -497, -29b, and let-7a were downregulated, while the anti-apoptotic miR-27a was upregulated. Whereas let-7a exerts its apoptotic function by inducing neurodegeneration via Toll-like receptor signaling, miR-16, -29b, and -497 negatively regulate the apoptosis regulator Bcl-2. These alterations in miRNA expression profiles suggest a shift towards a protective anti-apoptotic phenotype [48]. In a different mouse model of glaucoma, downregulation of miR-149 led to an increased RGC number and minimized ultrastructural RGC alterations [49]. In this study, betacellulin (*Btc*) was also identified as a miR-149 target. BTC is a mitogen influencing the activation of the PI3K/AKT signaling pathway, which mediates RGC protection via its pro-survival and anti-apoptotic effects. Further, in the N-methyl-D-aspartate (NMDA)-induced glaucoma mouse model, significant reductions in RGC viability were accompanied by miR-93-5p downregulation [50]. Reduced miR-93-5p levels in these mice, in turn, resulted in the elevated presence of its target phosphatase and tensin homolog (PTEN), which promotes autophagy of RGCs via the AKT/mTOR pathway. Confirming the central role of miR-93-5p in this context, the reduced viability of RGCs isolated from retinae of NMDA-induced glaucoma animals was counteracted either by overexpressing this miRNA species or by transfection with a miR-93-5p mimic.

In mouse models of optic nerve injury, increased expression of specific miRNAs has also been detected. miR-21 expression, for instance, correlated with reactive MG gliosis. Whereas activated MGs are neuroprotective after injury in the acute response phase, they later acquire a pro-inflammatory and pro-apoptotic phenotype. Modulating MG gliosis in both the acute and chronic post-injury phases in these mice resulted in enhanced RGC survival and functionality and led to improvements in retinal structural integrity [51]. Often, however, the protective roles of distinct miRNAs in RGCs have been assessed in vitro. In rat RGC-5 cells, for instance, overexpression of miR-187 was reported to suppress apoptosis and promote proliferation by targeting *Smad7* [52]. Similarly, upregulation of miR-211 was shown to downregulate *Frs2* and to decrease the extent of cell death in RGC-5 cells subjected to a high-pressure challenge [53]. These results hint at a protective effect of miR-187 and miR-211 on RGCs. On the other hand, lentivirus-mediated down-regulation of miR-100 has been described to reduce hydrogen peroxide-induced RGC apoptosis and to enhance neurite growth by activating the AKT/ERK and TRKB pathways through phosphorylation [54]. In a similar experimental approach, hydrogen peroxide-induced apoptosis of RGC was described to decrease upon miR-134 downregulation. In this case, a luciferase reporter assay confirmed that miR-134 directly interacts with the cyclic AMP-response element-binding protein (*Creb*), a transcription factor with central roles in neuronal protection that modulates the expression of the anti-apoptotic proteins BDNF and Bcl-2. Thus, inhibiting miR-134 effectively reduces apoptosis levels by allowing the enhanced translation of CREB and, consequently, the upregulation of its downstream targets BDNF and Bcl-2 [55].

7. The role of miRNAs in Müller Glia Development and Function

MiRNAs play an important role in retinal development as described in several studies using Dicer conditional knockouts [56–58] (summarized in [59]). One study in particular reported that the blockade of miRNA genesis in an αPax6-Cre mouse model prevented the development of late retinal progenitors and their progenies, including MG [60]. Specifically, three miRNAs have been identified as key regulators of the early to late developmental transition in retinal progenitors, namely let-7, miR-125, and miR-9 [61,62]. Thus, miRNAs may be involved in MG differentiation. As mentioned above, the miRNA expression of whole retinae has been previously profiled [63,64]. Since the vast majority of retinal cells are rod photoreceptors and MG account for only around 2% of them [65], the profiling and identification of MG-specific miRNAs requires FACS-purification or primary cultures. Two independent studies have so far aimed at identifying these miRNAs. The authors of the first study isolated MG from P8 retinae and cultured the cells before miRNA profiling. The culture period, however, was not clarified. In this study, miR-143, miR-145, miR-214, miR-199a, miR-199b*, and miR-29a were identified as highly expressed [66]. In the second study, miR-204, miR-125b, and miR-9 were identified as MG-specific miRNAs (mGliomiRs) in reporter-labelled (RlbpCreERT-dtTomato) FACS-purified P11/P12 murine MG [67]. These three miRNAs had high expression levels in MG, with increasing levels from P11 to adulthood. Moreover, besides these MG-specific miRNAs, a distinct set of miRNAs had similar expression levels in both neurons and glia (termed shared miRNAs). This set includes most members of the let-7 family and miR-29a. Thus, it is conceivable that miR-125, miR-9, and let-7 are not only key regulators in the early to late progenitor transition [61], but that they are also important for MG maturation and function.

A remaining question was whether miRNAs are required for proper MG function. This was addressed in a Dicer cKO study using a MG-specific Rlbp-CreERT:tdTomato:Dicer$^{fl/fl}$ reporter mouse [68]. Dicer deletion was induced in these mice by tamoxifen administration at P12, when MG are differentiated, as well as in one-month old animals. Over a period of 6–12 months, glia aggregated abnormally, leading in turn to massive structural disturbances. Although MG usually do not express the *Bcan* gene, which encodes a chondroitin sulfate proteoglycan, RNA-Seq showed this to be the most highly upregulated gene in these cells. Notably, this phenotype was primarily the consequence of miR-9 loss. miR-9 targets the 3'UTR of *Bcan*, and its administration in vitro or ex vivo prevented abnormal glia development and/or partially restored overall retinal structure. Although in these mice miRNAs were only deleted in MG and not in neurons, a massive loss of photoreceptors was also observed. More importantly, retinal remodeling also subsequently ensued. Remodeling generally occurs as a result of photoreceptor degeneration [69]. Interestingly, MG from human retinitis pigmentosa tissue displayed similar cell aggregation and were positive for Brevican (the protein encoded by *Bcan*). This suggests that not only loss of or disturbances in neuronal miRNAs, but also dysregulation of the glial miRNA biogenesis machinery could be causative of retinal diseases [68]. This hypothesis is further supported by MG ablation studies showing that the dysfunction of this cell population plays an important role in retinal diseases [70–73].

8. miRNAs in Müller Glia De-Differentiation and Their Potential Regeneration Capacity

Although there are miRNAs specific to retinal progenitors, neurons, and MG, and despite many of these miRNAs playing important roles in cell fate decisions, their capacity to alter the fate of mature, fully-differentiated cells remains controversial. In contrast to mammalian retinae, the fish retina can regenerate completely after injury. Remarkably, MG are the cells that mediate the regeneration process. MG de-differentiate to progenitors, proliferate, migrate, and differentiate de novo into all retinal cell types, including RGCs and photoreceptors. Key regulators in this regenerative process are the Acheate-scute family bHLH transcription factor 1 (*Ascl1*) and the RNA-binding protein Lin-28, which are both regulated by the miRNA let-7 [74,75]. Additional factors discovered to be involved in this process include Wnt [76] and Shh [77], which are regulated by the miRNA let-7 in fish and mouse. Notwithstanding, the mechanisms of MG reprogramming in mice, especially at adult ages, are more intricate and involve epigenetic alterations [78].

The brain-enriched miR-124 is known to regulate neurogenesis [39,41,67,79]. Accordingly, overexpression of miR-124 in MG-derived mouse progenitors in vitro results in twice as many βIII-Tubulin-positive cells as in wild-type control cells [66]. This indicates that this neuronal miRNA can be used to direct retinal progenitor like-cells towards a neuronal fate, as it has previously been observed on neural stem cells [80,81]. Moreover, when miR-124 alone or in combination with miR-9/9* was overexpressed in P12 mouse MG in vitro, MG de-differentiated into *Ascl1*-expressing progenitor-like cells that later on expressed mature neuronal markers including *Map2*, Calbindin, and Calretinin. The underlying mechanism for this process is known to require the RE1-silencing transcription factor (Rest) pathway [67], an evolutionarily conserved transcriptional regulator that inhibits neuronal gene expression in non-neuronal cells such as glia or fibroblasts [82–84], and whose inhibition by miR-124 enhances the expression of neuronal genes [85–87]. In addition, miR-124 has recently been described to promote axon growth in RGCs differentiated from young rat retinal stem cell-derived MG by silencing the REST complex [88]. Besides miR-124, miR-28 has also been reported to potentially play a role in photoreceptor differentiation. MG-derived progenitors treated with anti-miR-28 exhibited *Crx* and Rhodopsin expression while miR-28 overexpression did not [89]. In this case, however, the underlying mechanisms remain elusive.

9. Global miRNA Alterations in Retinal Diseases

Retinitis pigmentosa (RP) is a complex inherited retinal disease that emerges from a heterogeneous pool of mutations [90]. Yet, irrespective of the underlying mutation, clinical manifestations are often similar and include progressive photoreceptor loss and visual impairment. To determine if miRNA dysregulation is involved in the pathophysiology of RP, miRNA expression levels have been interrogated in multiple mouse models of retinal degeneration. One study examined the miRNA expression profile of two rhodopsin (*Rho*) mutants (recessive rho–/– knockout and dominant P347S-Rhodopsin, also known as R347) and two RDS/Peripherin mutants (recessive rds–/– null mutant and dominant Δ307-rds) [91]. The authors reported all four mouse models to exhibit miR-96, -182, and -183 downregulation, and miR-1, -133, and -142 upregulation. The dysregulated miRNA signature of isolated rods as well as of whole retinae of R347 and Δ307-rds mice were similar. These findings suggest that altered miRNA profiles are indeed associated with RP, irrespective of the causative mutation or of its dominant or recessive nature. However, the miR-183/96/182 cluster is highly expressed in photoreceptors and therefore its downregulation might be a consequence of the massive rod photoreceptor degeneration rather than causative of RP. In a follow-up study, C-terminal Binding Protein 2 (*Ctbp2*) was validated as a miR-1 target, with *Slc6a9* and *Rac1* being recognized by miR-9, -182, and -183 [36]. CTBP2, a major component of specialized synapses, was shown to be co-expressed with the miR-1/133 cluster in photoreceptors, and its levels were reported to decrease in photoreceptor synaptic regions of R347 retinae. The latter suggests that miR-1/133 may play a role in regulating synaptic remodeling at photoreceptor synapses by targeting *Ctbp2*. In contrast, *Slc6a9*, which encodes one of the two main transporters involved in removing glycine from the synaptic cleft, was co-expressed with miR-1/133 exclusively in cone photoreceptors.

The retinal degeneration 10 (rd10) mouse is a commonly used model of autosomal recessive retinitis pigmentosa and has been utilized to study miRNA expression patterns in early retinal degeneration [92]. In these mice, a spontaneous mutation in the rod phosphodiesterase (*Pde*) gene leads to photoreceptor death from post-natal day 16 on as a result of calcium dysregulation [93]. By using microarrays to profile the expression of over 1900 miRNAs in rd10 retinae, 152 differentially expressed miRNAs have been identified after (P17, P19, and P22), but also shortly before (P15) the initiation of photoreceptor apoptosis [92]. The miRNAs identified as differentially expressed prior to the onset of apoptosis include miR-6240, miR-6937-5p, miR-3473b, and miR-7035-5p, which are likely involved in the disease etiology. On the other hand, miR-155-5p, miR-142-5p, and miR-146a-5p were differentially expressed after the onset of apoptosis. Thus, it remains unclear whether these miRNAs counteract or enhance disease progression. By comparing differentially expressed miRNAs with inversely correlated mRNAs and performing gene ontology and biological pathway analyses, a large number of miRNA targets were revealed to encode factors involved in apoptosis, the inflammatory response, calcium signaling, visual perception, and phototransduction.

The differential expression of miRNAs in the context of retinal degenerative diseases has also been studied in canine models. Notably, the early onset retinal degeneration models Xlpra2 (RPGRORF15-microdeletion), Rcd1 (PDE6B-mutation), and Erd (STK38L-mutation), as well as the slowly progressing Prcd (PRCD-mutation) model, have been reported to exhibit similar miRNA expression profiles as healthy control dogs both prior to and at the peak of photoreceptor cell death [94]. Divergences were reported to arise only during the chronic cell death stage, with anti-apoptotic miRNAs such as miR-9, -19a, -20, -21, -29b, -146a, -155, and -221 being upregulated and pro-apoptotic miR-122 and miR-129 being downregulated. Although the miRNA species differentially expressed in canine and murine models of retinal degeneration are not identical, available reports hint at miRNAs playing a role in counteracting the degenerative processes characteristic of diseased retinae by delaying photoreceptor cell death.

A number of additional studies have interrogated the retinal miRNA expression profile in response to injury. Inducing photoreceptor death by ablating MG, for instance, leads to the differential expression of 16 miRNAs, with miR-142, miR-146, and the miR-1/133 cluster in particular exhibiting increased expression levels [95]. In this study, increased miR-133 expression was mainly detected within the outer nuclear layer, where it targets the anti-apoptotic gene cyclin D2. In fact, the cyclin D2 family has been reported to play a neuroprotective role in retinal degeneration [96]. Unexpectedly, a positive correlation between miR-133 and cyclin D2 was also reported, suggesting that miR-133 up-regulates the expression levels of its own target. Further, in models of light-induced photoreceptor death, 37 miRNAs have been described to increase in expression upon light damage, including seven that regulate the inflammatory response (miR-125, -155, -207, -347, -449, -351, -542). Among the latter, miR-155 is of particular interest as it is linked to the progression of the inflammatory response through the targeting of complement factor H (*Cfh*) [97], a major inhibitor of the alternative complement pathway [98]. Moreover, upregulation of miR-155 has been detected in both mouse and canine models of inherited retinal diseases [92,94], suggesting that the roles of certain miRNAs are conserved across species and, more notably, shared in different injury response contexts.

The miRNA profile of human retinae has been recently investigated via high-throughput sequencing [99]. The assessment of miRNA expression levels in 16 retinae from healthy donors led to the detection of 480 miRNA species with more than 3000 variants. Of note, the five most highly expressed miRNAs accounted for 70% and the top 20 miRNAs for almost 90% of the entire retinal miRNA profile. Moreover, the miRNAs miR-182 and miR-183 were the most prevalent miRNA species in retinal neurons and miR-204 was the most abundant miRNA in retinal pigment epithelium (RPE) cells. Some of these highly expressed human miRNAs coincide with those previously identified in murine retinae by microarray analyses and RNA in situ hybridization experiments [27,64,100,101], pointing to their potentially conserved retinal functions across mammalian species [102]. It is known from animal models that miRNA expression patterns change over the course of retinal development [64,101] and that such dynamic miRNA expression profiles are crucial to retinal cell differentiation (reviewed in [59]). Altogether, it is very likely that the impact miRNAs have in animal models is transferable to human retinal cell types in health and disease. This further implies that particular miRNAs may be used as disease biomarkers and, additionally, that the precise modulation of their expression levels might represent a valuable therapeutic strategy for the treatment of diverse retinal inherited disorders.

10. Conclusions

We are in the process of understanding the complex functions of miRNAs in retinal health and disease. Further studies are required to obtain coherent pictures of gene expression regulators in order to harness their potential use not only as biomarkers but also to treat and counteract retinal diseases. As individual miRNA species have the potential to orchestrate entire genetic programs, the possibility to use them as master regulators to stabilize or reset the cellular state of neurons and glial cells in the retina is highly promising.

Author Contributions: Conceptualization, M.Z. and V.B.; writing—original draft preparation, writing—review and editing, M.Z., J.E.R.A., S.G.W., and V.B.; visualization, M.Z.; funding acquisition, S.G.W. and V.B.

Acknowledgments: The authors would like to thank Sylvia J. Gasparini for critical feedback on the manuscript.

References

1. Ha, M.; Kim, V.N. Regulation of microRNA biogenesis. *Nat. Rev. Mol. Cell Biol.* **2014**, *15*, 509–524. [CrossRef]
2. Han, J.; Lee, Y.; Yeom, K.H.; Kim, Y.K.; Jin, H.; Kim, V.N. The Drosha-DGCR8 complex in primary microRNA processing. *Genes Dev.* **2004**, *18*, 3016–3027. [CrossRef]

3. Westholm, J.O.; Lai, E.C. Mirtrons: microRNA biogenesis via splicing. *Biochimie* **2011**, *93*, 1897–1904. [CrossRef]
4. Chiang, H.R.; Schoenfeld, L.W.; Ruby, J.G.; Auyeung, V.C.; Spies, N.; Baek, D.; Johnston, W.K.; Russ, C.; Luo, S.; Babiarz, J.E.; et al. Mammalian microRNAs: Experimental evaluation of novel and previously annotated genes. *Genes Dev.* **2010**, *24*, 992–1009. [CrossRef]
5. Bartel, D.P. MicroRNAs: Target recognition and regulatory functions. *Cell* **2009**, *136*, 215–233. [CrossRef]
6. Krol, J.; Loedige, I.; Filipowicz, W. The widespread regulation of microRNA biogenesis, function and decay. *Nat. Rev. Genet.* **2010**, *11*, 597–610. [CrossRef]
7. Tan, C.L.; Plotkin, J.L.; Veno, M.T.; von Schimmelmann, M.; Feinberg, P.; Mann, S.; Handler, A.; Kjems, J.; Surmeier, D.J.; O'Carroll, D.; et al. MicroRNA-128 governs neuronal excitability and motor behavior in mice. *Sci. (N.Y.)* **2013**, *342*, 1254–1258. [CrossRef] [PubMed]
8. Kutsche, L.K.; Gysi, D.M.; Fallmann, J.; Lenk, K.; Petri, R.; Swiersy, A.; Klapper, S.D.; Pircs, K.; Khattak, S.; Stadler, P.F.; et al. Combined Experimental and System-Level Analyses Reveal the Complex Regulatory Network of miR-124 during Human Neurogenesis. *Cell Syst.* **2018**, *7*, 438–452 e438. [CrossRef]
9. Kozomara, A.; Griffiths-Jones, S. miRBase: Annotating high confidence microRNAs using deep sequencing data. *Nucleic Acids Res.* **2014**, *42*, D68–D73. [CrossRef]
10. Ha, T.-Y. MicroRNAs in human diseases: From cancer to cardiovascular disease. *Immune. Netw.* **2011**, *11*, 135–154. [CrossRef]
11. Ebert, M.S.; Sharp, P.A. Roles for microRNAs in conferring robustness to biological processes. *Cell* **2012**, *149*, 515–524. [CrossRef]
12. Sundermeier, T.R.; Palczewski, K. The impact of microRNA gene regulation on the survival and function of mature cell types in the eye. *FASEB J.* **2016**, *30*, 23–33. [CrossRef]
13. Conte, I.; Hadfield, K.D.; Barbato, S.; Carrella, S.; Pizzo, M.; Bhat, R.S.; Carissimo, A.; Karali, M.; Porter, L.F.; Urquhart, J.; et al. MiR-204 is responsible for inherited retinal dystrophy associated with ocular coloboma. *Proc. Natl. Acad. Sci. USA* **2015**, *112*, E3236–E3245. [CrossRef]
14. Fire, A.; Xu, S.; Montgomery, M.K.; Kostas, S.A.; Driver, S.E.; Mello, C.C. Potent and specific genetic interference by double-stranded RNA in Caenorhabditis elegans. *Nature* **1998**, *391*, 806–811. [CrossRef]
15. Paddison, P.J.; Caudy, A.A.; Bernstein, E.; Hannon, G.J.; Conklin, D.S. Short hairpin RNAs (shRNAs) induce sequence-specific silencing in mammalian cells. *Genes Dev.* **2002**, *16*, 948–958. [CrossRef] [PubMed]
16. Brummelkamp, T.R.; Bernards, R.; Agami, R. A system for stable expression of short interfering RNAs in mammalian cells. *Sci. (N.Y.)* **2002**, *296*, 550–553. [CrossRef] [PubMed]
17. Busskamp, V.; Krol, J.; Nelidova, D.; Daum, J.; Szikra, T.; Tsuda, B.; Juttner, J.; Farrow, K.; Scherf, B.G.; Alvarez, C.P.; et al. miRNAs 182 and 183 are necessary to maintain adult cone photoreceptor outer segments and visual function. *Neuron* **2014**, *83*, 586–600. [CrossRef]
18. Michel, U.; Malik, I.; Ebert, S.; Bahr, M.; Kugler, S. Long-term in vivo and in vitro AAV-2-mediated RNA interference in rat retinal ganglion cells and cultured primary neurons. *Biochem. Biophys. Res. Commun.* **2005**, *326*, 307–312. [CrossRef] [PubMed]
19. Krutzfeldt, J.; Rajewsky, N.; Braich, R.; Rajeev, K.G.; Tuschl, T.; Manoharan, M.; Stoffel, M. Silencing of microRNAs in vivo with 'antagomirs'. *Nature* **2005**, *438*, 685–689. [CrossRef]
20. Ebert, M.S.; Neilson, J.R.; Sharp, P.A. MicroRNA sponges: Competitive inhibitors of small RNAs in mammalian cells. *Nat. Methods* **2007**, *4*, 721–726. [CrossRef] [PubMed]
21. Krol, J.; Busskamp, V.; Markiewicz, I.; Stadler, M.B.; Ribi, S.; Richter, J.; Duebel, J.; Bicker, S.; Fehling, H.J.; Schubeler, D.; et al. Characterizing light-regulated retinal microRNAs reveals rapid turnover as a common property of neuronal microRNAs. *Cell* **2010**, *141*, 618–631. [CrossRef]
22. Trapani, I.; Auricchio, A. Seeing the Light after 25 Years of Retinal Gene Therapy. *Trends Mol. Med.* **2018**, *24*, 669–681. [CrossRef] [PubMed]
23. Hudry, E.; Vandenberghe, L.H. Therapeutic AAV Gene Transfer to the Nervous System: A Clinical Reality. *Neuron* **2019**, *101*, 839–862. [CrossRef]
24. Sundermeier, T.R.; Zhang, N.; Vinberg, F.; Mustafi, D.; Kohno, H.; Golczak, M.; Bai, X.; Maeda, A.; Kefalov, V.J.; Palczewski, K. DICER1 is essential for survival of postmitotic rod photoreceptor cells in mice. *FASEB J.* **2014**, *28*, 3780–3791. [CrossRef]

25. Aldunate, E.Z.; Di Foggia, V.; Di Marco, F.; Hervas, L.A.; Ribeiro, J.C.; Holder, D.L.; Patel, A.; Jannini, T.B.; Thompson, D.A.; Martinez-Barbera, J.P.; et al. Conditional Dicer1 depletion using Chrnb4-Cre leads to cone cell death and impaired photopic vision. *Sci. Rep.* **2019**, *9*, 2314. [CrossRef]
26. Lagos-Quintana, M. New microRNAs from mouse and human. *RNA* **2003**, *9*, 175–179. [CrossRef]
27. Xu, S.; Witmer, P.D.; Lumayag, S.; Kovacs, B.; Valle, D. MicroRNA (miRNA) transcriptome of mouse retina and identification of a sensory organ-specific miRNA cluster. *J. Biol. Chem.* **2007**, *282*, 25053–25066. [CrossRef]
28. Weston, M.D.; Pierce, M.L.; Rocha-Sanchez, S.; Beisel, K.W.; Soukup, G.A. MicroRNA gene expression in the mouse inner ear. *Brain Res.* **2006**, *1111*, 95–104. [CrossRef] [PubMed]
29. Aldrich, B.T.; Frakes, E.P.; Kasuya, J.; Hammond, D.L.; Kitamoto, T. Changes in expression of sensory organ-specific microRNAs in rat dorsal root ganglia in association with mechanical hypersensitivity induced by spinal nerve ligation. *Neuroscience* **2009**, *164*, 711–723. [CrossRef]
30. Jin, Z.B.; Hirokawa, G.; Gui, L.; Takahashi, R.; Osakada, F.; Hiura, Y.; Takahashi, M.; Yasuhara, O.; Iwai, N. Targeted deletion of miR-182, an abundant retinal microRNA. *Mol. Vis.* **2009**, *15*, 523–533.
31. Dambal, S.; Shah, M.; Mihelich, B.; Nonn, L. The microRNA-183 cluster: The family that plays together stays together. *Nucleic Acids Res.* **2015**, *43*, 7173–7188. [CrossRef]
32. Zhu, Q.; Sun, W.; Okano, K.; Chen, Y.; Zhang, N.; Maeda, T.; Palczewski, K. Sponge transgenic mouse model reveals important roles for the microRNA-183 (miR-183)/96/182 cluster in postmitotic photoreceptors of the retina. *J. Biol. Chem.* **2011**, *286*, 31749–31760. [CrossRef] [PubMed]
33. Lumayag, S.; Haldin, C.E.; Corbett, N.J.; Wahlin, K.J.; Cowan, C.; Turturro, S.; Larsen, P.E.; Kovacs, B.; Witmer, P.D.; Valle, D.; et al. Inactivation of the microRNA-183/96/182 cluster results in syndromic retinal degeneration. *Proc. Natl. Acad. Sci. USA* **2013**, *110*, E507–E516. [CrossRef]
34. Krol, J.; Krol, I.; Alvarez, C.P.; Fiscella, M.; Hierlemann, A.; Roska, B.; Filipowicz, W. A network comprising short and long noncoding RNAs and RNA helicase controls mouse retina architecture. *Nat. Commun.* **2015**, *6*, 7305. [CrossRef] [PubMed]
35. Davari, M.; Soheili, Z.S.; Samiei, S.; Sharifi, Z.; Pirmardan, E.R. Overexpression of miR-183/-96/-182 triggers neuronal cell fate in Human Retinal Pigment Epithelial (hRPE) cells in culture. *Biochem. Biophys. Res. Commun.* **2017**, *483*, 745–751. [CrossRef] [PubMed]
36. Palfi, A.; Hokamp, K.; Hauck, S.M.; Vencken, S.; Millington-Ward, S.; Chadderton, N.; Carrigan, M.; Kortvely, E.; Greene, C.M.; Kenna, P.F.; et al. microRNA regulatory circuits in a mouse model of inherited retinal degeneration. *Sci. Rep.* **2016**, *6*, 31431. [CrossRef] [PubMed]
37. Lagos-Quintana, M.; Rauhut, R.; Yalcin, A.; Meyer, J.; Lendeckel, W.; Tuschl, T. Identification of tissue-specific microRNAs from mouse. *Curr. Biol.: Cb.* **2002**, *12*, 735–739. [CrossRef]
38. Landgraf, P.; Rusu, M.; Sheridan, R.; Sewer, A.; Iovino, N.; Aravin, A.; Pfeffer, S.; Rice, A.; Kamphorst, A.O.; Landthaler, M.; et al. A mammalian microRNA expression atlas based on small RNA library sequencing. *Cell* **2007**, *129*, 1401–1414. [CrossRef]
39. Karali, M.; Peluso, I.; Marigo, V.; Banfi, S. Identification and characterization of microRNAs expressed in the mouse eye. *Invest. Ophthalmol. Vis. Sci.* **2007**, *48*, 509–515. [CrossRef] [PubMed]
40. Sanuki, R.; Onishi, A.; Koike, C.; Muramatsu, R.; Watanabe, S.; Muranishi, Y.; Irie, S.; Uneo, S.; Koyasu, T.; Matsui, R.; et al. miR-124a is required for hippocampal axogenesis and retinal cone survival through Lhx2 suppression. *Nat. Neurosci.* **2011**, *14*, 1125–1134. [CrossRef]
41. Chu-Tan, J.A.; Rutar, M.; Saxena, K.; Aggio-Bruce, R.; Essex, R.W.; Valter, K.; Jiao, H.; Fernando, N.; Wooff, Y.; Madigan, M.C.; et al. MicroRNA-124 Dysregulation is Associated With Retinal Inflammation and Photoreceptor Death in the Degenerating Retina. *Invest. Ophthalmol. Vis. Sci.* **2018**, *59*, 4094–4105. [CrossRef]
42. Rutar, M.; Natoli, R.; Valter, K.; Provis, J.M. Early focal expression of the chemokine Ccl2 by Muller cells during exposure to damage-inducing bright continuous light. *Invest. Ophthalmol. Vis. Sci.* **2011**, *52*, 2379–2388. [CrossRef]
43. Newman, A.M.; Gallo, N.B.; Hancox, L.S.; Miller, N.J.; Radeke, C.M.; Maloney, M.A.; Cooper, J.B.; Hageman, G.S.; Anderson, D.H.; Johnson, L.V.; et al. Systems-level analysis of age-related macular degeneration reveals global biomarkers and phenotype-specific functional networks. *Genome Med.* **2012**, *4*, 16. [CrossRef] [PubMed]
44. Guo, C.; Otani, A.; Oishi, A.; Kojima, H.; Makiyama, Y.; Nakagawa, S.; Yoshimura, N. Knockout of ccr2 alleviates photoreceptor cell death in a model of retinitis pigmentosa. *Exp. Eye Res.* **2012**, *104*, 39–47. [CrossRef] [PubMed]

45. Rutar, M.; Natoli, R.; Provis, J.M. Small interfering RNA-mediated suppression of Ccl2 in Muller cells attenuates microglial recruitment and photoreceptor death following retinal degeneration. *J. Neuroinflammation* **2012**, *9*, 221. [CrossRef] [PubMed]
46. Sennlaub, F.; Auvynet, C.; Calippe, B.; Lavalette, S.; Poupel, L.; Hu, S.J.; Dominguez, E.; Camelo, S.; Levy, O.; Guyon, E.; et al. CCR2(+) monocytes infiltrate atrophic lesions in age-related macular disease and mediate photoreceptor degeneration in experimental subretinal inflammation in Cx3cr1 deficient mice. *Embo. Mol. Med.* **2013**, *5*, 1775–1793. [CrossRef]
47. Fu, Y.; Hou, B.; Weng, C.; Liu, W.; Dai, J.; Zhao, C.; Yin, Z.Q. Functional ectopic neuritogenesis by retinal rod bipolar cells is regulated by miR-125b-5p during retinal remodeling in RCS rats. *Sci. Rep.* **2017**, *7*, 1011. [CrossRef]
48. Jayaram, H.; Cepurna, W.O.; Johnson, E.C.; Morrison, J.C. MicroRNA Expression in the Glaucomatous Retina. *Invest. Ophthalmol. Vis. Sci.* **2015**, *56*, 7971–7982. [CrossRef]
49. Nie, X.G.; Fan, D.S.; Huang, Y.X.; He, Y.Y.; Dong, B.L.; Gao, F. Downregulation of microRNA-149 in retinal ganglion cells suppresses apoptosis through activation of the PI3K/Akt signaling pathway in mice with glaucoma. *Am. J. Physiol. Cell Physiol.* **2018**, *315*, C839–C849. [CrossRef]
50. Li, R.; Jin, Y.; Li, Q.; Sun, X.; Zhu, H.; Cui, H. MiR-93-5p targeting PTEN regulates the NMDA-induced autophagy of retinal ganglion cells via AKT/mTOR pathway in glaucoma. *Biomed. Pharm.* **2018**, *100*, 1–7. [CrossRef]
51. Li, H.J.; Sun, Z.L.; Pan, Y.B.; Sun, Y.Y.; Xu, M.H.; Feng, D.F. Inhibition of miRNA-21 promotes retinal ganglion cell survival and visual function by modulating Muller cell gliosis after optic nerve crush. *Exp. Cell Res.* **2019**, *375*, 10–19. [CrossRef]
52. Zhang, Q.L.; Wang, W.; Li, J.; Tian, S.Y.; Zhang, T.Z. Decreased miR-187 induces retinal ganglion cell apoptosis through upregulating SMAD7 in glaucoma. *Biomed. Pharm.* **2015**, *75*, 19–25. [CrossRef] [PubMed]
53. Yang, J.; Wang, N.; Luo, X. Intraocular miR-211 exacerbates pressure-induced cell death in retinal ganglion cells via direct repression of FRS2 signaling. *Biochem. Biophys. Res. Commun.* **2018**, *503*, 2984–2992. [CrossRef]
54. Kong, N.; Lu, X.; Li, B. Downregulation of microRNA-100 protects apoptosis and promotes neuronal growth in retinal ganglion cells. *BMC Mol. Biol.* **2014**, *15*, 25. [CrossRef] [PubMed]
55. Shao, Y.; Yu, Y.; Zhou, Q.; Li, C.; Yang, L.; Pei, C.G. Inhibition of miR-134 Protects Against Hydrogen Peroxide-Induced Apoptosis in Retinal Ganglion Cells. *J. Mol. Neurosci.* **2015**, *56*, 461–471. [CrossRef]
56. Damiani, D.; Alexander, J.J.; O'Rourke, J.R.; McManus, M.; Jadhav, A.P.; Cepko, C.L.; Hauswirth, W.W.; Harfe, B.D.; Strettoi, E. Dicer inactivation leads to progressive functional and structural degeneration of the mouse retina. *J. Neurosci.* **2008**, *28*, 4878–4887. [CrossRef] [PubMed]
57. Pinter, R.; Hindges, R. Perturbations of microRNA function in mouse dicer mutants produce retinal defects and lead to aberrant axon pathfinding at the optic chiasm. *Plos ONE* **2010**, *5*, e10021. [CrossRef]
58. Iida, A.; Shinoe, T.; Baba, Y.; Mano, H.; Watanabe, S. Dicer plays essential roles for retinal development by regulation of survival and differentiation. *Invest. Ophthalmol. Vis. Sci* **2011**, *52*, 3008–3017. [CrossRef] [PubMed]
59. Reh, T.A.; Hindges, R. MicroRNAs in Retinal Development. *Annu. Rev. Vis. Sci.* **2018**, *4*, 25–44. [CrossRef]
60. Georgi, S.A.; Reh, T.A. Dicer is required for the transition from early to late progenitor state in the developing mouse retina. *J. Neurosci.* **2010**, *30*, 4048–4061. [CrossRef]
61. La Torre, A.; Georgi, S.; Reh, T.A. Conserved microRNA pathway regulates developmental timing of retinal neurogenesis. *Proc. Natl. Acad. Sci. USA* **2013**, *110*, E2362–E2370. [CrossRef] [PubMed]
62. Xia, X.; Ahmad, I. let-7 microRNA regulates neurogliogenesis in the mammalian retina through Hmga2. *Dev. Biol.* **2016**, *410*, 70–85. [CrossRef] [PubMed]
63. Karali, M.; Manfredi, A.; Puppo, A.; Marrocco, E.; Gargiulo, A.; Allocca, M.; Corte, M.D.; Rossi, S.; Giunti, M.; Bacci, M.L.; et al. MicroRNA-restricted transgene expression in the retina. *Plos ONE* **2011**, *6*, e22166. [CrossRef]
64. Hackler, L., Jr.; Wan, J.; Swaroop, A.; Qian, J.; Zack, D.J. MicroRNA profile of the developing mouse retina. *Invest. Ophthalmol. Vis. Sci.* **2010**, *51*, 1823–1831. [CrossRef]
65. Jeon, C.J.; Strettoi, E.; Masland, R.H. The major cell populations of the mouse retina. *J. Neurosci.* **1998**, *18*, 8936–8946. [CrossRef]
66. Quintero, H.; Gomez-Montalvo, A.I.; Lamas, M. MicroRNA changes through Muller glia dedifferentiation and early/late rod photoreceptor differentiation. *Neuroscience* **2016**, *316*, 109–121. [CrossRef]

67. Wohl, S.G.; Reh, T.A. The microRNA expression profile of mouse Muller glia in vivo and in vitro. *Sci. Rep.* **2016**, *6*, 35423. [CrossRef]
68. Wohl, S.G.; Jorstad, N.L.; Levine, E.M.; Reh, T.A. Muller glial microRNAs are required for the maintenance of glial homeostasis and retinal architecture. *Nat. Commun.* **2017**, *8*, 1603. [CrossRef]
69. Jones, B.W.; Watt, C.B.; Frederick, J.M.; Baehr, W.; Chen, C.K.; Levine, E.M.; Milam, A.H.; Lavail, M.M.; Marc, R.E. Retinal remodeling triggered by photoreceptor degenerations. *J. Comp. Neurol.* **2003**, *464*, 1–16. [CrossRef]
70. Chung, S.H.; Shen, W.; Jayawardana, K.; Wang, P.; Yang, J.; Shackel, N.; Gillies, M.C. Differential gene expression profiling after conditional Muller-cell ablation in a novel transgenic model. *Invest. Ophthalmol. Vis. Sci.* **2013**, *54*, 2142–2152. [CrossRef]
71. Chung, S.H.; Gillies, M.; Sugiyama, Y.; Zhu, L.; Lee, S.R.; Shen, W. Profiling of microRNAs involved in retinal degeneration caused by selective Muller cell ablation. *Plos ONE* **2015**, *10*, e0118949. [CrossRef] [PubMed]
72. Byrne, L.C.; Khalid, F.; Lee, T.; Zin, E.A.; Greenberg, K.P.; Visel, M.; Schaffer, D.V.; Flannery, J.G. AAV-mediated, optogenetic ablation of Muller Glia leads to structural and functional changes in the mouse retina. *Plos ONE* **2013**, *8*, e76075. [CrossRef] [PubMed]
73. Shen, W.; Lee, S.R.; Araujo, J.; Chung, S.H.; Zhu, L.; Gillies, M.C. Effect of glucocorticoids on neuronal and vascular pathology in a transgenic model of selective Muller cell ablation. *Glia* **2014**, *62*, 1110–1124. [CrossRef]
74. Ramachandran, R.; Fausett, B.V.; Goldman, D. Ascl1a regulates Muller glia dedifferentiation and retinal regeneration through a Lin-28-dependent, let-7 microRNA signalling pathway. *Nat. Cell Biol.* **2010**, *12*, 1101–1107. [CrossRef] [PubMed]
75. Goldman, D. Muller glial cell reprogramming and retina regeneration. *Nat. Rev. Neurosci.* **2014**, *15*, 431–442. [CrossRef]
76. Yao, K.; Qiu, S.; Tian, L.; Snider, W.D.; Flannery, J.G.; Schaffer, D.V.; Chen, B. Wnt Regulates Proliferation and Neurogenic Potential of Muller Glial Cells via a Lin28/let-7 miRNA-Dependent Pathway in Adult Mammalian Retinas. *Cell Rep.* **2016**, *17*, 165–178. [CrossRef] [PubMed]
77. Kaur, S.; Gupta, S.; Chaudhary, M.; Khursheed, M.A.; Mitra, S.; Kurup, A.J.; Ramachandran, R. let-7 MicroRNA-Mediated Regulation of Shh Signaling and the Gene Regulatory Network Is Essential for Retina Regeneration. *Cell Rep.* **2018**, *23*, 1409–1423. [CrossRef] [PubMed]
78. Jorstad, N.L.; Wilken, M.S.; Grimes, W.N.; Wohl, S.G.; VandenBosch, L.S.; Yoshimatsu, T.; Wong, R.O.; Rieke, F.; Reh, T.A. Stimulation of functional neuronal regeneration from Muller glia in adult mice. *Nature* **2017**, *548*, 103–107. [CrossRef]
79. Papagiannakopoulos, T.; Kosik, K.S. MicroRNA-124: Micromanager of neurogenesis. *Cell Stem Cell* **2009**, *4*, 375–376. [CrossRef]
80. Cheng, L.C.; Pastrana, E.; Tavazoie, M.; Doetsch, F. miR-124 regulates adult neurogenesis in the subventricular zone stem cell niche. *Nat. Neurosci.* **2009**, *12*, 399–408. [CrossRef]
81. Maiorano, N.A.; Mallamaci, A. Promotion of embryonic cortico-cerebral neuronogenesis by miR-124. *Neural Dev.* **2009**, *4*, 40. [CrossRef]
82. Masserdotti, G.; Gillotin, S.; Sutor, B.; Drechsel, D.; Irmler, M.; Jorgensen, H.F.; Sass, S.; Theis, F.J.; Beckers, J.; Berninger, B.; et al. Transcriptional Mechanisms of Proneural Factors and REST in Regulating Neuronal Reprogramming of Astrocytes. *Cell Stem Cell* **2015**, *17*, 74–88. [CrossRef]
83. Abrajano, J.J.; Qureshi, I.A.; Gokhan, S.; Zheng, D.; Bergman, A.; Mehler, M.F. REST and CoREST modulate neuronal subtype specification, maturation and maintenance. *Plos ONE* **2009**, *4*, e7936. [CrossRef]
84. Visvanathan, J.; Lee, S.; Lee, B.; Lee, J.W.; Lee, S.K. The microRNA miR-124 antagonizes the anti-neural REST/SCP1 pathway during embryonic CNS development. *Genes Dev.* **2007**, *21*, 744–749. [CrossRef] [PubMed]
85. Conaco, C.; Otto, S.; Han, J.J.; Mandel, G. Reciprocal actions of REST and a microRNA promote neuronal identity. *Proc. Natl. Acad. Sci. USA* **2006**, *103*, 2422–2427. [CrossRef]
86. Nesti, E.; Corson, G.M.; McCleskey, M.; Oyer, J.A.; Mandel, G. C-terminal domain small phosphatase 1 and MAP kinase reciprocally control REST stability and neuronal differentiation. *Proc. Natl. Acad. Sci. USA* **2014**, *111*, E3929–E3936. [CrossRef] [PubMed]
87. Yeo, M.; Lee, S.K.; Lee, B.; Ruiz, E.C.; Pfaff, S.L.; Gill, G.N. Small CTD phosphatases function in silencing neuronal gene expression. *Sci. (N.Y.)* **2005**, *307*, 596–600. [CrossRef] [PubMed]

88. He, Y.; Li, H.B.; Li, X.; Zhou, Y.; Xia, X.B.; Song, W.T. MiR-124 Promotes the Growth of Retinal Ganglion Cells Derived from Muller Cells. *Cell Physiol. Biochem.* **2018**, *45*, 973–983. [CrossRef]
89. Ji, H.P.; Xiong, Y.; Song, W.T.; Zhang, E.D.; Gao, Z.L.; Yao, F.; Su, T.; Zhou, R.R.; Xia, X.B. MicroRNA-28 potentially regulates the photoreceptor lineage commitment of Muller glia-derived progenitors. *Sci. Rep.* **2017**, *7*, 11374. [CrossRef]
90. Hartong, D.T.; Berson, E.L.; Dryja, T.P. Retinitis pigmentosa. *Lancet* **2006**, *368*, 1795–1809. [CrossRef]
91. Loscher, C.J.; Hokamp, K.; Wilson, J.H.; Li, T.; Humphries, P.; Farrar, G.J.; Palfi, A. A common microRNA signature in mouse models of retinal degeneration. *Exp. Eye Res.* **2008**, *87*, 529–534. [CrossRef]
92. Anasagasti, A.; Ezquerra-Inchausti, M.; Barandika, O.; Munoz-Culla, M.; Caffarel, M.M.; Otaegui, D.; Lopez de Munain, A.; Ruiz-Ederra, J. Expression Profiling Analysis Reveals Key MicroRNA-mRNA Interactions in Early Retinal Degeneration in Retinitis Pigmentosa. *Invest. Ophthalmol. Vis. Sci.* **2018**, *59*, 2381–2392. [CrossRef]
93. Chang, B.; Hawes, N.L.; Hurd, R.E.; Davisson, M.T.; Nusinowitz, S.; Heckenlively, J.R. Retinal degeneration mutants in the mouse. *Vis. Res.* **2002**, *42*, 517–525. [CrossRef]
94. Genini, S.; Guziewicz, K.E.; Beltran, W.A.; Aguirre, G.D. Altered miRNA expression in canine retinas during normal development and in models of retinal degeneration. *BMC Genom.* **2014**, *15*, 172. [CrossRef]
95. Vasudevan, S.; Tong, Y.; Steitz, J.A. Switching from repression to activation: microRNAs can up-regulate translation. *Sci. (N.Y.)* **2007**, *318*, 1931–1934. [CrossRef] [PubMed]
96. Ma, C.; Papermaster, D.; Cepko, C.L. A unique pattern of photoreceptor degeneration in cyclin D1 mutant mice. *Proc. Natl. Acad. Sci. USA* **1998**, *95*, 9938–9943. [CrossRef] [PubMed]
97. Kutty, R.K.; Nagineni, C.N.; Samuel, W.; Vijayasarathy, C.; Hooks, J.J.; Redmond, T.M. Inflammatory cytokines regulate microRNA-155 expression in human retinal pigment epithelial cells by activating JAK/STAT pathway. *Biochem. Biophys. Res. Commun.* **2010**, *402*, 390–395. [CrossRef]
98. Lukiw, W.J.; Surjyadipta, B.; Dua, P.; Alexandrov, P.N. Common micro RNAs (miRNAs) target complement factor H (CFH) regulation in Alzheimer's disease (AD) and in age-related macular degeneration (AMD). *Int. J. Biochem. Mol. Biol.* **2012**, *3*, 105–116.
99. Karali, M.; Persico, M.; Mutarelli, M.; Carissimo, A.; Pizzo, M.; Singh Marwah, V.; Ambrosio, C.; Pinelli, M.; Carrella, D.; Ferrari, S.; et al. High-resolution analysis of the human retina miRNome reveals isomiR variations and novel microRNAs. *Nucleic Acids Res* **2016**, *44*, 1525–1540. [CrossRef]
100. Ryan, D.G.; Oliveira-Fernandes, M.; Lavker, R.M. MicroRNAs of the mammalian eye display distinct and overlapping tissue specificity. *Mol. Vis.* **2006**, *12*, 1175–1184.
101. Karali, M.; Peluso, I.; Gennarino, V.A.; Bilio, M.; Verde, R.; Lago, G.; Dolle, P.; Banfi, S. miRNeye: A microRNA expression atlas of the mouse eye. *BMC Genom.* **2010**, *11*, 715. [CrossRef] [PubMed]
102. Berezikov, E. Evolution of microRNA diversity and regulation in animals. *Nat. Rev. Genet.* **2011**, *12*, 846–860. [CrossRef] [PubMed]

7

Selective Ablation of Dehydrodolichyl Diphosphate Synthase in Murine Retinal Pigment Epithelium (RPE) Causes RPE Atrophy and Retinal Degeneration

Marci L. DeRamus [1], Stephanie J. Davis [1], Sriganesh Ramachandra Rao [2], Cyril Nyankerh [1], Delores Stacks [1], Timothy W. Kraft [1], Steven J. Fliesler [2] and Steven J. Pittler [1,*]

1 Department of Optometry and Vision Science, Vision Science Research Center, University of Alabama at Birmingham, Birmingham, AL 35294, USA; marcismith1952@gmail.com (M.L.D.); stephanie.davis@bison.howard.edu (S.J.D.); cyrilnya@uab.edu (C.N.); delorez@uab.edu (D.S.); twkraft@uab.edu (T.W.K.)

2 Departments of Ophthalmology and Biochemistry, State University of New York-University at Buffalo, Buffalo, NY 14209, USA; and Research Service, VA Western NY Healthcare System, Buffalo, NY 14215, USA; sramacha@buffalo.edu (S.R.R.); fliesler@buffalo.edu (S.J.F.)

* Correspondence: pittler@uab.edu;

Abstract: Patients with certain defects in the dehydrodolichyl diphosphate synthase (DHDDS) gene (RP59; OMIM #613861) exhibit classic symptoms of retinitis pigmentosa, as well as macular changes, suggestive of retinal pigment epithelium (RPE) involvement. The DHDDS enzyme is ubiquitously required for several pathways of protein glycosylation. We wish to understand the basis for selective ocular pathology associated with certain DHDDS mutations and the contribution of specific ocular cell types to the pathology of mutant *Dhdds*-mediated retinal degeneration. To circumvent embryonic lethality associated with *Dhdds* knockout, we generated a Cre-dependent knockout allele of murine *Dhdds* (*Dhdds*$^{flx/flx}$). We used targeted Cre expression to study the importance of the enzyme in the RPE. Structural alterations of the RPE and retina including reduction in outer retinal thickness, cell layer disruption, and increased RPE hyper-reflectivity were apparent at one postnatal month. At three months, RPE and photoreceptor disruption was observed non-uniformly across the retina as well as RPE transmigration into the photoreceptor layer, external limiting membrane descent towards the RPE, and patchy loss of photoreceptors. Functional loss measured by electroretinography was consistent with structural loss showing scotopic a- and b-wave reductions of 83% and 77%, respectively, at three months. These results indicate that RPE dysfunction contributes to DHDDS mutation-mediated pathology and suggests a more complicated disease mechanism than simply disruption of glycosylation.

Keywords: retinal degeneration; retinitis pigmentosa; retinal pigment epithelium dystrophy; RPE transmigration; Cre-Lox technology; mouse models

---

1. Introduction

Retinitis pigmentosa (RP) and related disorders are characterized by degeneration and loss of photoreceptors, attenuation of retinal blood vessels, pigment deposits, and a waxy pallor of the optic disc that result in impaired night vision and peripheral and central vision loss [1]. Defective protein glycosylation in the retinal pigment epithelium (RPE) has been associated with retinal degeneration elicited by photoreceptor abnormalities and impaired phagocytosis of aging photoreceptor outer segment (OS) membranes [2–5]. One such example, dehydrodolichyl diphosphate synthase (DHDDS; OMIM #608172), is an essential enzyme in the mevalonate pathway where it functions ubiquitously in isoprenoid chain elongation to form dolichols that comprise 17–20 isoprene units. The phosphorylated form of dolichol, dolichol pyrophosphate is necessary for N-glycosylation at specific residues in many membrane proteins [6]. There is no known unique function for DHDDS in the retina, or in any other ocular tissue. There are numerous N-glycosylated proteins in the retina and photoreceptors, such as rhodopsin [7] and the cGMP-gated cation channel in rods. Additionally, in the RPE, there are several glycosylated structural proteins, ion channels and transport proteins that contribute to the transepithelial potential of the polarized RPE monolayer [8–10].

Mutations in the gene encoding DHDDS lead to a recessive form of RP called RP59 (OMIM #613861, DHDDS, K42E), which was first identified in several families of Ashkenazi Jewish origin [11–13]. RP59 is considered to belong to the family of human genetic diseases known as "congenital disorders of glycosylation" (CDGs) [14]. Two other mutations in the DHDDS gene (T206A and R98W), which occur heterozygously with the K42E mutation, were also reported, but have not been studied in detail [15,16]. Patients with the K42E mutation in DHDDS exhibit all the cardinal features of RP as well as macular changes [12], suggesting possible RPE involvement. While the K42E, T206A, and R98W mutations are only associated with known RP symptoms, another mutation in the DHDDS gene has led to infant morbidity at seven months of age [17].

As a first step to assess the role of DHDDS in specific retinal cell types and to understand the molecular mechanism of RP59, we created a Cre-lox dependent line of mice that allows targeted, cell type-specific deletion of *Dhdds* in cells of interest. Using a conditional knockout was necessary to circumvent embryonic lethality associated with global knockout of *Dhdds* [18,19]. Here, we describe the generation and characterization of a *Dhdds*$^{flx/flx}$ CreRPE mouse line (i.e., RPE-specific *Dhdds* knockout) and its validation as a model of RPE atrophy and retinal degeneration. We show that RPE-specific deletion of *Dhdds* induces structural and functional deficits in the RPE and the photoreceptors, which suggests that RPE pathology may be a significant contributor to the retinal degeneration observed in patients with RP59 mutations.

2. Materials and Methods

2.1. Generation of *Dhdds*$^{flx/flx}$ CreRPE Mice

A construct containing lacZ flanked by FLP-FRT and *Dhdds* exon 3 flanked by loxP sites from the Knockout Mouse Project (KOMP, UC Davis, Davis, CA, USA) was linearized and introduced into mouse ES cells (C57Bl/6J background) at the Roswell Park Cancer Institute (RPCI) Gene Targeting and Transgenic Facility (Buffalo, NY, USA) using standard technology. To confirm the correctly targeted cells, polymerase chain reaction (PCR) was performed with the primers listed below (see *PCR Genotyping*, below). The lacZ cassette was excised with FLP-FRT recombinase, and excision was confirmed by PCR. Mouse lines that carried the *Dhdds* loxP conditional knockout allele were crossed to generate homozygotes and the latter were also crossed to a mouse line (on a C57Bl/6J background) carrying a homozygous transgene expressing Cre recombinase under the control of the RPE-specific VMD2 (vitelliform macular degeneration 2) promoter [20,21]. RPE-specific expression of Cre in the VMD2 promoter-driven mouse line was confirmed by crossing those mice with a ZsGreen reporter mouse line (B6.Cg-*Gt(ROSA)26Sor*$^{tm6(CAG-ZsGreen1)Hze}$/J, The Jackson Laboratory, Bar Harbor, ME, USA) and examining the retinas by confocal fluorescence microscopy. Genotypes of offspring were confirmed by PCR with *Dhdds*- and Cre RPE-specific primer pairs. All mice used in this study were treated following the ARVO *Statement on the Use of Animals in Ophthalmic and Vision Research* and the policies of the University of Alabama at Birmingham (UAB) Institutional Animal Care and Use Committee (IACUC). This project was approved for animal use on April 2019 by the UAB IACUC and requires updated approvals each year (protocol number IACUC-21270). All animals were maintained on a standard 12/12-h light/dark cycle, fed standard rodent chow, provided water *ad libitum*, and housed in plastic cages with standard rodent bedding.

2.2. PCR Genotyping

Mouse genomic DNA samples obtained from tail snips were verified by PCR using primers *Dhdds*-FWD: 5′-GTGTCATCCCCTGCTGCAGAT-3′ and *Dhdds*-REV: 5′-TGGGTGTAGTGGCTCAGGTC-3′ for genotype identification of floxed *Dhdds* alleles designed in a region which was conserved in both wild type (WT) and floxed alleles and also in the region flanking the loxP sites. The expected PCR product sizes for the WT and floxed alleles are 393 and 517 bp, respectively, thus differentiating WT, heterozygous floxed, and homozygous floxed alleles. PCR verification of Cre transgene modification was carried out using the following forward and reverse primer sets for Cre RPE 5′-AGGTGTAGAGAAGGCACTTAGC-3′ and 5′-CTAATCGCCATCT-TCCAGCAGG-3′, respectively, yielding a 411 bp product. RPE specific expression and activity of Cre-recombinase in VMD2-RPE Cre was verified by breeding these mouse lines against an ZsGreen reporter mouse strain (B6.Cg-*Gt(ROSA)26Sor*$^{tm6(CAG\text{-}ZsGreen1)Hze}$/J, Stock# 007906; The Jackson Laboratory, Bar Harbor, ME, USA) and monitoring ZsGreen expression in the retina.

2.3. Spectral-Domain Optical Coherence Tomography

Spectral-domain optical coherence tomography (SD-OCT) (840 nm; Bioptigen, Inc./Leica, Durham, NC, USA) was used to obtain in vivo images of the retina at one, two, and three months of age. OCT images were collected with Bioptigen InVivoVue® 1.4 software and Bioptigen Diver® 2.0 software was used to analyze outer nuclear layer (ONL) thickness and full retinal thickness (F.R.T.) across all retinal layers at five eccentricities spanning two-thirds of the retina centered at the optic nerve head. A detailed description of this procedure has been reported previously [22]. F.R.T. was calculated from the difference of markers 1 and 10 and ONL thickness was calculated from the difference between 5 and 6.

2.4. Fundus Examination and Fluorescein Angiography

Fundus examination was performed with a Micron IV digital fundus microscope (Phoenix Technology Group, Pleasanton, CA, USA), using the mouse objective and hydroxypropylmethyl cellulose 2.5% on the surface of the cornea. Digital images of the fundus were captured with dedicated StreamPix® 6 digital software (NorPix, Inc., Montreal, Quebec, Canada) and processed using Adobe® Photoshop® 6 (Adobe Systems, Inc., San Jose, CA, USA).

2.5. Visual Function Testing

Full-field scotopic and photopic electroretinograms (ERGs) were obtained as described in detail previously using an OcuScience® HMsERG instrument (OcuScience, Henderson, NV, USA) [22]. Response amplitudes and implicit times of a-waves and b-waves representing the activity of photoreceptors and bipolar cells, respectively, were quantified. In brief, mice were dark-adapted overnight, anesthetized, and then placed on a heating pad to maintain body temperature. Following pupil dilation with 2.5% phenylephrine and 1% tropicamide ophthalmic solutions, a thin silver wire electrode was placed on the cornea (interfaced with methylcellulose and covered with a specially designed contact lens) and referenced to a needle ground electrode in the cheek. The responses to Ganzfeld flash stimuli, spanning a range of five log units, were measured and recorded; following light adaptation to background illumination, cone-driven responses also were recorded.

2.6. Histology/Immunohistochemistry

The methodologies used in this study have been described in detail previously [23]. Briefly, for conventional histology, eyes ($n \geq 4$ per condition) were fixed by immersion in freshly prepared 4% paraformaldehyde in 0.125 M Na-phosphate buffer, pH 7.4, at 4 °C overnight, embedded in paraffin, and tissue sections (toluidine blue-stained) were viewed with an Olympus BH2 photomicroscope equipped with a Nikon digital camera. Digitized images were collected and further analyzed with ImagePro

Plus® software, Version 4.1 (Media Cybernetics; Rockville, MD, USA). For immunohistochemistry, frozen sections of retinal tissue (embedded in Tissue-Plus™ Optimal Cutting Temperature (O.C.T.) compound; Thermo Fisher Scientific, Waltham, MA, USA), obtained with a cryostat and collected on glass microscope slides were incubated with suitable primary antibodies, with detection by application of species-specific, fluor-conjugated secondary antibodies, counterstaining nuclei with DAPI, followed by laser confocal immunofluorescence microscopy (Leica TCS SPE scanning confocal microscope; Leica Microsystems Inc., Buffalo Grove, IL, USA), as previously reported [24].

2.7. Fluorescein Angiography

Fluorescein angiography was performed following intraperitoneal injection (i.p., 10 μL/gram body weight) of a 10 mg/mL solution of AK-Fluor 10% (Sigma Pharmaceuticals; Liberty, IA, USA) in PBS. Uptake of fluorescein and fundus imaging was monitored with a Micron IV Retinal Imaging Microscope (Phoenix Technology Group, Inc., Pleasanton, CA, USA).

2.8. Electron Microscopy

Mouse eyes were processed for plastic embedment, ultramicrotomy, and EM analysis essentially as described in detail previously [23]. Immediately after sacrifice, eyes were orientated by marking the superior hemisphere along the vertical meridian at the limbus with a hot needle, before starting the dissection. A cut was made in the superior cornea and the eyes were fixed for 2 h at 4 °C in fresh 0.1 M sodium phosphate buffer (pH 7.4), containing 2.5% (v/v) glutaraldehyde, 2.0% formaldehyde and 0.025% $CaCl_2$. After a 20–30 min primary fixation, the superior cornea and lens were removed, and fixation was continued overnight. The fixed eyes were then rinsed with 0.1 M sodium cacodylate buffer (pH 7.4) containing 0.025% $CaCl_2$, and then post-fixed for 1 h in 1% osmium tetroxide in 0.1 M sodium cacodylate buffer. After post-fixation, the eyes were rinsed twice in 0.1 M sodium cacodylate buffer and once in distilled water, then dehydrated in graded ethanol series followed by propylene oxide and infiltration overnight in Spurr's resin. The eyes were then embedded in resin-filled BEEM® capsules (Polysciences, Warrington, PA, USA) and allowed to polymerize in a 70 °C oven for 48 h. Tissue sections were obtained with a Reichert–Jung Ultracut E® microtome using a diamond knife. Thin (60–80 nm thickness) sections were collected on copper 75/300 mesh grids and stained with 2% (v/v) uranyl acetate and Reynolds' lead citrate. Sections were viewed with a JEOL 100CX electron microscope at an accelerating voltage of 60 keV.

2.9. Serial Block-Face Scanning Electron Microscopy (SBF-SEM)

Samples prepared for TEM as described above were further processed by Thermo Fisher Scientific (Waltham, MA, USA) using an Apreo VolumeScope™ serial block-face scanning electron microscope (SBF-SEM). Excess resin was removed from the tissue using a Leica ultramicrotome. The trimmed blocks were then glued to a SEM stub (Agar Scientific, AGG1092450) using a two-component silver conductive epoxy, H20E EPO-TEK (Ted Pella, Inc.; Redding, CA, USA). To minimize charging of the block by the electron beam, the bottom and sides of the block were sputter-coated with a 30 nm thick gold film layer. The samples were then imaged on the VolumeScope™ operating in low vacuum mode at 50 Pa and using a lens mounted backscattered detector. All of the data sets were imaged with an accelerating voltage of 2.2 kV and a beam current of 100 pA using 1-μs dwell time combined with two-line integration. Two regions of interest (ROIs) were acquired on the knock-out sample (KO-148). For ROI1, 738 sections were collected with the internal microtome set to a 40 nm cutting thickness (z resolution) with an area of 92.9 μm × 89.1 μm at 10 nm/pixel. For ROI2, 745 sections were collected with an area of 97.6 μm × 96.3 μm using the same imaging condition as ROI1. For the wild type sample (WT-146), an area of 92.9 μm × 89.1 μm was imaged at 10 nm/pixel using a cutting thickness (z resolution) of 40 nm. The acquired data sets were finally aligned and visualized using 3D volume rendering to highlight the RPE anomalies using Amira software (Thermo Fisher Scientific).

2.10. Statistical Analysis

For ERG analyses, we evaluated differences between genetically modified vs. WT control mice across flash intensities by performing repeated measures two-way ANOVA with Holm–Sidak post-hoc analysis at each time point. To evaluate functional (visual acuity, a-wave and b-wave amplitudes and implicit times) and structural (SD-OCT retinal layer thickness) parameters across time, we used a two-way repeated measures ANOVA (time X treatment conditions) with Holm–Sidak post-hoc analysis. For biochemical and quantitative immunohistochemical data, binary statistical comparisons between specific genetically modified vs. WT control group data were analyzed using an unpaired Student's *t*-test.

3. Results

3.1. Generation of a Floxed Dhdds Mouse Line

The scheme used for the generation of a *Dhdds* conditional allele, employing a validated *Dhdds* construct (from KOMP) and mouse embryonic stem cells (ESCs), is shown in Figure 1 (see *Materials and Methods*, above). Clones from confirmed flippase recognition target (FRT)-excised alleles were used to generate *Dhdds* heterozygous and homozygous mouse lines on a C57Bl/6J background.

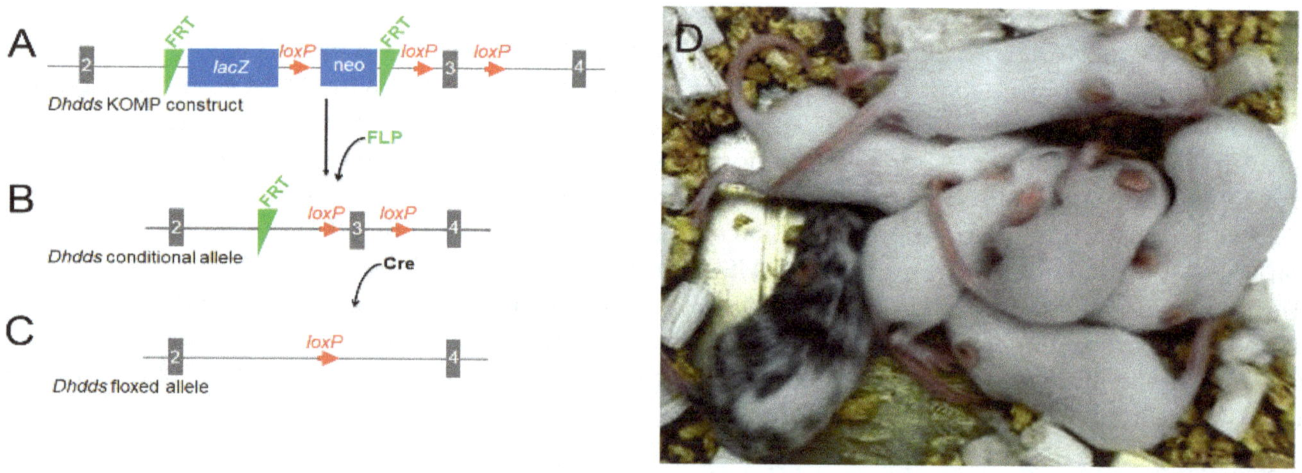

Figure 1. Generation of Cre-dependent *Dhdds* conditional knockout (KO) mice. (**A**) A validated *Dhdds* construct from the Knockout Mouse Project (KOMP) (U.C. Davis) was linearized and introduced into mouse ESCs. (**B**) Transformed cells were treated with FLP-FRT recombinase and PCR was used to verify lacZ cassette excision. (**C**) Clones from confirmed FRT-excised alleles were used to generate *Dhdds*$^{flx/flx-}$ mice. (**D**) Pups carrying the *Dhdds* floxed allele were identified by coat appearance.

3.2. Validation of Retinal Cell Type-Specific Cre-Expressing Mouse Lines

To assess the specificity and efficiency of the Cre recombinase in the RPE, we cross-bred transgenic mice expressing Cre recombinase (bred to homozygosity) with a ZsGreen Ai6 reporter mouse line, and then evaluated ZsGreen expression in the retina by confocal fluorescence microscopy. As expected, WT mouse retinas (a negative control) did not exhibit ZsGreen expression (Figure 2A). However, ZsGreen fluorescence was detected in Cre recombinase-positive mice specifically in the RPE layer by 1 postnatal (PN) month (Figure 2B), with >90% of the RPE cells being labeled. We subsequently confirmed that Cre recombinase continued to be expressed robustly and specifically in the RPE for >3 months (data not shown).

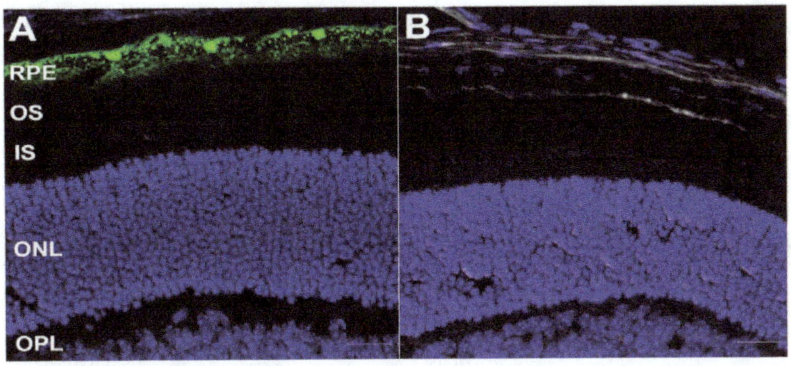

Figure 2. Cre recombinase-dependent ZsGreen expression (green) in mouse retina. (**A**) Retina from a postnatal (PN) one-month old CreRPE × ZsGreen reporter mouse, demonstrating ZsGreen expression specifically in retinal pigment epithelium (RPE) cells. (**B**) Retina from an age-matched, wild type (WT) mouse retina, demonstrating lack of ZsGreen expression. Nuclei counterstained with DAPI (blue). Abbreviations: IS, photoreceptor inner segment layer; OS, photoreceptor outer segment layer; ONL, outer nuclear layer; OPL, outer plexiform layer. Scale bars (both panels): 20 µm.

3.3. RPE-Specific Ablation of Dhdds Causes a Geographic Atrophy-Like Phenotype and Retinal Degeneration, Involving Photoreceptors

In vivo retinal imaging using SD-OCT (Figure 3) showed comparable normal layer stratification in WT, CreRPE and *Dhdds*$^{+/flx}$ CreRPE age-matched mice in each group. However, *Dhdds*$^{flx/flx}$ CreRPE mice showed altered hyper-reflectivity at all ages (indicated by red arrows, Figure 3), indicative of pathologic changes and a reduction in outer retinal layer thickness.

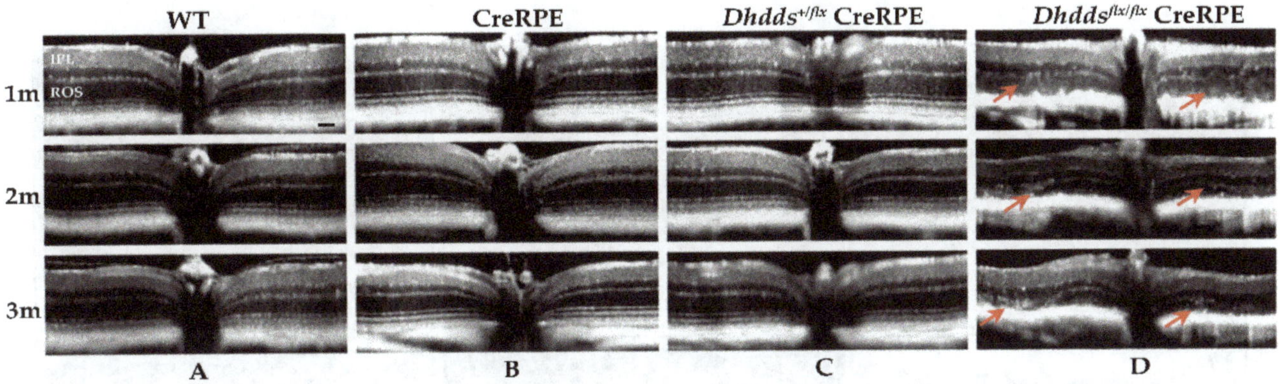

Figure 3. SD-OCT revealed structural changes in *Dhdds*$^{flx/flx}$ CreRPE mice at all ages. OCT scans were performed at 1, 2, and 3 months (m) postnatal for each genotype. (**A**) WT, (**B**) CreRPE, (**C**) *Dhdds*$^{+/flx}$ CreRPE all showed normal layer stratification. (**D**) *Dhdds*$^{flx/flx}$ CreRPE showed alterations of hyper-reflectivity at all ages, indicative of pathologic changes (red arrows) and reduction in layer thickness, particularly in the outer retina. IPL, inner plexiform layer, ROS, rod outer segment. Scale bar (shown in WT 1 m panel): 50 µm, applies to all panels.

"Spidergram" plots of average thickness values (in mm) vs. retinal eccentricity (distance from the optic nerve head (ONH) along with vertical meridian) for the outer nuclear layer (ONL) and FRT are shown in Figure 4. No significant differences were observed when comparing WT, heterozygous, or Cre-only mice for both ONL and FRT measurements. However, *Dhdds*$^{flx/flx}$ CreRPE mice showed a significant reduction (vs. WT) in ONL and F.R.T. values at all ages analyzed ($n \geq 4$, all $p < 0.001$).

Histologically, at PN 3 months, light micrograph images revealed that all retina layers in mice lacking Cre expression appeared normal (Figure 5A and Supplementary Materials, Figure S1A). In contrast, the age-matched Dhdds$^{flx/flx}$ Cre RPE mice displayed a geographic atrophy-like RPE appearance with the most degeneration observed mid-centrally throughout the retina (Supplementary Materials, Figure S1B). There were regions of well-preserved Dhdds$^{flx/flx}$ Cre RPE retina that showed severe RPE pathology (Figure 5B). Notably, the descent of the external limiting membrane (ELM) [25] towards Bruch's membrane was also observed (Figure 5C,E). There was a near-total loss of photoreceptors and RPE within the most affected regions (Figure 5D). Very well-preserved regions were also observed in the periphery (Figure 5F).

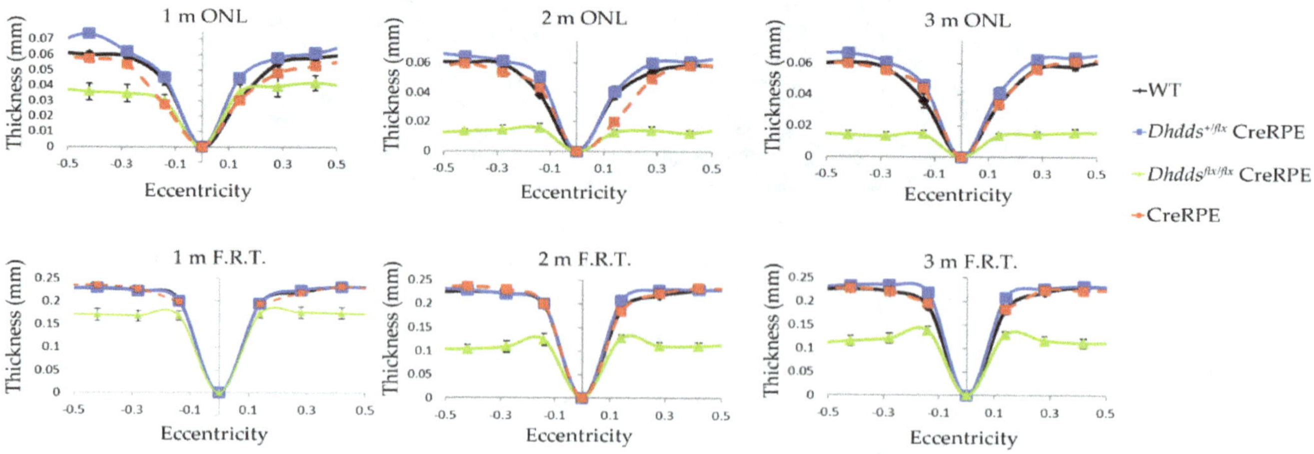

Figure 4. Quantitative morphometric analysis of WT, CreRPE, *Dhdds*$^{+/flx}$ CreRPE, and *Dhdds*$^{flx/flx}$ CreRPE mice SD-OCT data. Average OCT measurements at each eccentricity revealed no significant differences when comparing WT, CreRPE and *Dhdds*$^{+/flx}$ CreRPE mice for both outer nuclear layer (ONL) and F.R.T. thickness measurements (n = 4 for all genotypes, except for WT at one month (1 m; n = 8) and two months (2 m; n = 5). However, significant changes were observed when comparing WT and *Dhdds*$^{flx/flx}$ CreRPE mice at any age with respect to both ONL and F.R.T. values.

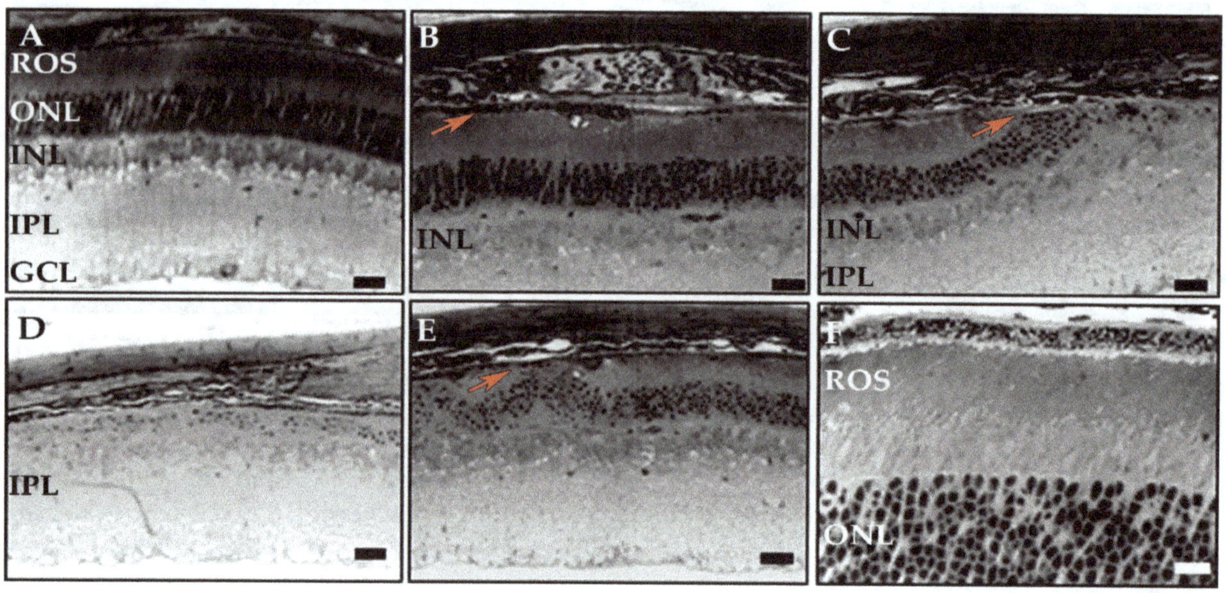

Figure 5. Pathology observed in *Dhdds*$^{flx/flx}$ Cre RPE mouse retina. (**A**) *Dhdds*$^{flx/flx}$ retina without Cre expression appears normal. (**B–F**) Five regions of a retina from a *Dhdds*$^{flx/flx}$ CreRPE mouse expressing Cre in RPE are shown. (**B**,**F**) Relatively well-preserved peripheral retina with some photoreceptor loss, outer segment (OS) shortening, and differing severity of RPE pathology are shown (arrow in panel **B** points to severely compromised RPE. (**C**,**E**) Transition zones of severe to mild retinal pathology showing loss of photoreceptors, severe compromise of RPE and external limiting membrane (ELM) descent (arrows). (**D**) A more central region of the retina showing severe cell loss in both the retina and RPE. Scale bars (all panels, except **F**): 20 μm; scale bar, panel **F**: 10 μm. ROS, rod outer segments; ONL, outer nuclear layer, INL, inner nuclear layer; IPL, inner plexiform layer, GCL, ganglion cell layer.

Additional pathology was revealed by higher magnification EM analysis (Figure 6, panels C–O). In contrast, *Dhdds*$^{flx/flx}$ retinas without Cre expression were indistinguishable from WT retinas (Figure 6A,B). The two areas most affected showed severe RPE dystrophy with concomitant degeneration and loss of photoreceptor cells (Figure 6C,D,F,G,J,M–O). ELM descent was apparent in areas where there was a transition from milder to more severe pathology (* in panels D–F,J). RPE cell transmigration was apparent in the outer retina (arrows, panels G,J,O,L). Thus, compared to WT neural retina and RPE, the observed RPE anomalies including migration of nucleus and RPE melanosomes, displacement of the ELM, and shortened misshaped outer segments throughout the retina were seen in the *Dhdds*$^{flx/flx}$ *CreRPE* mice.

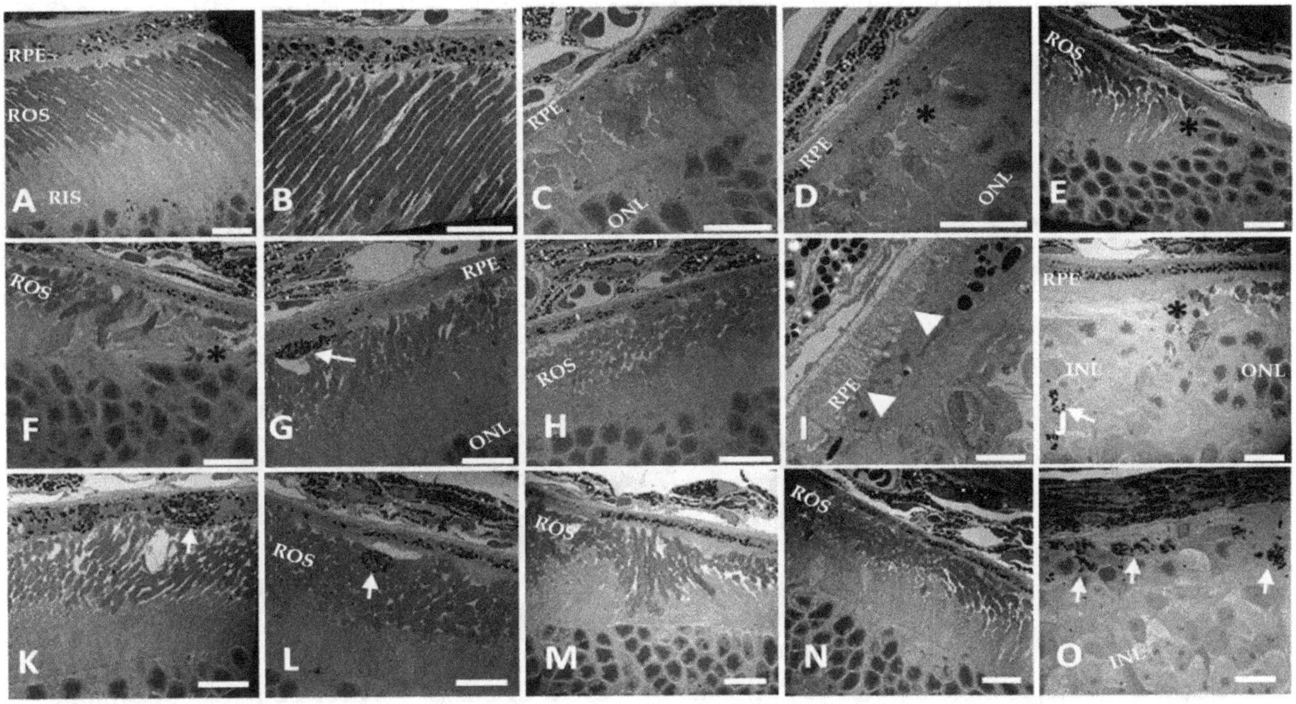

Figure 6. High magnification observation of *Dhdds*$^{flx/flx}$ CreRPE retina. EM images of 3m (**A**,**B**) *Dhdds*$^{flx/flx}$ and (**C**–**O**) *Dhdds*$^{flx/flx}$ CreRPE mice. Mice homozygous for the floxed *Dhdds* allele (*Dhdds*$^{flx/flx}$) are not distinguishable from WT. (**A**) Rod outer segments are properly aligned and all retinal layers are intact (only rod inner and outer segments and the outer nuclear layer are shown). (**B**) The RPE shows normal thickness and melanin distribution. (**C**–**O**) Examples of mildly and severely compromised RPE and retina in *Dhdds*$^{flx/flx}$ CreRPE mice. Severe RPE and outer retina degeneration is concentrated mid-centrally on both sides of the optic nerve head (see histology, Figure 5, and Supplementary Materials, Figure S1). Severe RPE/PR atrophy is observed in the most affected central regions (**C**–**F**,**I**,**J**,**O**). External limiting membrane (ELM) descent (*) towards the RPE is apparent in the transition regions from severely affected to more intact regions (**D**–**F**,**J**). Transmigration of RPE cellular material into the ROS space (arrows) is also seen (**G**,**J**,**L**,**O**). Extended RPE basal fenestrations (arrowheads, **I**) are apparent in the most affected regions (**D**,**I**). Outside of the central region of severe degeneration are regions with compromised but still apparent retinal and RPE layers (**K**–**N**). Scale bars (all panels, except **I**): 10 μm; panel **I**, 2.5 μm.

To further examine the effects of *Dhdds* deletion in the RPE, serial block face-scanning electron microscopy was used to examine a ~100 μ^3 region of the *Dhdds*$^{flx/flx}$ retina across an area of transition from milder to more severe pathology (Supplementary Materials, Videos S1–3). In WT mice, the retina appeared normal in all layers across the entire block. Examination of two regions of the *Dhdds*$^{flx/flx}$ Cre RPE retina showed areas of severe compromise as well as areas where retinal histology was more well-preserved. Transmigration of RPE nuclei and melanosomes into the photoreceptor region (subretinal space and photoreceptor outer segment layer, and even deeper, into the ONL) was also apparent.

3.4. Altered Scotopic and Photopic ERG Amplitudes in *Dhdds$^{flx/flx}$* CreRPE Mice

Analysis by ERG (Figure 7) showed that both homozygous and heterozygous *Dhdds$^{flx/flx}$* CreRPE mice exhibited reduced scotopic ERG a- and b-wave responses. At PN 1 month, scotopic a-wave responses (289 ± 42 μV; n = 5) were significantly reduced in *Dhdds$^{flx/flx}$* CreRPE mice compared to WT mice (395 ± 14 μV; n = 8; $p < 0.05$). Scotopic b-wave responses also were reduced for both *Dhdds$^{+/flx}$* CreRPE (772 ± 42 μV; n = 20) and *Dhdds$^{flx/flx}$* CreRPE (479 ± 69 μV; n = 5) mice, compared to WT mice (934 ± 38 μV; n = 8; $p < 0.01$). At PN 2 months of age, *Dhdds$^{flx/flx}$* CreRPE scotopic ERG a-wave (223 ± 48 μV; n = 10) and b-wave (477 ± 88 μV; n = 10) responses and *Dhdds$^{+/flx}$* CreRPE a-wave (305 ± 19 μV; n = 10) and b-wave (557 ± 64 μV; n = 10) responses were significantly reduced compared to the WT a-wave (366 ± 10 μV; n = 15) and b-wave (935 ± 27 μV; n = 15) responses ($p < 0.005$ for all comparisons). At PN 3 months, scotopic a-wave amplitudes were reduced only in *Dhdds$^{flx/flx}$* CreRPE (60 ± 48 μV; n = 6) compared to WT mice (354 ± 16 μV; n = 18; $p < 0.001$); b-wave responses were reduced in both *Dhdds$^{+/flx}$* CreRPE (662 ± 88 μV; n = 6) and *Dhdds$^{flx/flx}$* CreRPE (150 ± 105 μV; n = 6) mice compared to WT mice (914 ± 35 μV; n = 18) $p < 0.05$ and $p < 0.01$, respectively).

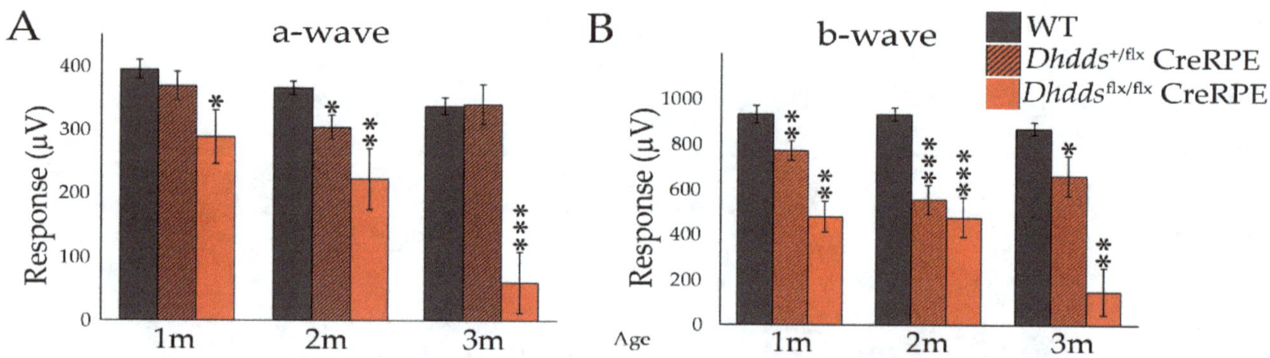

Figure 7. Scotopic ERG analysis of WT, *Dhdds$^{+/flx}$* CreRPE, *Dhdds$^{flx/flx}$* CreRPE mice. Maximum responses to saturating light stimuli showed significant decreases in (**A**) a-wave and (**B**) b-wave amplitudes for *Dhdds$^{+/flx}$* CreRPE and *Dhdds$^{flx/flx}$* CreRPE when compared to WT mice at 1, 2 and 3 postnatal months. Statistical significance: * $p < 0.05$, ** $p < 0.01$, *** $p < 0.001$.

The photopic a-wave and b-wave responses (Figure 8) at PN 1 month were not different when comparing WT (n = 5) and *Dhdds$^{+/flx}$* CreRPE (n = 13) mice, however the photopic responses of *Dhdds$^{flx/flx}$* CreRPE mice (n = 4) were significantly lower. Photopic ERG responses were significantly different only for *Dhdds$^{+/flx}$* CreRPE a-wave (29 ± 2 μV; n = 4; $p < 0.01$), but not b-wave, responses at PN 2 months of age. In *Dhdds$^{flx/flx}$* CreRPE mice, b-wave (86 ± 19 μV; n = 6) amplitudes were significantly reduced ($p < 0.01$), compared to WT mice (n = 13), but not the a-wave responses. At PN 3 months, *Dhdds$^{flx/flx}$* CreRPE mice exhibited significant functional impairment in the photopic a-wave (2 ± 1 μV; n = 4) and b-wave (7 ± 1 μV; n = 4) responses compared to WT a-wave (14 ± 1 μV; n = 9) and b-wave responses (144 ± 8 μV; n = 9; $p < 0.001$ for all comparisons).

Optokinetic reflex (OKR) analysis (Supplementary Materials, Figure S3), a measure of retina-to-brain transmission (i.e., visual capacity), showed reductions in photopic (4–31%) and scotopic (8–29%) contrast sensitivity over the range of 0.031 to 0.272 c/d in PN 3-month old *Dhdds$^{flx/flx}$* CreRPE mice ($p < 0.05$), compared to WT controls of the same age. However, no differences in spatial frequency (a measure of visual acuity) were observed between the different mouse lines. This is partly evident in the OKR scotopic and photopic plots, which show a similar high-frequency cut-off for all three mouse lines examined.

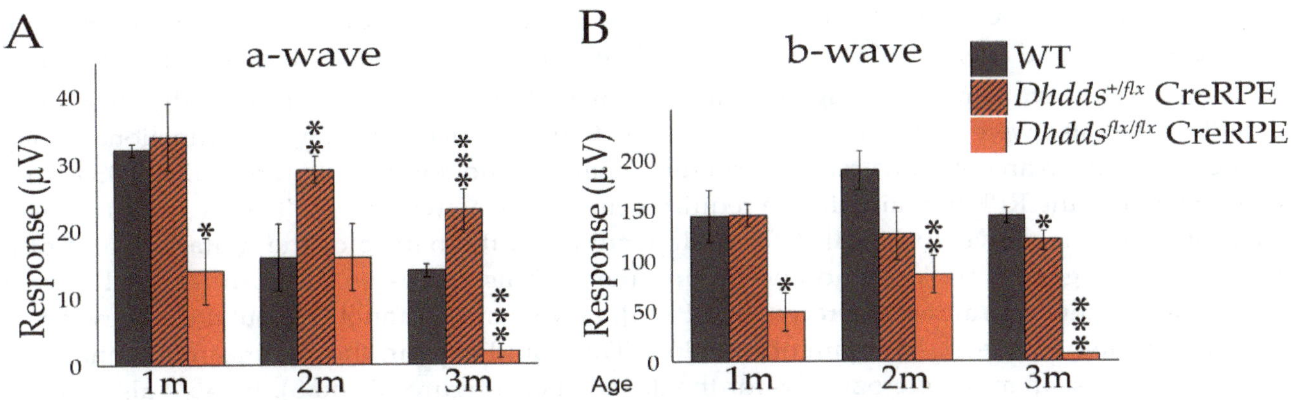

Figure 8. Photopic ERG analysis of WT, CreRPE *Dhdds*$^{+/flx}$, CreRPE *Dhdds*$^{flx/flx}$ mice. (**A**) a-wave responses were significantly lower in CreRPE *Dhdds*$^{-/-}$ at 1 (n = 4) and 3 (n = 4) months postnatal compared to WT (one month (1 m), n = 5; three months (3 m), n = 9) mice. (**B**) Photopic b-wave amplitudes for *Dhdds*$^{+/flx}$ CreRPE mice showed no statistically significant differences when compared to WT mice at 1 (n = 13) and 2 (n = 4) postnatal months, but were reduced by 3 months (n = 4). In contrast, the responses of *Dhdds*$^{flx/flx}$ CreRPE mice (two months (2 m), n = 6) were significantly lower when compared to WT mice at all postnatal ages examined. Statistical significance: * $p < 0.05$, ** $p < 0.01$, *** $p < 0.001$.

4. Discussion

Studies involving genetic screening of families with autosomal recessive retinitis pigmentosa have implicated a founder missense mutation (K42E) in the gene encoding DHDDS [12,26]. DHDDS is required for N-glycosylation of proteins by adding multiple copies of isopentenyl pyrophosphate (IPP) to farnesyl pyrophosphate (FPP) to produce dehydrodolichyl diphosphate (Dedol-PP), a precursor of dolichol, which is utilized as a sugar carrier in protein glycosylation in the endoplasmic reticulum [6]. Even though the generation of isoprenoid chains is complex, involving multiple enzymes and enzyme complexes [27], only DHDDS and Nogo-B receptor are required for long-chain isoprenoid synthesis (C_{70}-C_{120}) [28]. Previous studies have reported that mutations in the opsin gene that abolish N-linked glycosylation cause retinal degeneration [28–30]. To understand the basis for the ocular pathology associated with DHDDS mutation, we utilized a Cre recombinase conditional knockout (*Dhdds*$^{flx/flx}$ CreRPE) driven under the control of the RPE-specific VMD2 promoter to achieve RPE-targeted excision of the loxP-modified *Dhdds* gene, which renders the enzyme non-functional.

The VMD2 construct was originally generated to be conditional on the presence of doxycycline; however, we found that the mice displayed a phenotype in the absence of doxycycline induction. While we cannot rule out the presence of some level of doxycycline in the standard chow mouse diet, it is more likely that Cre expression was due to "leaky" expression, which bypassed doxycycline control, as confirmed in Figure 2. Since the promoters used for cell-specific targeting of Cre expression turn on after development is complete, developmental changes that would otherwise preempt retina/RPE development were not observed.

The expression of Cre recombinase in the Cre lines was confirmed using a ZsGreen reporter strategy. The *Dhdds*$^{flx/flx}$ CreRPE mice exhibited about 90% coverage of Cre expression by PN 1 month (Figure 2) which persisted up to 3 months at least. We crossed the conditional *Dhdds*$^{flx/flx}$ lines with heterozygous VMD2 Cre lines to generate homozygous *Dhdds*$^{flx/flx}$ mice with RPE-specific knockout of DHDDS expression as the model for our study.

In vivo imaging suggested that ONL thickness and F.R.T. were comparable between age-matched WT and *Dhdds*$^{+/flx}$ CreRPE mice, but significantly reduced in *Dhdds*$^{flx/flx}$ CreRPE mice. While the specific pathology is observed in much greater detail in the histological (light microscopy; Figure 5) and ultrastructural (electron microscopy; Figure 6) images provided, it is clear that the pathology indicated in the SD-OCT tomograms (Figure 3D) is consistent with the histological observations. This altered structural integrity of *Dhdds*$^{flx/flx}$ CreRPE retinas also corresponded to a significant decrease in a-wave and b-wave compared to age-matched WT at all flash intensities. Unexpectedly, the scotopic a- and b-waves also were reduced in *Dhdds*$^{+/flx}$ CreRPE mice, which may suggest a functional change that occurs prior to any obvious retinal structural changes and suggests that 50% DHDDS activity is insufficient in the RPE to maintain the required enzymatic activity level. Thus, carriers of *Dhdds* mutations also may develop visual defects, depending on the nature of the mutation, and other factors, such as genetic background and environment. This agrees with the rod-cone dystrophy reported in patients with autosomal recessive RP [16]. However, we cannot rule out the expression of a truncated protein that leads to a gain of function. This could explain the significant attenuation of the photoresponse in mice heterozygous for the floxed allele (Figures 7 and 8). It could also possibly explain the manifestation of the disease only in ocular tissues, if the gain of function is due to specific targeting of retina-specific protein complexes. Further experimentation will be required to sort this out.

We carried out further experiments to examine the fundus of older *Dhdds*$^{flx/flx}$ CreRPE mice at 6, 8 and 10 months PN. These fundus images obtained with fluorescein angiography showed the classical signs of RP including abnormal pigmentation in 8-month old *Dhdds*$^{flx/flx}$ CreRPE mice; vascular changes, including microaneurysms, increased vessel tortuosity and attenuation, were also observed by 6 months of age (Supplementary Materials, Figure S2).

Originally it was proposed that the cause of the pathology in DHDDS-related RP patients (RP59) is defective glycosylation of rod opsin because of reduced DHDDS enzyme activity [12,26]. While this assumption may explain the classic RP symptoms observed, it fails to explain the AMD-like macular involvement. Interestingly, Lam and colleagues [11] found no N-glycosylation deficiency in RP59 patients, based upon isoelectric focusing gel analysis of plasma transferrin (a systemic glycoprotein). In addition, in a related study (Rao et al., manuscript submitted for publication), utilizing a rod photoreceptor-specific knockout of *Dhdds* in mice, we found no evidence for a resulting lack of protein glycosylation in the retina; yet, there was a rapidly progressing photoreceptor degeneration, resulting in complete loss of photoreceptors by PN 6 weeks of age. Also, in a companion article in this Special Issue [31], we generated a mouse model harboring the global K42E homozygous *Dhdds* mutation associated with RP59 patients, but observed no retinal degeneration, even out to 9 postnatal months of age. Clearly, mutations that only partially diminish enzymatic activity would be far less severe than a complete ablation of the gene encoding the enzyme.

5. Conclusions

From these observations, we conclude that targeted ablation of *Dhdds* selectively in RPE cells results in perturbation of DHDDS-dependent processes, resulting in structural and functional deficits in both the RPE and photoreceptors, in a manner resembling geographic atrophy. The degeneration progresses relatively slowly (compared to the rod-specific *Dhdds* ablation model) over the course of a few months, rather than weeks.

Author Contributions: Conceptualization, S.J.P., S.R.R., S.J.F. and M.L.D.; methodology, S.J.D., M.L.D., S.J.F., and S.J.P.; software, S.J.P., M.L.D., and T.W.K; validation, S.J.D., M.L.D., D.S., S.R.R., and S.J.P.; data curation, M.L.D., C.N., S.R.R., S.J.F. and S.J.P.; writing—original draft preparation, M.L.D., C.N., and S.J.P.; writing—review and editing, S.J.F., S.J.P., S.R.R., M.L.D., and D.S., visualization, S.J.P., S.R.R., and S.J.F.; supervision, T.W.K., S.J.F., and S.J.P.; project administration, S.J.F. and S.J.P.; funding acquisition, S.J.P. and S.J.F. All authors have read and agreed to the published version of the manuscript.

Acknowledgments: We thank Jeffrey Messinger for expert technical assistance with light level histology and TEM, Isaac Cobb for technical assistance with some of the experiments, Amy Stablewski (Roswell Park Cancer Institute (RPCI) Gene Targeting and Transgenic Facility) for the generation of *Dhdds*$^{flx/flx}$ mice, and Yun Le (University of Oklahoma Health Sciences Center) for generously providing the CreRPE mouse line. The opinions expressed herein do not reflect those of the Department of Veteran Affairs or the U.S. Government.

References

1. Dryja, T.P.; McGee, T.L.; Reichel, E.; Hahn, L.B.; Cowley, G.S.; Yandell, D.W.; Sandberg, M.A.; Berson, E.L. A point mutation of the rhodopsin gene in one form of retinitis pigmentosa. *Nature* **1990**, *343*, 364–366. [CrossRef] [PubMed]
2. Bok, D.; Hall, M.O. The role of the pigment epithelium in the etiology of inherited retinal dystrophy in the rat. *J. Cell Biol.* **1971**, *49*, 664–682. [CrossRef] [PubMed]
3. Clark, V.M.; Hall, M.O. RPE cell surface proteins in normal and dystrophic rats. *Investig. Ophthalmol. Vis. Sci.* **1986**, *27*, 136–144.
4. Clark, V.M.; Zhou, X.Y.; Pfeffer, B.A. Partial characterization of fucosylated cell surface glycoproteins of cultured RPE. *Curr. Eye Res.* **1990**, *9*, 977–986. [CrossRef] [PubMed]
5. Edwards, R.B.; Szamier, R.B. Defective phagocytosis of isolated rod outer segments by RCS rat retinal pigment epithelium in culture. *Science* **1977**, *197*, 1001–1003. [CrossRef]
6. Buczkowska, A.; Swiezewska, E.; Lefeber, D.J. Genetic defects in dolichol metabolism. *J. Inherit. Metab. Dis.* **2015**, *38*, 157–169. [CrossRef]
7. Giladi, M.; Edri, I.; Goldenberg, M.; Newman, H.; Strulovich, R.; Khananshvili, D.; Haitin, Y.; Loewenstein, A. Purification and characterization of human dehydrodolychil diphosphate synthase (DHDDS) overexpressed in E. coli. *Protein Expr. Purif.* **2017**, *132*, 138–142. [CrossRef]
8. Kean, E.L. The dolichol pathway in the retina and its involvement in the glycosylation of rhodopsin. *Biochim. Biophys. Acta* **1999**, *1473*, 272–285. [CrossRef]
9. Nowycky, M.C.; Wu, G.; Ledeen, R.W. Glycobiology of ion transport in the nervous system. *Adv. Neurobiol.* **2014**, *9*, 321–342. [CrossRef]
10. Wimmers, S.; Karl, M.O.; Strauss, O. Ion channels in the RPE. *Prog. Retin. Eye Res.* **2007**, *26*, 263–301. [CrossRef]
11. Lam, B.L.; Zuchner, S.L.; Dallman, J.; Wen, R.; Alfonso, E.C.; Vance, J.M.; Pericak-Vance, M.A. Mutation K42E in dehydrodolichol diphosphate synthase (DHDDS) causes recessive retinitis pigmentosa. *Adv. Exp. Med. Biol.* **2014**, *801*, 165–170. [CrossRef] [PubMed]
12. Zelinger, L.; Banin, E.; Obolensky, A.; Mizrahi-Meissonnier, L.; Beryozkin, A.; Bandah-Rozenfeld, D.; Frenkel, S.; Ben-Yosef, T.; Merin, S.; Schwartz, S.B.; et al. A missense mutation in DHDDS, encoding dehydrodolichyl diphosphate synthase, is associated with autosomal-recessive retinitis pigmentosa in Ashkenazi Jews. *Am. J. Hum. Genet.* **2011**, *88*, 207–215. [CrossRef] [PubMed]
13. Venturini, G.; Koskiniemi-Kuendig, H.; Harper, S.; Berson, E.L.; Rivolta, C. Two specific mutations are prevalent causes of recessive retinitis pigmentosa in North American patients of Jewish ancestry. *Genet. Med.* **2015**, *17*, 285–290. [CrossRef] [PubMed]
14. Ng, B.G.; Freeze, H.H. Perspectives on Glycosylation and Its Congenital Disorders. *Trends Genet.* **2018**, *34*, 466–476. [CrossRef]
15. Biswas, P.; Duncan, J.L.; Maranhao, B.; Kozak, I.; Branham, K.; Gabriel, L.; Lin, J.H.; Barteselli, G.; Navani, M.; Suk, J.J.; et al. Genetic analysis of ten pedigrees with inherited retinal degeneration (IRD) by exome sequencing and phenotype-genotype association. *Physiol. Genom.* **2017**, *49*, 216–229. [CrossRef]
16. Kimchi, A.; Khateb, S.; Wen, R.; Guan, Z.; Obolensky, A.; Beryozkin, A.; Kurtzman, S.; Blumenfeld, A.; Pras, E.; Jacobson, S.G.; et al. Nonsyndromic Retinitis Pigmentosa in the Ashkenazi Jewish Population: Genetic and Clinical Aspects. *Ophthalmology* **2018**, *125*, 725–734. [CrossRef]
17. Sabry, S.; Vuillaumier-Barrot, S.; Mintet, E.; Fasseu, M.; Valayannopoulos, V.; Heron, D.; Dorison, N.; Mignot, C.; Seta, N.; Chantret, I.; et al. A case of fatal Type I congenital disorders of glycosylation (CDG I) associated with low dehydrodolichol diphosphate synthase (DHDDS) activity. *Orphanet J. Rare Dis.* **2016**, *11*, 84. [CrossRef]

18. Ferrara, N.; Carver-Moore, K.; Chen, H.; Dowd, M.; Lu, L.; O'Shea, K.S.; Powell-Braxton, L.; Hillan, K.J.; Moore, M.W. Heterozygous embryonic lethality induced by targeted inactivation of the VEGF gene. *Nature* **1996**, *380*, 439–442. [CrossRef]
19. Rucker, E.B., 3rd; Dierisseau, P.; Wagner, K.U.; Garrett, L.; Wynshaw-Boris, A.; Flaws, J.A.; Hennighausen, L. Bcl-x and Bax regulate mouse primordial germ cell survival and apoptosis during embryogenesis. *Mol. Endocrinol.* **2000**, *14*, 1038–1052. [CrossRef]
20. Le, Y.Z.; Zheng, W.; Rao, P.C.; Zheng, L.; Anderson, R.E.; Esumi, N.; Zack, D.J.; Zhu, M. Inducible expression of cre recombinase in the retinal pigmented epithelium. *Investig. Ophthalmol. Vis. Sci.* **2008**, *49*, 1248–1253. [CrossRef] [PubMed]
21. Le, Y.Z.; Zhu, M.; Anderson, R.E. Cre Recombinase: You Can't Live with It, and You Can't Live Without It. *Adv. Exp. Med. Biol.* **2016**, *854*, 725–730. [CrossRef] [PubMed]
22. DeRamus, M.L.; Stacks, D.A.; Zhang, Y.; Huisingh, C.E.; McGwin, G.; Pittler, S.J. GARP2 accelerates retinal degeneration in rod cGMP-gated cation channel beta-subunit knockout mice. *Sci. Rep.* **2017**, *7*, 42545. [CrossRef] [PubMed]
23. Stricker, H.M.; Ding, X.Q.; Quiambao, A.; Fliesler, S.J.; Naash, M.I. The Cys214–>Ser mutation in peripherin/rds causes a loss-of-function phenotype in transgenic mice. *Biochem. J.* **2005**, *388*, 605–613. [CrossRef] [PubMed]
24. Tu, C.; Li, J.; Jiang, X.; Sheflin, L.G.; Pfeffer, B.A.; Behringer, M.; Fliesler, S.J.; Qu, J. Ion-current-based proteomic profiling of the retina in a rat model of Smith-Lemli-Opitz syndrome. *Mol. Cell. Proteom.* **2013**, *12*, 3583–3598. [CrossRef] [PubMed]
25. Zanzottera, E.C.; Ach, T.; Huisingh, C.; Messinger, J.D.; Spaide, R.F.; Curcio, C.A. Visualizing retinal pigment epithelium phenotypes in the transition to geographic atrophy in age-related macular degeneration. *Retina* **2016**, *36*, S12–S25. [CrossRef]
26. Zuchner, S.; Dallman, J.; Wen, R.; Beecham, G.; Naj, A.; Farooq, A.; Kohli, M.A.; Whitehead, P.L.; Hulme, W.; Konidari, I.; et al. Whole-exome sequencing links a variant in DHDDS to retinitis pigmentosa. *Am. J. Hum. Genet.* **2011**, *88*, 201–206. [CrossRef]
27. Grabińska, K.A.; Park, E.J.; Sessa, W.C. cis-Prenyltransferase: New insights into protein glycosylation, rubber synthesis, and human diseases. *J. Biol. Chem.* **2016**, *291*, 18582–18590. [CrossRef]
28. Park, E.J.; Grabinska, K.A.; Guan, Z.; Stranecky, V.; Hartmannova, H.; Hodanova, K.; Baresova, V.; Sovova, J.; Jozsef, L.; Ondruskova, N.; et al. Mutation of Nogo-B receptor, a subunit of cis-prenyltransferase, causes a congenital disorder of glycosylation. *Cell Metab.* **2014**, *20*, 448–457. [CrossRef]
29. Murray, A.R.; Fliesler, S.J.; Al-Ubaidi, M.R. Rhodopsin: The functional significance of asn-linked glycosylation and other post-translational modifications. *Ophthalmic Genet.* **2009**, *30*, 109–120. [CrossRef]
30. White, D.A.; Fritz, J.J.; Hauswirth, W.W.; Kaushal, S.; Lewin, A.S. Increased sensitivity to light-induced damage in a mouse model of autosomal dominant retinal disease. *Investig. Ophthalmol. Vis. Sci.* **2007**, *48*, 1942–1951. [CrossRef]
31. Ramachanra Rao, S.; Fliesler, S.J.; Nguyen, M.N.; Kotla, P.; Pittler, S.J. Lack of overt retinal degeneration in K42E DHDDS knock-in mouse model of RP59. *Cells* **2020**. submitted.

8

Balancing the Photoreceptor Proteome: Proteostasis Network Therapeutics for Inherited Retinal Disease

Siebren Faber and Ronald Roepman *

Department of Human Genetics and Radboud Institute for Molecular Life Sciences, Radboud University Medical Center, Geert Grooteplein Zuid 10, 6525 GA Nijmegen, The Netherlands
* Correspondence: ronald.roepman@radboudumc.nl

Abstract: The light sensing outer segments of photoreceptors (PRs) are renewed every ten days due to their high photoactivity, especially of the cones during daytime vision. This demands a tremendous amount of energy, as well as a high turnover of their main biosynthetic compounds, membranes, and proteins. Therefore, a refined proteostasis network (PN), regulating the protein balance, is crucial for PR viability. In many inherited retinal diseases (IRDs) this balance is disrupted leading to protein accumulation in the inner segment and eventually the death of PRs. Various studies have been focusing on therapeutically targeting the different branches of the PR PN to restore the protein balance and ultimately to treat inherited blindness. This review first describes the different branches of the PN in detail. Subsequently, insights are provided on how therapeutic compounds directed against the different PN branches might slow down or even arrest the appalling, progressive blinding conditions. These insights are supported by findings of PN modulators in other research disciplines.

Keywords: protein trafficking; protein folding; protein degradation; chaperones; chaperonins; heat shock response; unfolded protein response; autophagy; therapy

---

1. Introduction

The rod and cone photoreceptor (PR) cells are the most abundant cell types in the human retina, with ~6.4 million cones and up to 125 million rods per adult retina [1]. PRs are highly specialized, polarized neurons of neuroepithelial origin, consisting of morphologically and functionally distinct cellular compartments, including a synaptic terminal, an inner segment (IS), an outer segment (OS), and a connecting cilium bridging the IS and OS. The classical division into rods and cones is based on their different OS morphology and differential expression of subtypes of opsin. The rod outer segments are long, thin, rod-shaped organelles containing rhodopsin in large stacks of membranous discs, allowing to process variations in dim-light conditions, but they lose this ability in bright light conditions. The OSs of cones represent a shorter conical organelle containing either S-opsin, M-opsin, or L-opsin, which are less sensitive compared to rhodopsin, but are perfectly suited to process bright light of different wavelengths, allowing color vision [2].

Despite the difference in photosensitivity, the process of converting light stimuli into biochemical signals, the phototransduction cascade, is almost indistinguishable between rods and cones [3,4]. In rods, upon capture of a photon, the chromophore 11-*cis* retinal, which is conjugated to a rhodopsin molecule, undergoes a conformational change that isomerizes it to all-*trans* retinal leading to the activation of rod opsin. The activated opsin molecule is now able to bind and subsequently activate the G-protein, transducin. Transducin consists of three subunits: G_α, G_β, and G_γ. In its inactive state, G_α is bound to a GDP. When transducin gets activated by rhodopsin, this GDP is replaced by a GTP and subsequently G_α dissociates from the $G_{\beta\gamma}$ subunit. The GTP bound G_α is now able to displace one of the two inhibitory γ-subunits of cGMP-specific 3′,5′-cyclic phosphodiesterase (PDE6) causing the exposure of one of the two catalytic sites of the $PDE6_{\alpha\beta}$ heterodimer ($PDE6_{\alpha'}$ for cones). The exposed catalytic sites are now able to hydrolyze multiple cGMP molecules to 5′-GMP. In the dark state, cGMP binds to its specific cation channel allowing a steady movement of cations into the OS, which is compensated by the efflux of cations from the OS by Na^+/Ca^{2+}, K^+ exchangers (NCKXs) [5]. Due to the hydrolysis of cGMP, its levels decrease causing the closure of cation channels in the OS. The resulting hyperpolarization of the OS membrane spreads throughout the cell, eventually reaching the synaptic terminal. Here, the hyperpolarization causes closure of calcium channels and subsequently a decrease in calcium-dependent synaptic glutamate release [3,4], which activates the glutamate receptors of the bipolar cells postsynaptically, transducing the brain-bound electrical signal [6].

The phototransduction cascade, carried out in only a few milliseconds, is based on capture of one single photon in dim light. However, in bright daylight conditions, immense amounts of photons are caught by the human PRs, mainly cones, every second, which causes toxic photo-oxidative damage to the OS components. These components, which include most proteins involved in the phototransduction cascade, are therefore continuously renewed (~10% every day for human PRs), by incorporating newly synthesized PR discs at the OS base, and shedding the oldest membrane discs at the cell's tip [7,8]. The shed OS tips are subsequently phagocytosed by the retinal pigment epithelium (RPE) cells, which is the highest active phagocytic process in our body [9,10]. Because of this highly active protein turnover, a mutation in a gene encoding a protein involved in this machinery most often leads to PR cell death, a classical hallmark of many inherited retinal diseases (IRDs).

IRDs are a genetically heterogeneous group of rare eye disorders with a progressive manifestation causing vision loss or even complete blindness [11]. Mutations in many genes that are required for PR function were found to be causative for IRDs. These include genes encoding proteins involved in protein trafficking, splicing, energy metabolism, and photoreceptor structure [12]. The compartments of PRs most prominently implicated in IRDs are the OS and the connecting cilium. The connecting cilium correlates with the transition zone of a primary cilium and functions as a gatekeeper to regulate the molecular composition of the OS. Thus, the OS, connecting cilium, and the immediately adjacent basal body, form the photoreceptor sensory cilium, one of the most highly specialized primary cilia, fully optimized for photoreception and transduction [13,14]. Hence, IRDs with defects in these compartments are referred to as retinal ciliopathies [11].

Defects in the conserved ciliary processes mostly manifest as syndromic ciliopathy conditions, affecting multiple organs. The most prominent ciliopathies in which the retina is affected are Bardet–Biedl syndrome (BBS), Joubert syndrome (JS), Meckel–Gruber syndrome (MKS), and Senior–Løken syndrome (SLS) [4,11]. Because PRs are highly specialized, polarized neurons, retinal ciliopathies often also occur in a nonsyndromic fashion, affecting ciliary proteins specific to rods and/or cones. Based on the PR cell type affected, different IRDs can be categorized, including retinitis pigmentosa (RP), Leber congenital amaurosis (LCA), cone-rod dystrophy (CRD), and achromatopsia (ACHM) [4,11].

RP is the most common form of inherited blindness worldwide, with a prevalence of about 1:4000 people. The cells that are affected initially in RP are the rods leading to night blindness and loss of peripheral vision. Secondary, cones are most often also affected as the disease progresses [15].

LCA is the most severe form of inherited retinal degeneration, causing patients to suffer from severe visual impairment to complete blindness before the first year of life. With LCA, both rods and cones are affected at early stages often leading to complete blindness [16].

Another early onset form of hereditary retinal dystrophy is CRD, which manifest in the opposite order compared to RP, since in CRD cones are initially affected, followed by the loss of rods [17].

A disease in which specifically the cones deteriorate is ACHM, most often leading to complete color blindness [18].

Apart from some specific exceptions, most of the above described blinding conditions are still considered incurable. However, significant and promising progress has been made with therapeutic studies targeting specific genes and/or mutations, most prominently by employing gene augmentation and antisense-oligo nucleotide (AON)-based techniques [19,20]. Yet, a major disadvantage of these treatments is that they are complex and invasive for the patient. On top of that, for nearly every mutation, a personalized approach needs to be developed. Therefore, there is a high interest in pharmacological agents with a broad range of disease targets. To discover such agents, a growing number of studies have focused on a common phenomenon seen in many IRDs before the actual death of rods and cones: the accumulation and/or misfolding of proteins in the inner segment of the photoreceptors [21].

This phenomenon can be explained by the malfunction of several processes, all involved in protein homeostasis or proteostasis. A first process is the disruption of protein transport from the IS to the OS (Figure 1A). As the OS lacks the biosynthesis machinery for proteins and lipids, all of the components required for OS morphogenesis, maintenance, and sensory functions must be transported from the endoplasmic reticulum (ER), located in the IS, to the OS [2], across the connective connecting cilium stalk. Therefore, defects in this transport most often lead to the accumulation of proteins in the IS. Another process involved in the accumulation of proteins in the IS is the dysregulation of pathways involved in protein degradation, including ER-associated degradation (ERAD) and autophagy (Figure 1C). Finally, also incorrect folding of specific proteins due to loss-of-function mutations can results in protein accumulation in the IS (Figure 1B). An accumulation of misfolded proteins in the ER membrane or in the cytoplasm of the PRs can induce the heat shock response (HSR) and/or the unfolded protein response (UPR). Continuous activation of these responses will ultimately lead to death of PRs [21].

In this review the above mentioned branches of the proteostasis network will be described in detail. Subsequently, we will explain how potential therapeutic agents directed against these branches might slow down or even arrest the dramatic blinding conditions, supported by findings of PN modulators in other research disciplines.

2. The Different Branches of the Proteostasis Network

2.1. *Pathways Involved in Protein Trafficking*

2.1.1. Chaperones Involved in Lipid-Dependent Trafficking

Many PR-specific proteins depend on post-translational lipid modifications, including prenylation and myristoylation, for correct localization to the OS and their anchoring at one of the OS membranes [22]. Protein prenylation involves the transfer of either a farnesyl or a geranylgeranyl moiety to the C-terminal cysteine(s) of the target protein by farnesyltransferase (FTase) and geranylgeranyltransferase (GGTase-I), respectively [23]. Several chaperones are involved in this prenylation process, including AIPL1, PDE6D, and UNC119.

Aryl hydrocarbon receptor (AhR)-interacting protein-like 1 (AIPL1) was first discovered in association with Leber congenital amaurosis (LCA) [24]. Mutations in the *AIPL1* gene encoding for AIPL1 results in LCA4, one of the most severe forms of LCA leading to blindness in early childhood [25]. Since then, studies were set up to unravel the function of the AIPL1 protein. Studies in AIPL1 knockdown and knockout mouse models revealed that AIPL1 functions as a chaperone for PDE6 [26,27]. In these mouse models protein levels and activity of PDE6 were severely reduced, whereas other photoreceptor proteins were unaffected. Other studies suggest that AIPL1 is also necessary for the maintenance of PRs by enhancing the essential farnesylation reaction [28,29]. Several retinal proteins, including PDE, transducin, and rhodopsin kinase (GRK1) are known to be farnesylated [30]. These findings are in line with the observed rapid degeneration of rods and cones in the animal models, as well as in LCA4 patients.

Another chaperone, mainly involved in the trafficking of prenylated proteins, is PDE6D [8,31]. In mice, knockout of PDE6D results in mislocalization of prenylated PR proteins, including PDE6, GRK1, and Gγ [32]. In human, mutations in PDE6D are associated with Joubert syndrome (JS) [33,34]. This syndromic condition can be explained by mislocalization of other critical cargos of PDE6D important for the development and stability of the primary cilium. These cargos include inositol polyphosphate

5-phosphatase E (INPP5E) and retinitis pigmentosa GTPase regulator (RPGR) [33,35]. The trafficking of these cargos comprises of several steps [36,37]. First, PDE6D solubilizes the prenylated protein from the ER by sequestering the hydrophobic farnesyl or geranylgeranyl tail. Subsequently, PDE6D targets the cargo to the destination membrane by association with a peripherally membrane bound docking protein. Finally, binding of the displacement factor ARL3 to PDE6D causes a reduction in size of the hydrophobic cavity resulting in the release of the cargo [38]. PDE6D can now travel back to repeat its cycle.

UNC119 shares significant sequence and structural homology with the prenyl-binding protein PDE6D [37]. Similar to PDE6D, UNC119 is also a subject of ARL3-dependent cargo release, and therefore the transport mechanism of PDE6D and UNC119 are highly identical. However, a remarkable difference between PDE6D and UNC119 is the ARL3-dependent release of their cargo. In contrast to PDE6D, the hydrophobic pocket of UNC119 is expanded upon binding of ARL3, thereby weakening the interaction with the cargo instead of squeezing the lipid out of the hydrophobic pocket [39]. This might be partly explained by the binding of different lipid moieties of both chaperones. Whereas PDE6D sequesters prenylated proteins, UNC119 is known to bind myristoylated cargo [31,40]. UNC119 has been shown to be important in the trafficking of transducin, which is myristoylated on its α-subunit [41]. In UNC119 knockout mice, the trafficking of transducin to the OS during dark adaptation was significantly impaired, contributing to the observed slow retinal degeneration [42]. The observed mislocalization of transducin in these mice is not complete, supporting the fact that transducin is trafficked by other proteins, including PDE6D. Interestingly, a study performed in *Pde6d;Unc119* double-knockout mice showed partially improved rhodopsin kinase (GRK1) expression and trafficking in cones compared to *Pde6d* single-knockout mice [43]. Based on these findings, the authors suggest that the transport by PDE6D and UNC119 in cones might be interdependent. The improvement found in only cones is in line with the relatively mild phenotype seen in patients with a truncating mutation in UNC119, which is associated with late onset CRD [44].

2.2. *Pathways Involved in Protein Folding*

2.2.1. Chaperonins, Phosducins and Ric8A

In addition to the classic and ubiquitous molecular chaperones from the heat shock protein superfamily (discussed below), various studies have focused on chaperones and co-chaperones involved in folding and assembly of PR-specific proteins.

One of the PR-specific proteins that needs targeted guidance for its correct folding and assembly is transducin. The folding and assembly of the full transducin protein complex is performed in two distinct steps. In the first step, the so-called chaperonins or CCTs (chaperonins containing TCP-1) are involved. CCTs are protein-folding ATPase complexes consisting of two stacked rings, which form a central cavity [45]. The β-subunit of transducin (G_β) is able to enter this cavity. Once transducin enters, ATP binding occurs, resulting in the closure of the cavity by hydrolysis of the just bound ATP molecule [46]. In addition to ATP, the folding of G_β requires a co-chaperone, phosducin-like protein 1 (PhLP1). Binding of PhLP1 induces conformational changes of CCT that lock the β-propeller structure of G_β. Subsequently, G_β rotates inside the cavity followed by its release in complex with PhLP1. PhLP1 is required for the formation of the $G_{\beta\gamma}$ dimer [47].

The second step involves the trafficking of the $G_{\beta\gamma}$ dimer to the OS by phosducin, another member of the phosducin family of proteins. Phosducin forms a complex with $G_{\beta\gamma}$ by sequestering the hydrophobic farnesyl residue of G_γ [48]. The farnesyl residue serves as a membrane anchor, which targets $G_{\beta\gamma}$ to the OS [49]. Another speculated function of phosducin is the protection of $G_{\beta\gamma}$ against ubiquitination and degradation by the proteasome [50].

CCTs are also involved in the folding and assembly of the BBSome [51], a protein complex that regulates the ciliary import, export, and intraciliary trafficking of molecules [52]. Mutations in genes coding for BBSome proteins most often result in the development of Bardet–Biedl syndrome, one of the syndromic ciliopathy conditions in which the retina is affected [53], as indicated in the introduction. For some of the BBSome proteins it was shown that these proteins contain a β-propeller fold, similar to G_β [54]. Whether or not the folding and assembly of the BBSome proteins is comparable to the situation of G_β remains to be elucidated.

It remains largely unknown if the α-subunit of transducin also needs assistance in correct folding and trafficking to the OS before it forms a heterotrimeric complex with $G_{\beta\gamma}$. However, evidence is emerging that resistance to inhibitors of cholinesterase 8 (RIC8) proteins function as ubiquitous chaperones for G_α [55]. The two known isoforms—RIC8A and RIC8B—each regulate specific classes of G_α [56]. Although the specific PR class of Gα and its relation to RIC8 has not been investigated, it has been shown that a closely related form interacts with RIC8A [57]. The proposed mode of action of RIC8A is to positively regulate G_α by acting as a guanine nucleotide exchange factor (GEF). RIC8A preferentially binds GDP-bound G_α and causes GDP release. Subsequently, RIC8A assists in organizing a de novo nucleotide-binding pocket for binding of GTP. The RIC8A-G_α complex breaks apart when a GTP molecule binds. Subsequent hydrolysis of GTP results in the binding of G_α to the $G_{\beta\gamma}$ yielding the fully assembled heterotrimeric complex [58]. Taken together, CCT together with PhLP1 regulate the folding of the transducin β-subunit. Subsequently, G_β forms a dimer with G_γ by guidance of PhLP1. Finally, the $G_{\beta\gamma}$ dimer is trafficked to the OS by phosducin, where it can bind to G_α. RIC8A has been proposed as the chaperone of G_α and its assembly to the $G_{\beta\gamma}$ dimer.

2.2.2. Heat Shock Response (HSR)

The HSR is known to be present in every living organism, and functions as an essential survival mechanism against extracellular challenges, such as increased temperatures, and intracellular stressors such as oxidative stress, that lead to protein misfolding [21,59]. The HSR is featured by an extremely rapid activation of gene expression, leading to a remarkable increase in molecular chaperones, including heat shock proteins (HSPs) [60]. In vertebrates, the HSR is regulated by a family of transcription factors, which includes six members (HSF1-4, HSFX, and HSFY) [59]. HSF1 is believed to be the master regulator of molecular chaperone synthesis upon protein misfolding [61]. Under normal physiological conditions, monomeric HSF1 is repressed and localized in the cytosol by interacting with molecular chaperones, including HSP90, HSP70, and the chaperonin CCT. When a threshold of misfolded proteins is reached, the chaperones dissociate from HSF1 leading to trimerization and nuclear accumulation of HSF1 followed by transcriptional activation of HSPs. The major HSPs involved in the HSR include HSP90, HSP70, and HSP60 [61].

HSP90 and HSP70 are able to associate with the hydrophobic regions of the protein, and thereby preventing binding to other hydrophobic moieties [61]. Subsequently, they assist in the folding of these hydrophobic regions in such a way that the hydrophobic groups are not exposed. Furthermore, they aid in overcoming the energy thresholds of the intermediate folding states of the protein [62]. Similar to HSP90 and HSP70, the chaperonin HSP60 is also able to bind hydrophobic residues of proteins. In contrast, the barrel-shaped HSP60 is more passively involved in the folding of proteins by creating a favorable microenvironment for the hydrophobic regions in its central cavity [63].

2.2.3. Unfolded Protein Response (UPR)

A more specific cellular stress response related to the ER is the UPR. The UPR is activated in response to an accumulation of unfolded and/or misfolded proteins in the lumen of the ER [64]. The activation of the UPR aims to reduce ER stress and restore proteostasis in three distinct ways: an initial response to reduce protein synthesis, a second wave of increased production of molecular chaperones involved in protein folding to increase folding capacity, and finally the degradation of misfolded proteins when the folding capacity is insufficient to restore functional protein balance. It is generally accepted that a member of the HSP70 family, BiP/GRP78, is the key regulator in the activation of the UPR [65]. BiP has been shown to associate with all three transmembrane sensors of the UPR, including inositol requiring enzyme-1 (IRE1) α and β, protein kinase RNA (PKR)-like ER kinase

(PERK), and activating transcription factor 6 (ATF6) α and β. Under normal physiological conditions, BiP associates with the ER luminal domain of IRE1 and PERK via its ATPase domain, maintaining them in an inactive monomeric state.

The interaction of BiP with ATF6 masks a binding site to coat protein-II (COP-II) vesicles, thereby preventing ATF6 translocation to the Golgi. Upon ER stress, BiP dissociates from the sensors and binds to misfolded proteins. Subsequently, IRE1 and PERK are able to oligomerize followed by their trans-autophosphorylation and ATF6 traffics to the Golgi for further processing and activation.

Dissociation of BiP from IRE1 results in the activation of its RNase domain. This activation is sustained by binding of HSP47 to the luminal domain of IRE1, thereby hindering the binding of BiP [66]. Subsequently, a single mRNA encoding for X-box binding protein 1 (XBP1) is targeted for non-conventional splicing [67].

These spliced XBP1s trigger the expression of molecular chaperones and components of ERAD in order to relieve the load on the ER and eventually restore protein balance [68]. One of the upregulated chaperones is the ER resident co-chaperone ERdj4, which eases and stabilizes the binding of BiP [69]. Furthermore, it has been shown that protein disulfide isomerase A6 (PDIA6) plays an important role in the conversion of IRE1 to its monomeric state [70]. Based on these findings, it is speculated that ERdj4 and PDIA6 are important regulators of the IRE1 negative feedback loop. Activation of PERK leads to phosphorylation of the α-subunit of eukaryotic translation initiation factor 2 (eIF2α), thereby hindering the conversion of eIF2-GDP to eIF2-GTP by the GEF eIF2B [71]. The inactivation of eIF2α leads to overall decrease in mRNA translation and thus protein synthesis. Although, global mRNA translation is reduced, some specific mRNAs are favored to be translated, including activation transcription factor 4 (ATF4) [72]. ATF4 is able to activate the transcription of various genes involved in protein folding, autophagy, and apoptosis, including CCAAT/enhancer-binding protein (C/EBP) homologous protein (*CHOP*), ER oxidoreductin 1 (*ERO1*), and growth arrest and DNA damage-inducible protein (*GADD34*). GADD34 plays a role in the negative feedback loop for PERK by acting as a cofactor in the dephosphorylation of eIF2α [73]. CHOP and ERO1 mainly play a role in prolonged PERK activation [74], which will be discussed below.

Under ER stress, ATF6 binds to COP-II vesicles and traffics to the Golgi [75]. Here, it is cleaved by proteases S1P and S2P resulting in a cytosolic fragment [76]. This fragment travels into the nucleus to regulate transcription of specific UPR genes, including *CHOP* and *XBP1*. Interestingly, XBP1s and ATF6 are able to heterodimerize, and subsequently induce the expression of genes involved in ERAD [77].

2.3. *Pathways Involved in Protein Degradation*

2.3.1. ER-associated Degradation (ERAD)

Folding and maturation of proteins is a complicated process that is highly susceptible to errors. Up to 30% of all newly synthesized proteins are affected by such errors and are therefore degraded by the proteasome before they reach their defective mature state [78]. An important player in proteasomal-dependent protein degradation is ERAD. The process of ERAD can be divided into three consecutive steps: recognition of misfolded proteins in the ER, retrotranslocation of these proteins into the cytosol, and ubiquitin-dependent degradation by the ubiquitin–proteasome system (UPS) [79].

The recognition of misfolded proteins depends on the detection of substructures within proteins, including exposed hydrophobic regions, unpaired cysteine residues, and immature glycans [80]. The latter involves the lectin-type chaperones calnexin and calreticulin, which can bind to glycans possessing the $Glc_3Man_9GlcNAc_2$ structure produced by deglucosylation [81]. Incompletely or misfolded proteins undergo multiple rounds of reglucosylation by uridine diphosphate (UDP)-glucose:glycoprotein glucosyltransferase (UGGT) and subsequent folding by reassociation with calnexin or calreticulin, eventually resulting in the mature protein conformation [82].

On the other hand, terminally misfolded proteins must be extracted from this calnexin/calreticulin cycle. This extraction is regulated by the removal of terminal mannose residues from core glycans by mannosidases, including ER mannosidase I (ERMANI), ER degradation-enhancing α-mannosidase-like protein 1 (EDEM1), EDEM3, or Golgi-resident mannosidase α class 1C member 1 (MAN1C1) [83–85]. In this way, ERAD can discriminate between terminally misfolded proteins and their fully functional counterparts.

Since the ubiquitin-dependent degradation by the UPS is performed in the cytosol, terminally misfolded proteins subjected to ERAD have to be transported through the ER membrane via a transmembrane channel, called the retrotranslocon [86]. The exact composition of this channel is yet unknown. However, it has been shown that the membrane protein Derlin-1 and various E3 ubiquitin ligases are part of the retrotranslocon complex [87]. Once a small part of the substrate for ERAD is exposed to the surface of the ER, the substrate becomes a subject for poly-ubiquitination. Subsequently, the p97/valosin-containing protein (VCP), which is a member of the type II AAA+ protein family of ATPases, together with its cofactors, possessing ubiquitin-binding domains (UBDs), cooperatively produce a driving force for the retrotranslocation [88].

Retrotranslocated substrates for ERAD often possess exposed hydrophobic domains. Therefore, it is important that these substrates should be rapidly transported to the UPS for degradation to prevent aggregation. A chaperone complex consisting of BCL-2-associated athanogene 6 (BAG6), ubiquitin-like protein 4A (UBL4A), transmembrane domain recognition complex 35 (TRC35), and co-chaperone small glutamine-rich TPR-containing protein α (SGTA) has been shown to play an important role in the trafficking of ERAD substrates to the UPS by binding to the hydrophobic domains [89].

2.3.2. Autophagy

Another very important process involved in protein degradation is autophagy. Multiple forms of autophagy are known, including macroautophagy, chaperone-mediated autophagy (CMA), and microautophagy [90].

Macroautophagy is the most common form of autophagy and therefore often referred to simply as autophagy. Autophagy consists of multiple consecutive phases, including initiation, nucleation, elongation, closure, and fusion to the lysosome. The initiation phase is tightly regulated by AMP-activated protein kinase (AMPK) and mammalian target of rapamycin complex I (mTORC1) [91]. In addition, factors expressed resulting from ER stress are also able to trigger the initiation phase.

It all starts with the formation of the Unc-51-like kinase 1 (ULK1) complex followed by the phosphorylation of the class III phosphoinositide 3-kinase (PI3KC3) complex I leading to the nucleation of the phagophore [91,92]. Subsequently, autophagosome elongation and closure requires two ubiquitin-like conjugation systems, including an ATG7 dependent system and an ATG5-ATG12 dependent system. Together they are responsible for the lipidation, by phosphatidyethanolamine (PE), from cleavage of microtubule-associated protein 1 light chain 3 (LC3). Membrane sources in form of lipids needed for the elongation of the autophagosomal membrane are provided by ATG9-dependent vesicle trafficking. After closure of the autophagosomal membrane, the autophagosome has to fuse with the lysosome to form an autolysosome in order to degrade its enclosed cargo [93].

A selective form of autophagy is CMA, which to date is only identified in mammals [94]. This form of autophagy is specific for proteins containing a KFERQ motif in their amino acid sequence [95]. Heat shock cognate of the HSP70 family, HSC70, is able to recognize this motif and subsequently targets these proteins to the lysosome [96]. Here, it binds to the lysosomal receptor LAMP-2A and facilitates, together with its co-chaperones, in the unfolding process of the substrate in order to translocate it into the lysosome [97].

Microautophagy is a process in which cytoplasmic cargo is directly engulfed into the lysosome [98]. This process is triggered by the same stimuli compared to common autophagy, but in contrast it mainly facilitates the degradation of smaller substrates, including misfolded proteins. Similar to CMA, Hsc70 is involved in the protein cargo selection for degradation [99].

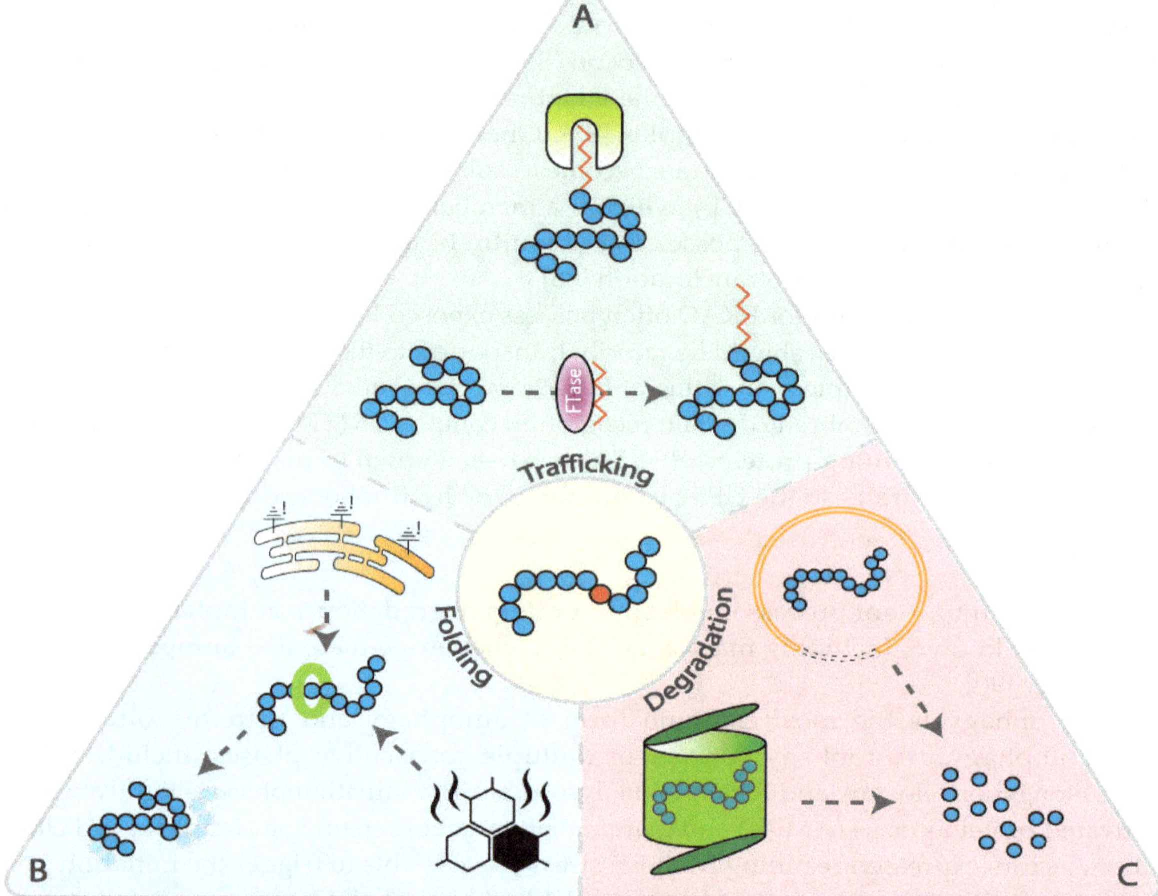

Figure 1. Schematic representation of the different branches of the proteostasis network, divided into trafficking, folding and degradation. (A) Trafficking: Protein prenylation involves the transfer of either a farnesyl or a geranylgeranyl moiety to the C-terminal cysteine(s) of the target protein by farnesyltransferase (FTase) and geranylgeranyltransferase (GGTase-I), respectively. Chaperones involved in regulation of this prenylation process and trafficking of prenylated proteins, include AIPL1, PDE6D, and UNC119 (depicted in green). (B) Folding: Two responses that are activated upon protein misfolding are the unfolded protein response (UPR) and the heat shock response (HSR). Both responses result in enhanced expression of chaperones (depicted in green) in order to restore the correct folding of proteins. (C) Degradation: ER-associated degradation (ERAD) results in the degradation of proteins by the ubiquitin–proteasome system (UPS). Another pathway of protein degradation is autophagy. Background colors in figure (green, blue, and red) correspond with background colors of Table 1.

Table 1. Therapeutic compounds directed against the different branches of the proteostasis network (PN). Therapeutic compounds are divided based on which branch of the PN they target, including trafficking (green), folding (blue), and degradation (red). Subgroups include compounds directed against protein lipid-modifications, (co-)chaperonins, HSR, UPR, ERAD, and autophagy. * Compounds that are not yet available.

Target	Compounds *	Function	Effect on PRs	References
Protein lipid-modifications	FTase inhibitors	Inhibits the farnesylation of proteins	(Proposed) underprenylation and mislocalization of many PR proteins	[100,101]
	GGTase-I inhibitors	Inhibits the geranylgeranylation of proteins	(Proposed) underprenylation and mislocalization of many PR proteins	[102]
(Co-)chaperonins	CCT inducers *	Improves folding of transducin and possibly other PR proteins	Undetermined	[103]
	PhLP1 inducers *	Improves function of CCTs and possibly CCT-independent functions	Malformation of OS by transgenic expression of a PhLP1 dominant-negative mutant	[47,103,104]
	CCT-BBSome stabilizers *	Stabilizes BBSome formation and thereby the export of molecules from the OS	Undetermined	[105]
	Small molecule Ric8 inhibitors *	Prevents folding of disease-causing Gα	Undetermined	[106,107]
Heat shock response (HSR)	geldanamycin, tanespimycin, alvespimycin	1st generation HSP90 inhibitors	Geldanamycin not suitable for future experiments because of poor applicability and toxicity; Tanespimycin reduced mutant protein accumulation in rat RP model (R135L); prolonged treatment with alvespimycin leads to PR cell death	[108–112]
	luminespib, onalespib, ganetespib, HSP990	Newer generation HSP90 inhibitors	HSP990 treatment in a RP rat model (P23H) enhances visual function and delayed PR degeneration, but prolonged treatment led to visual impairment by GRK1 and PDE6 reduction; prolonged treatment with ganetespib led to PR cell death	[109,111,112]
	AAV-*HSF-1*	Overexpressing HSF-1 and thereby transcriptional activation of HSPs	Subretinal injection of AAV-*Hsf-1* in a RP rat model (P23H) improved visual reponse	[113]
	Arimoclomol	Induces HSR and UPR, only in stressed cells	Prolonged PR survival and improved visual responses in P23H transgenic rats	[114]
Unfolded protein response (UPR)	AAV-BiP	Relieves ER stress by reducing cleaved ATF6, phosphorylated eIF2α and CHOP	Subretinal delivery of AAV5-BiP reduced PR cell death and improved visual responses in P23H transgenic rats	[115,116]
	CHOP inhibitors *	Inhibits proapoptotic transcription activity of CHOP	CHOP knockout in a trangenic mouse model of RP (T17M) led to PR cell death and strong impairment in visual function; CHOP knockout in P23H RHO mice had no effect on PR survival in young mice, but partly protected PR degeneration in older mice	[117–119]
	ATF4 inhibitors *	Inhibits downstream transcription activation of Chop, Ero1, and Gadd34	ATF4 knockdown in T17M RHO mice decreased retinal degeneration and improved PR survival	[120]
	GSK2606414A	Specific PERK inhibitor	Treatment with GSK2606414A in P23H RHO rats accelerated PR cell death and further impaired visual function	[121]
	Salubrinal	Inhibitor of eIF2α dephosphorylation	Treatment with salubrinal in P23H RHO rats improved PR survival	[121]

Table 1. *Cont.*

Target	Compounds *	Function	Effect on PRs	References
	KIRA6	Allosterically inhibits IRE1α RNase activity	Intravitreal injection of KIRA6 in P23H RHO rats increased PR survival	[122]
	Reactive electrophilic species (RES) modulators *	Modulate the effects of RES on IRE1	Undetermined	[123–128]
	Ceapins	Selective inhibitors of ATF6α	Undetermined	[129,130]
ER-associated degradation (ERAD)	Kyoto University Substances (KUSs)	Inhibits VCP's ATPase activity, without affecting the cellular functions of VCP	Individual treatment with KUS121 and KUS187 in a *rd10* mouse model preserved ONL thickness and improved visual function	[131]
	AAA+ protein derivatives *	Unfolding of misfolded proteins	Transgenic expression of PAN in Gy-/- mice increased PR survival and preserved visual function	[132]
	DUB/USP modulators	Modulating the ubiquitin cleavage from proteins, thereby modulating proteosomal degradation	Undetermined	[133–135]
Autophagy	Rapamycin, everolimus, temsirolimus, ridaforolimus	Inhibiting mTOR pathway by directly binding to mTORC1	Improved rod survival in P23H-3 rats	[136]
	Metformin	Activation of AMP-activated protein kinase (AMPK)	Metformin treatment protected against retinal cell death in diabetic mice, whereas it accelerated PR degeneration in P23H RHO mice	[137,138]
	Valproic acid (VPA)	Upregulates autophagy by inhibiting inositol synthesis	VPA treatment in BBS12-/- mice, P23H RHO *Xenopus laevis*, and a *rd1* mouse model resulted in PR protection, whereas treatment in T17M RHO *X. laevis*, a P23H-1 rat model, and a *rd10* mouse model excerbated PR degeneration	[139–141]

3. Therapeutic Approaches to Restore Protein Balance

The light sensing OS of PRs requires renewal every ten days due to its high photoactivity, especially of the cones during daytime vision. This demands a high turnover of biosynthetic compounds, including membranes and proteins). Therefore, a well-balanced proteostasis network is of particular importance for the PRs. For many IRDs it has been shown that this balance in the PRs is disrupted, leading to protein accumulation in the IS and eventually the death of photoreceptors. For this reason, several studies have focused on therapeutically targeting the three main branches of the PR proteostasis network to restore the protein balance. The different therapeutic approaches and their effects on PRs are discussed below and summarized in Table 1.

3.1. Therapeutic Strategies Involved in Protein Trafficking

3.1.1. Targeting Protein Lipid Modifications

Agents targeting prenylation have been extensively studied in cancer research. The first agents tested were FTase inhibitors used to target the farnesylation of K-Ras, which was shown to induce several forms of cancer, including colorectal cancer and lung cancer [142]. Although some clinical improvements were seen for different forms of cancer, these improvements could not be related to inhibition of K-Ras. Subsequent experiments revealed that K-Ras was geranylgeranylated when farnesylation was blocked by FTase inhibitors [143]. Therefore, inhibitors of GGTase-I emerged as potential target for cancer therapy. However, a phase I clinical trial investigating a dual FTase and GGTase-I inhibitor showed dose-limiting side effects in patients with locally advanced pancreatic cancer, indicating that inhibition of prenylation has a broad detrimental effect on human health [102]. FTase inhibitors are also of particular interest in the Hutchinson–Gilford progeria syndrome (HGPS) research field. HGPS is a rare premature-aging disease caused by a dominant de novo point mutation in the *LMNA* gene, resulting in the expression of a mutant form of lamin A, also known as progerin [144]. Progerin remains persistently farnesylated, which makes it a suitable candidate for FTase inhibitors [100]. Although, promising improvements in bone structure, vascular stiffness, and hearing have been obtained using FTase inhibitors in HGPS patients, nothing is reported about possible dose-limiting side effects [101].

Despite the promising results of using FTase and GGTase-I inhibitors for targeting several forms of cancer and HGPS, the side effects are of major concern; especially in the highly compartmentalized PRs, where many proteins depend on prenylation for subcellular trafficking and anchoring. General inhibition of prenylation would probably lead to underprenylation of many PR proteins leading to mislocalization and accumulation of these proteins in the IS. Therefore, inhibition of prenylation in PRs will rather accelerate protein accumulation than decreasing it.

3.2. Therapeutic Strategies Involved in Protein Folding

3.2.1. Targeting Chaperonins and Their Co-chaperones

The type II chaperonin CCT is proposed to be involved in the folding of approximately 10% of newly translated cytosolic proteins [145]. Besides ATP, CCT also needs the co-chaperone PhLP1 for the correct folding of these proteins [47]. It has been shown that inhibition of CCT by the transgenic expression of a dominant-negative mutant of PhLP1 results in the malformation of the OS in mouse photoreceptors [103]. Proteomic analysis revealed that the expression of several important PR proteins was affected, including PDE6, rhodopsin, transducin, peripherin 2, ROM1, musashi-1, and UNC-119. It could be possible that CCT is responsible for the folding of these proteins. Yet, only transducin has been shown to be a direct substrate of CCT. Therefore, a more plausible explanation would be that PhLP1 regulates the expression of these proteins in a CCT-independent manner.

Besides transducin, the BBSome is also a substrate for CCT for its correct folding and assembly. It has been shown that some of the BBSome proteins, including BBS6, BBS10, and BBS12, can form a

CCT-like complex together with CCT subunits. Interestingly, 50% of clinically diagnosed BBS cases are caused by a mutation in one of these three genes. Furthermore, mutations in these genes result in a more severe phenotype compared to other BBS proteins [105].

These findings highlight the importance of chaperone defects as pathogenic factors and therefore as potential therapeutic targets. Surprisingly, chaperonins and their co-chaperones, such as PhLP1, have not been investigated in relation to therapy. Especially PhLP1 would be an interesting therapeutic target, because of its proposed CCT-dependent and CCT-independent regulation of important PR proteins [104].

In cancer research, RIC8, functioning as GEF and chaperone for G_α, has been proposed as a potential therapeutic target, since it has been shown that constitutive activation of G_α by somatic mutations leads to development of various cancers [106]. Therefore, inhibition of RIC8 by small molecules might reduce tumorigenesis. A constitutive active mutant of rod G_α has also been associated to a form of congenital stationary night blindness [107]. RIC8 inhibition might therefore also alleviate or delay this phenotype. However, as described earlier, the function of RIC8 in the PR has not been investigated and inhibition of RIC8 would only be applicable to this specific mutation.

3.2.2. Targeting the Heat Shock Response (HSR)

HSP90, a component involved in the HSR, is commonly overexpressed in multiple forms of cancer [146]. It has been proposed that cancer cells increase their HSP90 expression and thereby change their proteostasis network in order to adapt to dysregulated and misfolded protein synthesis as a consequence of rapid cell division [147]. For this reason, many studies have focused on investigating HSP90 inhibitors. The first HSP90 inhibitor identified was geldanamycin, but this never reached the clinical testing phase because of its poor applicability and toxicity [108]. Nevertheless, geldanamycin paved the way for production of geldanamycin analogs, including 17-AAG/tanespimycin and 17-DMAG/alvespimycin [109]. Although clinical testing was halted for these agents, it did provide proof-of-principle that HSP90 is a relevant target for cancer therapy. Now, a new generation of HSP90 inhibitors, including luminespib, onalespib, and ganetespib, show greater potency in clinical testing [109].

HSP90 inhibitors have also been tested in models for retinal degeneration. Systemic administration of 17-AAG accompanied by inner-blood retina barrier modulation in a mouse model of RP (RP10) protects against photoreceptor degeneration induced by aggregating RP10-associated mutant IMPDH1 protein [110]. Furthermore, HSP90 inhibition by 17-AAG in a transgenic rat model of RP (R135L) reduced the intracellular accumulation of the mutant protein and restored the localization of this protein comparable to wild type controls [111]. Administration of another HSP90 inhibitor, HSP990, in a different transgenic rat model of RP (P23H) resulted in enhanced visual function and delayed photoreceptor degeneration. However, prolonged treatment with HSP990 leads to a reduction in GRK1 and PDE6 protein levels followed by visual impairment [111]. The visual impairment caused by prolonged HSP90 inhibition is in line with findings from a study in which four HSP90 inhibitors were tested, including 17-AAG, 17-DMAG, luminespib, and ganetespib, in a rat retinal damage model. Here, it was shown that prolonged inhibition with 17-DMAG and ganetespib results in PR cell death, whereas there was no PR injury detected upon treatment with the other two agents [112].

These contradictory findings might be explained by the different modes of action of the HSP90 inhibitors, since the effect of 17-AAG was dependent on HSF1 in the P23H rat model, whereas its effect was HSF1-independent in the R135L model. This is further supported by the notion that HSP90 is known to facilitate the folding and assembly of more than 300 proteins [146]. Alternatively, agents that induce the HSR in other ways might be more suitable as potential treatments for IRDs. A direct way to target the HSR is by overexpressing the *HSF-1* gene. A study in the p23H RHO RD rat model showed a significant increase of scotopic electroretinogram (ERG) amplitudes compared to untreated controls upon ectopic overexpression of *HSF-1* by subretinal injection of AAV-*HSF-1* [113].

The hydroxylamine derivative arimoclomol might be a more indirect alternative agent to induce the HSR. Treatment of transgenic rats, carrying a P23H rhodopsin mutation, with arimoclomol resulted in improved PR OS structure and reduced rhodopsin accumulation in the IS, accompanied by prolonged PR survival and improved visual responses [114]. It was shown that these improvements were mediated by both the HSR and the UPR, thereby indicating that these responses are intertwined. Another great advantage of arimoclomol is that it only acts on stressed cells. In this way, potential side effects, as a consequence of inducing an HSR response in healthy cells present in the retina, are avoided.

3.2.3. Targeting the Unfolded Protein Response (UPR)

As described earlier, the UPR senses ER stress by using three transmembrane sensors, including IRE1, PERK, and ATF6. In IRDs, mutations causing defective proteins can result in prolonged ER stress. It has been shown that upon prolonged ER stress, downstream effectors of the PERK pathway, ATF4 and CHOP heterodimerize. This results in increased protein synthesis, protein misfolding, and oxidative stress, eventually leading to cell death [148]. Another branch of the UPR that gets hyperactivated upon prolonged ER stress is IRE1. Hyperactive IRE1 cleaves microRNAs that normally inhibit proapoptotic targets, thereby inducing apoptosis [149]. Because apoptosis as a consequence of ER stress is often seen in PRs of IRD patients, therapeutically targeting UPR regulators or pathways involved in one of the three branches of the UPR might promote PR survival and thereby visual function.

As discussed earlier, it is commonly accepted that BiP/GRP78 is the key regulator in the activation of the UPR. Therefore, BiP might be a potential therapeutic target for relieving ER stress. Indeed, studies have shown that subretinal delivery of AAV5-BiP to a transgenic rat model of RP (P23H) results in reduction of PR cell death and improved ERG amplitudes [115]. Furthermore, a study in primary human retinal pigmented epithelium cells (hRPE) showed that AAV2-BiP promotes the survival of these cells under ER stress [116]. Both studies suggest that these improvements are due to a suppression of apoptosis by downregulation of CHOP protein levels. For this reason, reducing CHOP levels might be a promising strategy to alleviate ER stress. This notion is supported by a large body of evidence in the field of Alzheimer's Disease, cardiac hypertrophy, and diabetes, wherein they link CHOP to these disease conditions [150].

Recently, several studies investigated the effect of CHOP reduction in the context of photoreceptor degeneration. A first study was performed in a transgenic mouse model of RP (T17M) [117]. Subsequently, these mice were crossed with CHOP knockout mice in order to get T17M RHO CHOPP$^{-/-}$ mice. Complete knockdown of CHOP in these mice resulted in photoreceptor cell death, indicated by significant thinning of the outer nuclear layer, accompanied by a strong impairment in visual function. In a similar experimental setup comparing P23H RHO CHOPP$^{-/-}$ mice with P23H RHO mice, they found no effect on PR survival in young animals. In older mice, however, the central retina of the CHOPP$^{-/-}$ mice was partly protected against degeneration [118]. Another study in transgenic mice expressing human P23H rhodopsin also showed that knockout of CHOP had no effect on the rescue of retinal degeneration [119]. These studies indicated that complete ablation of CHOP has no positive effect in early developmental stages. As already described earlier, CHOP is mainly involved in prolonged PERK activation. Therefore, reducing CHOP levels to physiological levels during prolonged ER stress might be a better solution. This notion is supported by above described findings in older mice.

Interestingly, knocking down the proapoptotic partner of CHOP, ATF4 in a T17M rhodopsin mutant mouse model resulted in decreased retinal degeneration and improved PR survival [120].

Further support that the PERK branch of the UPR might be a promising therapeutic target comes from studies investigating ER stress related diseases, including Alzheimer's Disease (AD), amyotrophic lateral disease (ALS), Parkinson's Disease, and prion diseases [151,152].

In an Alzheimer's disease mouse model it was shown that deletion of PERK resulted in decreased phosphorylation of eIF2α and prevented deficits in protein synthesis leading to an improvement of the AD phenotype in these mice [153]. Comparable results were obtained in prion-diseased mice by overexpressing GADD34, which plays a role in the negative feedback loop for PERK by acting as a cofactor in the dephosphorylation of eIF2α [154]. Treatment of the prion-diseased mice with salubrinal, an inhibitor of eIF2α dephosphorylation, had the opposite effect compared to GADD34 overexpression, thereby supporting the positive effects of eIF2α dephosphorylation. The positive effect of the inhibition of the PERK pathway is further supported by a study investigating the effect of the specific PERK inhibitor, GSK2606414A, in prion-diseased mice [155]. Treatment with this inhibitor showed reduced neuronal cell death leading to increased survival of these mice.

Surprisingly, opposing results were found for GSK2606414A and salubrinal treatment when administered in P23H RHO transgenic rats. GSK2606414A treatment resulted in accelerated photoreceptor cell death and further impaired visual function, whereas salubrinal treatment was found to improve photoreceptor survival [121]. It could be possible that in some disease conditions or models the PERK pathway is protective, whereas in other conditions it is rather a secondary effect of the disease process. Therefore, targeting other branches of the UPR might overcome this issue.

Targeting the IRE1 branch of the UPR has been shown to be beneficial in multiple rodent models, including a P23H RHO rat model [122]. In this model, intravitreal injection of KIRA6, which allosterically inhibits the RNase domain of IRE1, showed increased photoreceptor survival.

Recently, an emerging role of reactive electrophilic species (RES) as key regulators for the UPR, more specifically the IRE1 pathway, have been described [123]. Furthermore, RES have been reported to be involved in ER-stress related diseases, including neurodegenerative diseases, amyotrophic lateral sclerosis (ALS), and cancer [124–126]. The RES nitric oxide (NO) has been shown to modulate PDI and IRE1 through S-nitrosylation and thereby inhibiting the IRE1 branch of the UPR [127,128]. Therefore, modulation by RES might be a new potential therapeutic strategy for ER stress-associated diseases, including IRDs.

Maybe the most interesting sensor of the UPR, in context of IRDs, is ATF6, because mutations in ATF6 have been shown to cause autosomal recessive achromatopsia and early onset photoreceptor degeneration, also affecting the macula [156,157].

Until recently, no compounds were available that specifically target the ATF6 branch of the UPR. However, by cell-based screens a new class of pyrazole amides, named Ceapins, were identified as selective inhibitors of ATF6α [129,130]. Ceapins selectively prevent transport of AFT6α to the Golgi apparatus during ER stress. Interestingly, Ceapins have no toxic impact on unstressed cells, whereas they increase ER stress sensitivity upon ER stress induction.

3.3. Therapeutic Strategies Involved in Protein Degradation

3.3.1. Targeting the ER-associated Degradation (ERAD)

One of the essential players in ERAD is p97/VCP, belonging to the type II AAA+ protein family of ATPases. Because of its essential role in ERAD, VCP is proposed as a novel therapeutic target for the treatment of various diseases, including cystic fibrosis, cancer, and neurodegenerative disorders [131]. Besides its function in retrotranslocation and protein degradation, VCP is also involved in many other cellular processes, including mitosis, nuclear reformation, DNA/RNA repair, aggresome formation and inflammatory signaling [158]. Therefore, for therapeutic applicability, selective intervention of VCP is required to minimize the side effects. Small compounds, named Kyoto University Substances (KUSs), might fulfill these criteria. KUSs have been shown to specifically inhibit VCP's ATPase activity, without affecting the cellular functions of VCP [131]. Administering KUSs, more specifically KUS121 or KUS187, by intraperitoneal injection in a *rd10* mouse model resulted in preserved outer nuclear layer (ONL) thickness and improved visual function measured by ERG.

Because of the unfolding properties of VCP also other AAA+ proteins have been proposed as potent therapeutic agents, especially in solving protein misfolding and aggregation in neurodegenerative diseases. Although not functionally related to ERAD, the repurposing of two AAA+ proteins, including Hsp104 and proteasome-activating nucleotidase (PAN) were shown to protect from protein misfolding in several neurodegenerative animal models [159]. Furthermore, transgenic expression of PAN in rods of mice lacking the γ-subunit of transducin ($G\gamma^{-/-}$) resulted in increased photoreceptor survival accompanied by preserved visual function [132].

Another possible therapeutic target of ERAD could be the enhancement of proteosomal degradation. Important players in this process are the deubiquitination enzymes (DUBs), also known as ubiquitin-specific proteases (USPs). USPs are known to cleave ubiquitin moieties from proteins and thereby preventing these proteins from proteosomal degradation [133]. Therefore, inhibiting USPs might work as a therapeutic approach to stimulate the degradation of misfolded proteins by the proteasome. In cancer research inhibition of specific USPs, including USP7 and USP10, has already been shown to have beneficial effects, by acting on the tumor suppressor p53 [134].

Depending on the type of mutation, p53 can either gain oncogenic properties or lose its tumor suppressor ability [160]. Therefore, based on the mutant form of p53, either increasing or lowering the levels of p53 could be beneficial. Inhibiting USP7, a negative regulator of p53, leads to increased p53 levels, whereas inhibiting USP10, a positive regulator of p53, leads to reduction of p53 levels [134]. With this in mind, the causative mutation for the disease has to be known, as well as the specificity of the USP inhibitor before administering it to the patient. From discrepancies in findings of different studies it cannot be concluded whether p53 is involved in the pathogenesis of PR cell death [161,162]. However, a recent study found a biallelic mutation in *USP45* associated with LCA. This indicates that USPs can play important roles in the pathogenesis of PR degeneration [163].

Another important issue to address is that DUBs associated with VCP have been suggested to promote protein turnover by assisting in retrotranslocation instead of their traditional function in preventing proteasomal degradation. Therefore, inducing these specific VCP associated DUBs might have therapeutic potential [135].

3.3.2. Targeting Autophagy

One of the best known inducers of autophagy is rapamycin, which directly binds to mTORC1, thereby inhibiting the mTOR pathway [164]. Because of its limited absorption, studies have been focusing on investigating rapamycin analogs or rapalogs, including everolimus, temsirolimus, and ridaforolimus. These mTORC1 inhibitors were highlighted as promising therapeutic agents in various protein misfolding associated diseases, including neurodegenerative diseases and multiple forms of cancer [165,166]. Also, a study in an RP rat model has shown the therapeutic potential of rapamycin in treating blindness [136]. In this study, rod cell degeneration was slowed down, without affecting cones, in a P23H rat model upon systemic administration of rapamycin. In contrast, other studies showed that activation of the mTOR pathway promotes cone survival [167–169]. Taken together, these results indicate that activation of autophagy is particularly protective for rods, but can have opposing effects on cones.

Studies investigating other mTOR inhibitors, including ATP-competitive mTOR inhibitors, are emerging [170]. Furthermore, indirect modulators of the mTOR pathway, including metformin and nilotinib have also been shown to play a protective role in diabetes, cancer, and neurodegenerative diseases via indirect activation of AMPK [171–173]. Contradictory results are found in mouse models of retinal degeneration when treated with metformin. In diabetic mice, metformin treatment protected against retinal cell death, whereas in a P23H RHO mouse model it accelerated the photoreceptor degeneration, indicating different modes of action by metformin [137,138].

In addition to autophagy upregulators acting on the mTOR pathway, also mTOR-independent autophagy upregulators have been widely studied, mainly in Huntington's disease [174]. One such agent is valproic acid (VPA), which upregulates autophagy by inhibiting inositol synthesis. In line with findings in neurodegeneration models, VPA treatment in models for photoreceptor degeneration can be detrimental or protective [139,175]. In a mouse model for Bardet–Biedl syndrome ($BBS12^{-/-}$), as well as in a *Xenopus laevis* model for RP (P23H) treatment with VPA resulted in photoreceptor protection [139,140]. In contrast, a T17M *X. laevis* model of RP and the P23H-1 rat model showed exacerbated photoreceptor degeneration upon VPA treatment [15,139]. Even in mouse models with a different mutation in the same gene (PDE6) this discrepancy in outcome was observed: VPA treatment reduced photoreceptor loss in the *rd1* model, whereas VPA treatment slightly accelerated photoreceptor loss in the *rd10* model [141]. Taken together, these studies indicate that the outcome of VPA treatment depends on the genotype and even on the type of mutation. The conflicting results might be partly explained by the different modes of action by VPA, since VPA is also acting as a histone deacetylase (HDAC) inhibitor, thereby altering expression of different genes [176].

4. Discussion and Outlook

The OS of the PR can be considered as a highly specialized cilium responsible for the conversion of light stimuli into electrical signals, also known as the phototransduction cascade. This cascade requires a tremendous amount of energy as well as a continuous OS protein turnover to maintain cellular homeostasis. Therefore, a perfectly balanced proteostasis network is of particular importance for the PRs. In many IRDs this balance is disrupted leading to protein accumulation in the IS and ultimately to PR cell death. Several attempts were made to restore this balance by therapeutically targeting different branches of the proteostasis network, including protein trafficking, folding, and degradation. For therapeutic intervention, it has to be taken into account that these different branches consist of tightly intertwined processes, which depend on each other and influence each other's function and activation. For example, administration of the AMPK activator metformin to P23H RHO mice resulted in enhanced trafficking of rhodopsin to the rod OSs. However, it still led to reduced PR function and survival. Apparently, metformin did not succeed in full restoration of the correct folding of rhodopsin, leading to increased destabilization of the OSs [137]. Taken together, enhancing protein trafficking without improving protein folding will accelerate the disease progression rather than diminishing it. Recently, also an intimate cross-talk between the UPR, more specifically IRE1, and ERAD has been described [177]. On one hand, splicing of XBP1s by activated IRE1 promotes the expression of ERAD components, while on the other hand ERAD serves as a feedback loop for IRE1 by targeting it for degradation. This cross-talk is probably further extended to other branches of the UPR, since it has been shown that the turnover of ATF6 is also regulated by ERAD [178].

Another issue that has to be taken into account for therapeutic intervention is that in some disease conditions certain branches of the proteostasis network are protective, whereas in other disease conditions it is a consequence of the disease process. Therefore, it is often not clear which branch of the proteostasis network would be the most effective target to treat a certain disease type. Even different mutations in the same gene causing similar disease conditions can have an effect on the treatment outcome, indicated by contradictory findings in VPA treatment in the *rd1* and *rd10* mouse models [141]. This discrepancy might be partly explained by the severity of the gene mutations leading to different rates of disease progression, since *rd1* mice show rapid degeneration of PRs, whereas the *rd10* mouse model represents a more slowly progressive form of RP. With this in mind, therapeutic compounds that have an positive effect on slow progressing forms of RP might not be suitable for fast progressing forms of RP and early onset forms of blindness, such as LCA.

The animal model used for therapeutic testing, especially animals carrying a transgene, can also influence therapeutic outcome. One such animal model carrying a transgene is the P23H RHO rat model. Numerous different lines with various transgene expression exist [179–181]. It has been shown that the amount of expression of the transgene can have an effect on the disease phenotype. Even overexpression of wild type human rod opsin has been shown to induce PR degeneration [182]. In contrast, it has been shown that overexpression of wild type RHO partially rescues visual responses in a P23H RHO rat model [113]. Nevertheless, studies using the P23H RHO rat model presented in this review should be interpreted with caution, especially when translating therapeutic outcome to the patient situation.

Instead of directly targeting the different branches of the proteostasis network, mimicking the actions of these branches might also be a valuable therapeutic approach. The main action of the PERK pathway of the UPR is reducing the protein synthesis and thereby reducing the ER-stress load. This action can also be regulated by targeting the epigenome, including histone acetylation. Enzymes that play an important role in this acetylation process are the histone deacetylases (HDACs). Inhibiting these HDACs was shown to be protective for PR cell death. Administration of the HDAC6 inhibitor tubastatin A in an inherited blindness zebrafish model resulted in the rescue of retinal morphology and visual function [183]. However, further investigation of the underlying molecular mechanisms is necessary, since poor efficacy and safety have been reported for other HDAC inhibitors, including VPA [176,184].

Another way to influence protein synthesis is by the regulation of splicing. The importance of splicing in the retina is indicated by mutations found in the ubiquitously expressed pre-mRNA processing factors (PRPFs), which only cause retinal-specific degeneration [185]. In situ gene editing of a pathogenic, dominant mutation in PRPF31 resulted in the rescue of protein expression as well as the phenotype [186]. The proof-of-principle for targeting splicing as potential therapeutic strategy is further supported by the application of antisense oligonucleotides for the treatment of inherited retinal diseases, including CEP290 associated LCA [20,187].

In addition to influencing protein synthesis, degeneration of PRs, which is the ultimate consequence of sustained ER-stress and a key hallmark of IRDs, can also been seen as a therapeutic target. A broad range of therapeutic agents is available that can be protective for PR cell death, including cell death inhibitors, caspase modulators, and neurotrophic factors. Individual treatment of P23H-1 rats with the known cell death inhibitors calpeptin, N-acetylcysteine, and necrostatin-1s all resulted in improved photoreceptor function [188]. Furthermore, the chemical chaperone tauroursodeoxycholic acid (TUDCA), which inhibits apoptosis by preventing BAX from being transported to the mitochondria to initiate caspase release, has been shown to preserve cones in a LCA mouse model upon systemic injection [189]. On top of that, direct inhibition of caspases by subretinal AAV delivered X-linked inhibitor of apoptosis (XIAP) in two RP rat models protected PR structure and function [190]. Finally, neurotrophic factors, including CNTF, BDNF, GDNF, LEDGF, PEDF, and RdCVF were also found to have positive effects on PR survival [191]. However, the therapeutic potential of neurotrophic factors as a general treatment may not outweigh the plausible risk of side effects. These side effects can be reduced by carefully selecting the proper administration route, which accounts for every therapeutic agent described in this review. In general, there are three possible delivery methods to reach the eye: systemic, topical, and local. Each of these methods have their advantages and disadvantages [192]. Systemic delivery is often accompanied by systemic side effects and drugs need to pass the blood–retinal barrier first to perform their function, but it is less invasive compared to intraocular injections. Topical delivery in form of eye drops or ointments is not invasive, but the chance that the therapeutic compound reaches its destination is often an issue. Intraocular injection is the most invasive delivery method, but most often also the most effective one. Furthermore, with this method the involvement of the immune system is largely circumvented, as the eye is a largely immune-privileged organ, thereby further reducing the risk of potential side effects. Intraocular delivery can be performed by injecting the therapeutic compound by itself, but the cell penetrance and thus delivery efficiency is much higher when the compound is packed into nanoparticles, for example [192].

Immense progress has been made in optimizing the delivery methods in combination with the drug formulation, especially for gene augmentation and antisense-oligo nucleotide (AON)-based treatments. Now, an increasing number of studies are aimed at developing broader applicable treatments, and therefore are focused on therapies targetting the proteostatis network. Many of these studies show hopeful results in delaying blinding conditions [111,114,121,122,131]. However, much effort has still to be made to first efficiently halt the progression of IRD, let alone fully restore vision.

Acknowledgments: The authors would like to acknowledge Marius Ueffing for valuable advice on P23H RHO models.

References

1. Osterberg, G. Topography of the layer of rods and cones in the human retina. *Acta Ophthalmol. Suppl.* **1935**, *6*, 1–103.
2. May-Simera, H.; Nagel-Wolfrum, K.; Wolfrum, U. Cilia-The sensory antennae in the eye. *Prog. Retin. Eye Res.* **2017**, *60*, 144–180. [CrossRef] [PubMed]
3. Arshavsky, V.Y.; Lamb, T.D.; Pugh, E.N., Jr. G proteins and phototransduction. *Annu. Rev. Physiol.* **2002**, *64*, 153–187. [CrossRef] [PubMed]
4. Sokolov, M.; Yadav, R.P.; Brooks, C.; Artemyev, N.O. Chaperones and retinal disorders. *Adv. Protein Chem. Struct. Biol.* **2019**, *114*, 85–117. [CrossRef] [PubMed]
5. Krizaj, D. Calcium regulation in photoreceptors. *Front. Biosci. A J. Virtual Libr.* **2002**, *7*, 2023–2044. [CrossRef]
6. Martemyanov, A.K. The Transduction Cascade in Retinal ON-Bipolar Cells: Signal Processing and Disease. *Annu. Rev. Vis. Sci.* **2017**, *3*, 25–51. [CrossRef] [PubMed]
7. Young, R.W.R. The renewal of photoreceptor cell outer segments. *J. Cell Biol.* **1967**, *33*, 61–72. [CrossRef] [PubMed]
8. Baehr, W. Membrane protein transport in photoreceptors: The function of PDEdelta: The Proctor lecture. *Investig. Ophthalmol. Vis. Sci.* **2014**, *55*, 8653–8666. [CrossRef]
9. Leveillard, T.; Sahel, J.A. Metabolic and redox signaling in the retina. *Cell Mol. Life Sci.* **2017**, *74*, 3649–3665. [CrossRef]
10. Narayan, D.S.; Chidlow, G.; Wood, J.P.; Casson, R.J. Glucose metabolism in mammalian photoreceptor inner and outer segments. *Clin. Exp. Ophthalmol.* **2017**, *45*, 730–741. [CrossRef]
11. Bujakowska, K.M.; Liu, Q.; Pierce, E.A. Photoreceptor Cilia and Retinal Ciliopathies. *Cold Spring Harb. Perspect. Biol.* **2017**, *9*. [CrossRef] [PubMed]
12. Daiger, S.P.; Sullivan, L.S.; Rossiter, B.J.F. Cloned and/or Mapped Human Genes Causing Retinal Degeneration or Related Diseases. Available online: https://sph.uth.edu/retnet/ (accessed on 23 July 2019).
13. Roepman, R. Protein networks and complexes in photoreceptor cilia. *Sub-Cell. Biochem.* **2007**, *43*, 209–235.
14. Liu, Q. The proteome of the mouse photoreceptor sensory cilium complex. *Mol. Cell. Proteom.* **2007**, *6*, 1299–1317. [CrossRef] [PubMed]
15. Athanasiou, D.; Aguila, M.; Bellingham, J.; Li, W.; McCulley, C.; Reeves, P.J.; Cheetham, M.E. The molecular and cellular basis of rhodopsin retinitis pigmentosa reveals potential strategies for therapy. *Prog. Retin. Eye Res.* **2018**, *62*, 1–23. [CrossRef] [PubMed]
16. den Hollander, A.I.; Koenekoop, R.K.; Mohamed, M.D.; Arts, H.H.; Boldt, K.; Towns, K.V.; Sedmak, T.; Beer, M.; Nagel-Wolfrum, K.; McKibbin, M.; et al. Mutations in LCA5, encoding the ciliary protein lebercilin, cause Leber congenital amaurosis. *Nat. Genet.* **2007**, *39*, 889–895. [CrossRef] [PubMed]
17. Hamel, C.P. Cone rod dystrophies. *Orphanet J. Rare Dis.* **2007**, *2*, 7. [CrossRef] [PubMed]
18. Hirji, N.; Aboshiha, J.; Georgiou, M.; Bainbridge, J.; Michaelides, M. Achromatopsia: Clinical features, molecular genetics, animal models and therapeutic options. *Ophthalmic Genet.* **2018**, *39*, 149–157. [CrossRef] [PubMed]
19. Song, J.Y.; Aravand, P.; Nikonov, S.; Leo, L.; Lyubarsky, A.; Bennicelli, J.L.; Pan, J.; Wei, Z.; Shpylchak, I.; Herrera, P.; et al. Amelioration of neurosensory structure and function in animal and cellular models of a congenital blindness. *Mol. Ther.* **2018**. [CrossRef]
20. Garanto, A.; Chung, D.C.; Duijkers, L.; Corral-Serrano, J.C.; Messchaert, M.; Xiao, R.; Bennett, J.; Vandenberghe, L.H.; Collin, R.W. In vitro and in vivo rescue of aberrant splicing in CEP290-associated LCA by antisense oligonucleotide delivery. *Hum. Mol. Genet.* **2016**, *25*, 2552–2563. [CrossRef]
21. Athanasiou, D.; Aguila, M.; Bevilacqua, D.; Novoselov, S.S.; Parfitt, D.A.; Cheetham, M.E. The cell stress machinery and retinal degeneration. *FEBS Lett.* **2013**, *587*, 2008–2017. [CrossRef]
22. Maurer-Stroh, S.; Koranda, M.; Benetka, W.; Schneider, G.; Sirota, F.L.; Eisenhaber, F. Towards complete sets of farnesylated and geranylgeranylated proteins. *PLoS Comput. Biol.* **2007**, *3*, e66. [CrossRef] [PubMed]
23. Casey, P.J.P. Protein prenyltransferases. *J. Biol. Chem.* **1996**, *271*, 5289–5292. [CrossRef] [PubMed]

24. Sohocki, M.M.M. Mutations in a new photoreceptor-pineal gene on 17p cause Leber congenital amaurosis. *Nat. Genet.* **2000**, *24*, 79–83. [CrossRef] [PubMed]
25. den Hollander, A.I. Leber congenital amaurosis: Genes, proteins and disease mechanisms. *Prog. Retin. Eye Res.* **2008**, *27*, 391–419. [CrossRef] [PubMed]
26. Liu, X. AIPL1, the protein that is defective in Leber congenital amaurosis, is essential for the biosynthesis of retinal rod cGMP phosphodiesterase. *Proc. Natl. Acad. Sci. USA* **2004**, *101*, 13903–13908. [CrossRef] [PubMed]
27. Ramamurthy, V. Leber congenital amaurosis linked to AIPL1: A mouse model reveals destabilization of cGMP phosphodiesterase. *Proc. Natl. Acad. Sci. USA* **2004**, *101*, 13897–13902. [CrossRef] [PubMed]
28. Ramamurthy, V. AIPL1, a protein implicated in Leber's congenital amaurosis, interacts with and aids in processing of farnesylated proteins. *Proc. Natl. Acad. Sci. USA* **2003**, *100*, 12630–12635. [CrossRef] [PubMed]
29. Yadav, R.P.; Artemyev, N.O. AIPL1: A specialized chaperone for the phototransduction effector. *Cell Signal.* **2017**, *40*, 183–189. [CrossRef] [PubMed]
30. Roosing, S.; Collin, R.W.; den Hollander, A.I.; Cremers, F.P.; Siemiatkowska, A.M. Prenylation defects in inherited retinal diseases. *J. Med. Genet.* **2014**, *51*, 143–151. [CrossRef] [PubMed]
31. Zhang, H.; Constantine, R.; Frederick, J.M.; Baehr, W. The prenyl-binding protein PrBP/delta: A chaperone participating in intracellular trafficking. *Vis. Res.* **2012**, *75*, 19–25. [CrossRef]
32. Zhang, H.H. Deletion of PrBP/delta impedes transport of GRK1 and PDE6 catalytic subunits to photoreceptor outer segments. *Proc. Natl. Acad. Sci. USA* **2007**, *104*, 8857–8862. [CrossRef] [PubMed]
33. Thomas, S. A homozygous PDE6D mutation in Joubert syndrome impairs targeting of farnesylated INPP5E protein to the primary cilium. *Hum. Mutat.* **2014**, *35*, 137–146. [CrossRef] [PubMed]
34. Megarbane, A.; Hmaimess, G.; Bizzari, S.; El-Bazzal, L.; Al-Ali, M.T.; Stora, S.; Delague, V.; El-Hayek, S. A novel PDE6D mutation in a patient with Joubert syndrome type 22 (JBTS22). *Eur. J. Med. Genet.* **2018**. [CrossRef]
35. Rao, K.N.; Zhang, W.; Li, L.; Anand, M.; Khanna, H. Prenylated retinal ciliopathy protein RPGR interacts with PDE6delta and regulates ciliary localization of Joubert syndrome-associated protein INPP5E. *Hum. Mol. Genet.* **2016**, *25*, 4533–4545. [CrossRef] [PubMed]
36. Qureshi, B.M.; Schmidt, A.; Behrmann, E.; Burger, J.; Mielke, T.; Spahn, C.M.T.; Heck, M.; Scheerer, P. Mechanistic insights into the role of prenyl-binding protein PrBP/delta in membrane dissociation of phosphodiesterase 6. *Nat. Commun.* **2018**, *9*, 90. [CrossRef] [PubMed]
37. Hanke-Gogokhia, C.; Frederick, J.M.; Zhang, H.; Baehr, W. Binary Function of ARL3-GTP Revealed by Gene Knockouts. *Adv. Exp. Med. Biol.* **2018**, *1074*, 317–325. [CrossRef] [PubMed]
38. Ismail, A.S. Arl2-GTP and Arl3-GTP regulate a GDI-like transport system for farnesylated cargo. *Nat. Chem. Biol.* **2011**, *7*, 942–949. [CrossRef]
39. Fansa, K.E. Sorting of lipidated cargo by the Arl2/Arl3 system. *Small GTPases* **2016**, *7*, 222–230. [CrossRef] [PubMed]
40. Constantine, R. Uncoordinated (UNC)119: Coordinating the trafficking of myristoylated proteins. *Vis. Res.* **2012**, *75*, 26–32. [CrossRef] [PubMed]
41. Zhang, H. UNC119 is required for G protein trafficking in sensory neurons. *Nat. Neurosci.* **2011**, *14*, 874–880. [CrossRef] [PubMed]
42. Ishiba, Y. Targeted inactivation of synaptic HRG4 (UNC119) causes dysfunction in the distal photoreceptor and slow retinal degeneration, revealing a new function. *Exp. Eye Res.* **2007**, *84*, 473–485. [CrossRef] [PubMed]
43. Zhang, H.; Frederick, J.M.; Baehr, W. Unc119 gene deletion partially rescues the GRK1 transport defect of Pde6d (-/-) cones. *Adv. Exp. Med. Biol.* **2014**, *801*, 487–493. [CrossRef]
44. Kobayashi, A.A. HRG4 (UNC119) mutation found in cone-rod dystrophy causes retinal degeneration in a transgenic model. *Investig. Ophthalmol. Vis. Sci.* **2000**, *41*, 3268–3277.
45. Zhang, J. Mechanism of folding chamber closure in a group II chaperonin. *Sci. Am.* **2010**, *463*, 379–383. [CrossRef] [PubMed]
46. Wells, A.C. Role of the chaperonin CCT/TRiC complex in G protein betagamma-dimer assembly. *J. Biol. Chem.* **2006**, *281*, 20221–20232. [CrossRef] [PubMed]
47. Lukov, L.G. Phosducin-like protein acts as a molecular chaperone for G protein betagamma dimer assembly. *EMBO J.* **2005**, *24*, 1965–1975. [CrossRef] [PubMed]

48. Loew, A.A. Phosducin induces a structural change in transducin β γ. *Structure* **1998**, *6*, 1007–1019. [CrossRef]
49. Brooks, C. Farnesylation of the Transducin G Protein γ Subunit Is a Prerequisite for Its Ciliary Targeting in Rod Photoreceptors. *Front. Mol. Neurosci.* **2018**, *11*, 16. [CrossRef]
50. Obin, M. Ubiquitylation of the transducin betagamma subunit complex. Regulation by phosducin. *J. Biol. Chem.* **2002**, *277*, 44566–44575. [CrossRef]
51. Zhang, Q. Intrinsic protein-protein interaction-mediated and chaperonin-assisted sequential assembly of stable bardet-biedl syndrome protein complex, the BBSome. *J. Biol. Chem.* **2012**, *287*, 20625–20635. [CrossRef]
52. Klink, B.U. A recombinant BBSome core complex and how it interacts with ciliary cargo. *eLife* **2017**, *6*, e27434. [CrossRef] [PubMed]
53. Forsythe, E. Bardet-Biedl syndrome. *Eur. J. Hum. Genet.* **2013**, *21*, 8–13. [CrossRef] [PubMed]
54. Jin, H. The conserved Bardet-Biedl syndrome proteins assemble a coat that traffics membrane proteins to cilia. *Cell* **2010**, *141*, 1208–1219. [CrossRef] [PubMed]
55. Chan, P. Molecular chaperoning function of Ric-8 is to fold nascent heterotrimeric G protein a subunits. *Proc. Natl. Acad. Sci. USA* **2013**, *110*, 3794–3799. [CrossRef] [PubMed]
56. Tall, G.G. Ric-8 regulation of heterotrimeric G proteins. *J. Recept. Signal Transduct.* **2013**, *33*, 139–143. [CrossRef]
57. Fenech, C. Ric-8A, a Gα protein guanine nucleotide exchange factor potentiates taste receptor signaling. *Front. Cell. Neurosci.* **2009**, *3*, 11. [CrossRef] [PubMed]
58. Sprang, R.S. Structural basis of effector regulation and signal termination in heterotrimeric Gα proteins. *Adv. Protein Chem.* **2007**, *74*, 1–65.
59. Joutsen, J.; Sistonen, L. Tailoring of Proteostasis Networks with Heat Shock Factors. *Cold Spring Harb. Perspect. Biol.* **2019**, *11*. [CrossRef]
60. Morimoto, R.I.R. The heat-shock response: Regulation and function of heat-shock proteins and molecular chaperones. *Essays Biochem.* **1997**, *32*, 17–29.
61. Vabulas, R.M.R.M. Protein folding in the cytoplasm and the heat shock response. *Cold Spring Harbor Perspect. Biol.* **2010**, *2*, a004390. [CrossRef]
62. Hartl, F.U.; Bracher, A.; Hayer-Hartl, M. Molecular chaperones in protein folding and proteostasis. *Nature* **2011**, *475*, 324–332. [CrossRef] [PubMed]
63. Apetri, C.A. Chaperonin chamber accelerates protein folding through passive action of preventing aggregation. *Proc. Natl. Acad. Sci. USA* **2008**, *105*, 17351–17355. [CrossRef] [PubMed]
64. Walter, P. The unfolded protein response: From stress pathway to homeostatic regulation. *Science* **2011**, *334*, 1081–1086. [CrossRef] [PubMed]
65. Bertolotti, A.A. Dynamic interaction of BiP and ER stress transducers in the unfolded-protein response. *Nat. Cell Biol.* **2000**, *2*, 326–332. [CrossRef] [PubMed]
66. Lamriben, L. Activating and Repressing IRE1a: The Hsp47 and BiP Tug of War. *Mol. Cell* **2018**, *69*, 159–160. [CrossRef] [PubMed]
67. Calfon, M. IRE1 couples endoplasmic reticulum load to secretory capacity by processing the XBP-1 mRNA. *Sci. Am.* **2002**, *415*, 92–96. [CrossRef] [PubMed]
68. Lee, A.H. XBP-1 regulates a subset of endoplasmic reticulum resident chaperone genes in the unfolded protein response. *Mol. Cell. Biol.* **2003**, *23*, 7448–7459. [CrossRef] [PubMed]
69. Fritz, M.J. Deficiency of the BiP cochaperone ERdj4 causes constitutive endoplasmic reticulum stress and metabolic defects. *Mol. Biol. Cell* **2014**, *25*, 431–440. [CrossRef]
70. Eletto, D. Protein disulfide isomerase A6 controls the decay of IRE1a signaling via disulfide-dependent association. *Mol. Cell* **2014**, *53*, 562–576. [CrossRef] [PubMed]
71. Harding, H.P.H. Protein translation and folding are coupled by an endoplasmic-reticulum-resident kinase. *Sci. Am.* **1999**, *397*, 271–274.
72. Vattem, M.K. Reinitiation involving upstream ORFs regulates ATF4 mRNA translation in mammalian cells. *Proc. Natl. Acad. Sci. USA* **2004**, *101*, 11269–11274. [CrossRef] [PubMed]
73. Novoa, I.I. Feedback inhibition of the unfolded protein response by GADD34-mediated dephosphorylation of eIF2α. *J. Cell Biol.* **2001**, *153*, 1011–1022. [CrossRef] [PubMed]
74. Marciniak, J.S. CHOP induces death by promoting protein synthesis and oxidation in the stressed endoplasmic reticulum. *Gen. Dev.* **2004**, *18*, 3066–3077. [CrossRef] [PubMed]

75. Shen, J. ER stress regulation of ATF6 localization by dissociation of BiP/GRP78 binding and unmasking of Golgi localization signals. *Dev. Cell* **2002**, *3*, 99–111. [CrossRef]
76. Haze, K.K. Mammalian transcription factor ATF6 is synthesized as a transmembrane protein and activated by proteolysis in response to endoplasmic reticulum stress. *Mol. Biol. Cell* **1999**, *10*, 3787–3799. [CrossRef] [PubMed]
77. Yamamoto, K. Transcriptional induction of mammalian ER quality control proteins is mediated by single or combined action of ATF6α and XBP1. *Dev. Cell* **2007**, *13*, 365–376. [CrossRef] [PubMed]
78. Schubert, U.U. Rapid degradation of a large fraction of newly synthesized proteins by proteasomes. *Sci. Am.* **2000**, *404*, 770–774. [CrossRef] [PubMed]
79. Olzmann, A.J. The mammalian endoplasmic reticulum-associated degradation system. *Cold Spring Harbor Perspect. Biol.* **2013**, *5*. [CrossRef] [PubMed]
80. Helenius, A. Roles of N-linked glycans in the endoplasmic reticulum. *Ann. Rev. Biochem.* **2004**, *73*, 1019–1049. [CrossRef]
81. Aebi, M. N-glycan structures: Recognition and processing in the ER. *Trends Biochem. Sci.* **2010**, *35*, 74–82. [CrossRef] [PubMed]
82. Hebert, N.D. ERAD substrates: Which way out? *Semin. Cell Dev. Biol.* **2010**, *21*, 526–532. [CrossRef] [PubMed]
83. Gonzalez, D.S.D. Identification, expression, and characterization of a cDNA encoding human endoplasmic reticulum mannosidase I, the enzyme that catalyzes the first mannose trimming step in mammalian Asn-linked oligosaccharide biosynthesis. *J. Biol. Chem.* **1999**, *274*, 21375–21386. [CrossRef] [PubMed]
84. Olivari, S. EDEM1 regulates ER-associated degradation by accelerating de-mannosylation of folding-defective polypeptides and by inhibiting their covalent aggregation. *Biochem. Biophys. Res. Commun.* **2006**, *349*, 1278–1284. [CrossRef] [PubMed]
85. Hirao, K. EDEM3, a soluble EDEM homolog, enhances glycoprotein endoplasmic reticulum-associated degradation and mannose trimming. *J. Biol. Chem.* **2006**, *281*, 9650–9658. [CrossRef] [PubMed]
86. Hampton, Y.R. Finding the will and the way of ERAD substrate retrotranslocation. *Curr. Opin. Cell Biol.* **2012**, *24*, 460–466. [CrossRef] [PubMed]
87. Ye, Y. A membrane protein complex mediates retro-translocation from the ER lumen into the cytosol. *Sci. Am.* **2004**, *429*, 841–847. [CrossRef] [PubMed]
88. Meyer, H. Emerging functions of the VCP/p97 AAA-ATPase in the ubiquitin system. *Nat. Cell Biol.* **2012**, *14*, 117–123. [CrossRef] [PubMed]
89. Xu, Y. SGTA recognizes a noncanonical ubiquitin-like domain in the Bag6-Ubl4A-Trc35 complex to promote endoplasmic reticulum-associated degradation. *Cell Rep.* **2012**, *2*, 1633–1644. [CrossRef] [PubMed]
90. Boya, P.; Esteban-Martinez, L.; Serrano-Puebla, A.; Gomez-Sintes, R.; Villarejo-Zori, B. Autophagy in the eye: Development, degeneration, and aging. *Prog. Retin. Eye Res.* **2016**, *55*, 206–245. [CrossRef] [PubMed]
91. Wong, P.M. The ULK1 complex: Sensing nutrient signals for autophagy activation. *Autophagy* **2013**, *9*, 124–137. [CrossRef] [PubMed]
92. Walker, S. Making autophagosomes: Localized synthesis of phosphatidylinositol 3-phosphate holds the clue. *Autophagy* **2008**, *4*, 1093–1096. [CrossRef] [PubMed]
93. Frost, L.S.; Mitchell, C.H.; Boesze-Battaglia, K. Autophagy in the eye: Implications for ocular cell health. *Exp. Eye Res.* **2014**, *124*, 56–66. [CrossRef] [PubMed]
94. Arias, E. Chaperone-mediated autophagy in protein quality control. *Curr. Opin. Cell Biol.* **2011**, *23*, 184–189. [CrossRef] [PubMed]
95. Dice, J.F.J. Peptide sequences that target cytosolic proteins for lysosomal proteolysis. *Trends Biochem. Sci.* **1990**, *15*, 305–309. [CrossRef]
96. Chiang, H.L.H. A role for a 70-kilodalton heat shock protein in lysosomal degradation of intracellular proteins. *Science* **1989**, *246*, 382–385. [CrossRef] [PubMed]
97. Cuervo, A.M.A. A receptor for the selective uptake and degradation of proteins by lysosomes. *Science* **1996**, *273*, 501–503. [CrossRef] [PubMed]
98. Sahu, R. Microautophagy of cytosolic proteins by late endosomes. *Dev. Cell* **2011**, *20*, 131–139. [CrossRef] [PubMed]
99. Morozova, K. Structural and Biological Interaction of hsc-70 Protein with Phosphatidylserine in Endosomal Microautophagy. *J. Biol. Chem.* **2016**, *291*, 18096–18106. [CrossRef]

100. Capell, C.B. Inhibiting farnesylation of progerin prevents the characteristic nuclear blebbing of Hutchinson-Gilford progeria syndrome. *Proc. Natl. Acad. Sci. USA* **2005**, *102*, 12879–12884. [CrossRef]
101. Gordon, B.L. Clinical Trial of the Protein Farnesylation Inhibitors Lonafarnib, Pravastatin, and Zoledronic Acid in Children With Hutchinson-Gilford Progeria Syndrome. *Circ. J. Am. Heart Assoc.* **2016**, *134*, 114–125. [CrossRef]
102. Martin, E.N. A phase I trial of the dual farnesyltransferase and geranylgeranyltransferase inhibitor L-778,123 and radiotherapy for locally advanced pancreatic cancer. *Clin. Cancer Res.* **2004**, *10*, 5447–5454. [CrossRef] [PubMed]
103. Posokhova, E. Disruption of the chaperonin containing TCP-1 function affects protein networks essential for rod outer segment morphogenesis and survival. *Mol. Cell. Proteom.* **2011**, *10*. [CrossRef] [PubMed]
104. Willardson, M.B. Function of phosducin-like proteins in G protein signaling and chaperone-assisted protein folding. *Cell Signal.* **2007**, *19*, 2417–2427. [CrossRef] [PubMed]
105. Álvarez-Satta, M. Bardet-Biedl Syndrome as a Chaperonopathy: Dissecting the Major Role of Chaperonin-Like BBS Proteins (BBS6-BBS10-BBS12). *Front. Mol. Biosci.* **2017**, *4*, 55. [CrossRef] [PubMed]
106. Papasergi, M.M. The G protein a chaperone Ric-8 as a potential therapeutic target. *Mol. Pharmacol.* **2015**, *87*, 52–63. [CrossRef] [PubMed]
107. Szabo, V. p.Gln200Glu, a putative constitutively active mutant of rod α-transducin (*GNAT1*) in autosomal dominant congenital stationary night blindness. *Hum. Mutat.* **2007**, *28*, 741–742. [CrossRef] [PubMed]
108. Supko, J.G.J. Preclinical pharmacologic evaluation of geldanamycin as an antitumor agent. *Cancer Chemother. Pharmacol.* **1995**, *36*, 305–315. [CrossRef]
109. Jhaveri, K. Advances in the clinical development of heat shock protein 90 (Hsp90) inhibitors in cancers. *Biochim. Biophys. Acta* **2012**, *1823*, 742–755. [CrossRef]
110. Tam, C.S.L. Prevention of autosomal dominant retinitis pigmentosa by systemic drug therapy targeting heat shock protein 90 (Hsp90). *Hum. Mol. Genet.* **2010**, *19*, 4421–4436. [CrossRef]
111. Aguilà, M. Hsp90 inhibition protects against inherited retinal degeneration. *Hum. Mol. Genet.* **2014**, *23*, 2164–2175. [CrossRef]
112. Zhou, D. A rat retinal damage model predicts for potential clinical visual disturbances induced by Hsp90 inhibitors. *Toxicol. Appl. Pharmacol.* **2013**, *273*, 401–409. [CrossRef] [PubMed]
113. Gorbatyuk, S.M. Functional rescue of P23H rhodopsin photoreceptors by gene delivery. *Adv. Exp. Med. Biol.* **2012**, *723*, 191–197. [PubMed]
114. Parfitt, D.A.; Aguila, M.; McCulley, C.H.; Bevilacqua, D.; Mendes, H.F.; Athanasiou, D.; Novoselov, S.S.; Kanuga, N.; Munro, P.M.; Coffey, P.J.; et al. The heat-shock response co-inducer arimoclomol protects against retinal degeneration in rhodopsin retinitis pigmentosa. *Cell Death Dis.* **2014**, *5*, e1236. [CrossRef] [PubMed]
115. Gorbatyuk, S.M. Restoration of visual function in P23H rhodopsin transgenic rats by gene delivery of BiP/Grp78. *Proc. Natl. Acad. Sci. USA* **2010**, *107*, 5961–5966. [CrossRef] [PubMed]
116. Ghaderi, S.; Ahmadian, S.; Soheili, Z.S.; Ahmadieh, H.; Samiei, S.; Kheitan, S.; Pirmardan, E.R. AAV delivery of GRP78/BiP promotes adaptation of human RPE cell to ER stress. *J. Cell Biochem.* **2018**, *119*, 1355–1367. [CrossRef] [PubMed]
117. Nashine, S. Ablation of C/EBP homologous protein does not protect T17M RHO mice from retinal degeneration. *PLoS ONE* **2013**, *8*. [CrossRef] [PubMed]
118. Adekeye, A. Ablation of the proapoptotic genes CHOP or Ask1 does not prevent or delay loss of visual function in a P23H transgenic mouse model of retinitis pigmentosa. *PLoS ONE* **2014**, *9*. [CrossRef] [PubMed]
119. Chiang, W.C. Ablation of Chop Transiently Enhances Photoreceptor Survival but Does Not Prevent Retinal Degeneration in Transgenic Mice Expressing Human P23H Rhodopsin. *Adv. Exp. Med. Biol.* **2016**, *854*, 185–191.
120. Bhootada, Y.; Kotla, P.; Zolotukhin, S.; Gorbatyuk, O.; Bebok, Z.; Athar, M.; Gorbatyuk, M. Limited ATF4 Expression in Degenerating Retinas with Ongoing ER Stress Promotes Photoreceptor Survival in a Mouse Model of Autosomal Dominant Retinitis Pigmentosa. *PLoS ONE* **2016**, *11*, e0154779. [CrossRef]
121. Athanasiou, D.; Aguila, M.; Bellingham, J.; Kanuga, N.; Adamson, P.; Cheetham, M.E. The role of the ER stress-response protein PERK in rhodopsin retinitis pigmentosa. *Hum. Mol. Genet.* **2017**, *26*, 4896–4905. [CrossRef]
122. Ghosh, R. Allosteric inhibition of the IRE1a RNase preserves cell viability and function during endoplasmic reticulum stress. *Cell* **2014**, *158*, 534–548. [CrossRef]

123. Takasugi, N. The Emerging Role of Electrophiles as a Key Regulator for Endoplasmic Reticulum (ER) Stress. *Int. J. Mol. Sci.* **2019**, *20*, 1783. [CrossRef] [PubMed]
124. Nakamura, T. Aberrant protein S-nitrosylation contributes to the pathophysiology of neurodegenerative diseases. *Neurobiol. Dis.* **2015**, *84*, 99–108. [CrossRef] [PubMed]
125. Groeger, L.A. Signaling actions of electrophiles: Anti-inflammatory therapeutic candidates. *Mol. Interv.* **2010**, *10*, 39–50. [CrossRef] [PubMed]
126. Sakanyan, V. Reactive Chemicals and Electrophilic Stress in Cancer: A Minireview. *High-Throughput* **2018**, *7*, 12. [CrossRef]
127. Uehara, T. S-nitrosylated protein-disulphide isomerase links protein misfolding to neurodegeneration. *Sci. Am.* **2006**, *441*, 513–517. [CrossRef] [PubMed]
128. Nakato, R. Regulation of the unfolded protein response via S-nitrosylation of sensors of endoplasmic reticulum stress. *Sci. Rep.* **2015**, *5*, 14812. [CrossRef]
129. Gallagher, M.C. Ceapins are a new class of unfolded protein response inhibitors, selectively targeting the ATF6a branch. *eLife* **2016**, *5*, e11878. [CrossRef]
130. Gallagher, M.C. Ceapins inhibit ATF6a signaling by selectively preventing transport of ATF6a to the Golgi apparatus during ER stress. *eLife* **2016**, *5*, e11880. [CrossRef]
131. Kakizuka, A. VCP, a Major ATPase in the Cells, as a Novel Drug Target for Currently Incurable Disorders. In *Innovative Medicine: Basic Research and Development*; Nakao, K., Minato, N., Uemoto, S., Eds.; Springer: Tokyo, Japan, 2015.
132. Brooks, C. Archaeal Unfoldase Counteracts Protein Misfolding Retinopathy in Mice. *J. Neurosci.* **2018**, *38*, 7248–7254. [CrossRef]
133. Wilkinson, K.D.K. Regulation of ubiquitin-dependent processes by deubiquitinating enzymes. *FASEB J.* **1997**, *11*, 1245–1256. [CrossRef] [PubMed]
134. Zhang, W. Generation and Validation of Intracellular Ubiquitin Variant Inhibitors for USP7 and USP10. *J. Mol. Biol.* **2017**, *429*, 3546–3560. [CrossRef] [PubMed]
135. Liu, Y. Roles of p97-associated deubiquitinases in protein quality control at the endoplasmic reticulum. *Curr. Protein Pept. Sci.* **2012**, *13*, 436–446. [CrossRef] [PubMed]
136. Sizova, S.O. Modulation of cellular signaling pathways in P23H rhodopsin photoreceptors. *Cell. Signal.* **2014**, *26*, 665–672. [CrossRef] [PubMed]
137. Athanasiou, D.; Aguila, M.; Opefi, C.A.; South, K.; Bellingham, J.; Bevilacqua, D.; Munro, P.M.; Kanuga, N.; Mackenzie, F.E.; Dubis, A.M.; et al. Rescue of mutant rhodopsin traffic by metformin-induced AMPK activation accelerates photoreceptor degeneration. *Hum. Mol. Genet.* **2017**, *26*, 305–319. [CrossRef] [PubMed]
138. Kim, Y.S. Metformin protects against retinal cell death in diabetic mice. *Biochem. Biophys. Res. Commun.* **2017**, *492*, 397–403. [CrossRef] [PubMed]
139. Vent-Schmidt, R.Y.J.; Wen, R.H.; Zong, Z.; Chiu, C.N.; Tam, B.M.; May, C.G.; Moritz, O.L. Opposing Effects of Valproic Acid Treatment Mediated by Histone Deacetylase Inhibitor Activity in Four Transgenic, X. laevis Models of Retinitis Pigmentosa. *J. Neurosci.* **2017**, *37*, 1039–1054. [CrossRef] [PubMed]
140. Mockel, A.; Obringer, C.; Hakvoort, T.B.; Seeliger, M.; Lamers, W.H.; Stoetzel, C.; Dollfus, H.; Marion, V. Pharmacological modulation of the retinal unfolded protein response in Bardet-Biedl syndrome reduces apoptosis and preserves light detection ability. *J. Biol. Chem.* **2012**, *287*, 37483–37494. [CrossRef] [PubMed]
141. Mitton, P.K. Different effects of valproic acid on photoreceptor loss in Rd1 and Rd10 retinal degeneration mice. *Mol. Vis.* **2014**, *20*, 1527–1544.
142. Reuter, C.W.C. Targeting the Ras signaling pathway: A rational, mechanism-based treatment for hematologic malignancies? *Blood* **2000**, *96*, 1655–1669.
143. Whyte, D.B.D. K- and N-Ras are geranylgeranylated in cells treated with farnesyl protein transferase inhibitors. *J. Biol. Chem.* **1997**, *272*, 14459–14464. [CrossRef] [PubMed]
144. Eriksson, M. Recurrent de novo point mutations in lamin A cause Hutchinson-Gilford progeria syndrome. *Sci. Am.* **2003**, *423*, 293–298. [CrossRef] [PubMed]
145. Thulasiraman, V.V. In vivo newly translated polypeptides are sequestered in a protected folding environment. *EMBO J.* **1999**, *18*, 85–95. [CrossRef] [PubMed]
146. Butler Lisa, M.L. Maximizing the Therapeutic Potential of HSP90 Inhibitors. *Mol. Cancer Res.* **2015**, *13*, 1445–1451. [CrossRef] [PubMed]

147. Workman, P. Drugging the cancer chaperone HSP90: Combinatorial therapeutic exploitation of oncogene addiction and tumor stress. *Ann. N. Y. Acad. Sci.* **2007**, *1113*, 202–216. [CrossRef] [PubMed]
148. Han, J. ER-stress-induced transcriptional regulation increases protein synthesis leading to cell death. *Nat. Cell Biol.* **2013**, *15*, 481–490. [CrossRef] [PubMed]
149. Upton, J.P. IRE1a cleaves select microRNAs during ER stress to derepress translation of proapoptotic Caspase-2. *Science* **2012**, *338*, 818–822. [CrossRef] [PubMed]
150. Yang, Y. Transcription Factor C/EBP Homologous Protein in Health and Diseases. *Front. Immunol.* **2017**, *8*, 1612. [CrossRef] [PubMed]
151. Milisav, I. Unfolded Protein Response and Macroautophagy in Alzheimer's, Parkinson's and Prion Diseases. *Molecules* **2015**, *20*, 22718–22756. [CrossRef] [PubMed]
152. Wang, L. The unfolded protein response in familial amyotrophic lateral sclerosis. *Hum. Mol. Genet.* **2011**, *20*, 1008–1015. [CrossRef] [PubMed]
153. Ma, T. Suppression of eIF2a kinases alleviates Alzheimer's disease-related plasticity and memory deficits. *Nat. Neurosci.* **2013**, *16*, 1299–1305. [CrossRef] [PubMed]
154. Moreno, A.J. Sustained translational repression by eIF2a-P mediates prion neurodegeneration. *Sci. Am.* **2012**, *485*, 507–511.
155. Moreno, A.J. Oral treatment targeting the unfolded protein response prevents neurodegeneration and clinical disease in prion-infected mice. *Sci. Transl. Med.* **2013**, *5*, 206ra138. [CrossRef] [PubMed]
156. Xu, M. ATF6 Is Mutated in Early Onset Photoreceptor Degeneration With Macular Involvement. *Investig. Ophthalmol. Vis. Sci.* **2015**, *56*, 3889–3895. [CrossRef] [PubMed]
157. Ansar, M. Mutation of ATF6 causes autosomal recessive achromatopsia. *Hum. Genet.* **2015**, *134*, 941–950. [CrossRef] [PubMed]
158. Bug, M. Expanding into new markets–VCP/p97 in endocytosis and autophagy. *J. Struct. Biol.* **2012**, *179*, 78–82. [CrossRef] [PubMed]
159. March, Z.M.; Mack, K.L.; Shorter, J. AAA+ Protein-Based Technologies to Counter Neurodegenerative Disease. *Biophys. J.* **2019**. [CrossRef] [PubMed]
160. Rivlin, N. Mutations in the p53 Tumor Suppressor Gene: Important Milestones at the Various Steps of Tumorigenesis. *Genes Cancer* **2011**, *2*, 466–474. [CrossRef] [PubMed]
161. Vuong, L. p53 selectively regulates developmental apoptosis of rod photoreceptors. *PLoS ONE* **2013**, *8*, e67381. [CrossRef]
162. Yoshizawa, K. N-methyl-N-nitrosourea-induced retinal degeneration in mice is independent of the p53 gene. *Mol. Vis.* **2009**, *15*, 2919–2925. [PubMed]
163. Yi, Z. Biallelic mutations in USP45, encoding a deubiquitinating enzyme, are associated with Leber congenital amaurosis. *J. Med. Genet.* **2019**, *56*, 325–331. [CrossRef] [PubMed]
164. Ballou, M.L. Rapamycin and mTOR kinase inhibitors. *J. Chem. Biol.* **2008**, *1*, 27–36. [CrossRef] [PubMed]
165. Walters, E.H. mTORC Inhibitors as Broad-Spectrum Therapeutics for Age-Related Diseases. *Int. J. Mol. Sci.* **2018**, *19*, 2325. [CrossRef] [PubMed]
166. Meng, L.H. Toward rapamycin analog (rapalog)-based precision cancer therapy. *Acta Pharmacol. Sin.* **2015**, *36*, 1163–1169. [CrossRef] [PubMed]
167. Venkatesh, A. Activated mTORC1 promotes long-term cone survival in retinitis pigmentosa mice. *J. Clin. Investig.* **2015**, *125*, 1446–1458. [CrossRef] [PubMed]
168. Rajala, A. Constitutive Activation Mutant mTOR Promote Cone Survival in Retinitis Pigmentosa Mice. *Adv. Exp. Med. Biol.* **2018**, *1074*, 491–497. [PubMed]
169. Punzo, C.; Kornacker, K.; Cepko, C.L. Stimulation of the insulin/mTOR pathway delays cone death in a mouse model of retinitis pigmentosa. *Nat. Neurosci.* **2009**, *12*, 44–52. [CrossRef] [PubMed]
170. Benjamin, D. Rapamycin passes the torch: A new generation of mTOR inhibitors. *Nat. Rev. Drug Discov.* **2011**, *10*, 868–880. [CrossRef] [PubMed]
171. Rotermund, C. The Therapeutic Potential of Metformin in Neurodegenerative Diseases. *Front. Endocrinol.* **2018**, *9*, 400. [CrossRef] [PubMed]
172. Buzzai, M. Systemic treatment with the antidiabetic drug metformin selectively impairs p53-deficient tumor cell growth. *Cancer Res.* **2007**, *67*, 6745–6752. [CrossRef]
173. Kurelac, I. The multifaceted effects of metformin on tumor microenvironment. *Semin. Cell Dev. Biol.* **2019**. [CrossRef] [PubMed]

174. Williams, A. Novel targets for Huntington's disease in an mTOR-independent autophagy pathway. *Nat. Chem. Biol.* **2008**, *4*, 295–305. [CrossRef] [PubMed]
175. Campello, L.; Esteve-Rudd, J.; Cuenca, N.; Martin-Nieto, J. The ubiquitin-proteasome system in retinal health and disease. *Mol. Neurobiol.* **2013**, *47*, 790–810. [CrossRef] [PubMed]
176. Chuang, D.M. Multiple roles of HDAC inhibition in neurodegenerative conditions. *Trends Neurosci.* **2009**, *32*, 591–601. [CrossRef] [PubMed]
177. Hwang, J.; Qi, L. Quality Control in the Endoplasmic Reticulum: Crosstalk between ERAD and UPR pathways. *Trends Biochem. Sci.* **2018**, *43*, 593–605. [CrossRef] [PubMed]
178. Horimoto, S. The unfolded protein response transducer ATF6 represents a novel transmembrane-type endoplasmic reticulum-associated degradation substrate requiring both mannose trimming and SEL1L protein. *J. Biol. Chem.* **2013**, *288*, 31517–31527. [CrossRef] [PubMed]
179. Orhan, E. Genotypic and phenotypic characterization of P23H line 1 rat model. *PLoS ONE* **2015**, *10*, e0127319. [CrossRef] [PubMed]
180. Monai, N. Characterization of photoreceptor degeneration in the rhodopsin P23H transgenic rat line 2 using optical coherence tomography. *PLoS ONE* **2018**, *13*, e0193778. [CrossRef]
181. Machida, S.S. P23H rhodopsin transgenic rat: Correlation of retinal function with histopathology. *Investig. Ophthalmol. Vis. Sci.* **2000**, *41*, 3200–3209.
182. Olsson, J.E.J. Transgenic mice with a rhodopsin mutation (Pro23His): A mouse model of autosomal dominant retinitis pigmentosa. *Neuron* **1992**, *9*, 815–830. [CrossRef]
183. Leyk, J.; Daly, C.; Janssen-Bienhold, U.; Kennedy, B.N.; Richter-Landsberg, C. HDAC6 inhibition by tubastatin A is protective against oxidative stress in a photoreceptor cell line and restores visual function in a zebrafish model of inherited blindness. *Cell Death Dis.* **2017**, *8*, e3028. [CrossRef] [PubMed]
184. Daly, C. Histone Deacetylase: Therapeutic Targets in Retinal Degeneration. *Adv. Exp. Med. Biol.* **2016**, *854*, 455–461. [PubMed]
185. Tanackovic, G. PRPF mutations are associated with generalized defects in spliceosome formation and pre-mRNA splicing in patients with retinitis pigmentosa. *Hum. Mol. Genet.* **2011**, *20*, 2116–2130. [CrossRef] [PubMed]
186. Buskin, A. Disrupted alternative splicing for genes implicated in splicing and ciliogenesis causes PRPF31 retinitis pigmentosa. *Nat. Commun.* **2018**, *9*, 4234. [CrossRef] [PubMed]
187. Collin, W.J.R. Applications of antisense oligonucleotides for the treatment of inherited retinal diseases. *Curr. Opin. Ophthalmol.* **2017**, *28*, 260–266. [CrossRef] [PubMed]
188. Viringipurampeer, I.A.; Metcalfe, A.L.; Bashar, A.E.; Sivak, O.; Yanai, A.; Mohammadi, Z.; Moritz, O.L.; Gregory-Evans, C.Y.; Gregory-Evans, K. NLRP3 inflammasome activation drives bystander cone photoreceptor cell death in a P23H rhodopsin model of retinal degeneration. *Hum. Mol. Genet.* **2016**, *25*, 1501–1516. [CrossRef] [PubMed]
189. Zhang, T.; Baehr, W.; Fu, Y. Chemical chaperone TUDCA preserves cone photoreceptors in a mouse model of Leber congenital amaurosis. *Investig. Ophthalmol. Vis. Sci.* **2012**, *53*, 3349–3356. [CrossRef] [PubMed]
190. Leonard, C.K. XIAP protection of photoreceptors in animal models of retinitis pigmentosa. *PLoS ONE* **2007**, *2*, e314. [CrossRef]
191. Thanos, C. Delivery of neurotrophic factors and therapeutic proteins for retinal diseases. *Exp. Opin. Biol. Ther.* **2005**, *5*, 1443–1452. [CrossRef]
192. Himawan, E.; Ekstrom, P.; Buzgo, M.; Gaillard, P.; Stefansson, E.; Marigo, V.; Loftsson, T.; Paquet-Durand, F. Drug delivery to retinal photoreceptors. *Drug Discov. Today* **2019**. [CrossRef]

9

Diurnal Rhythmicity of Autophagy is Impaired in the Diabetic Retina

Xiaoping Qi [1], Sayak K. Mitter [1], Yuanqing Yan [2], Julia V. Busik [3], Maria B. Grant [1] and Michael E. Boulton [1,*]

1 Department of Ophthalmology and Visual Sciences, University of Alabama at Birmingham, AL 35294, USA; xqi@uabmc.edu (X.Q.); sayakmitter@gmail.com (S.K.M.); mariagrant@uabmc.edu (M.B.G.)
2 Department of Neurosurgery, The University of Texas Health Science Center, Houston, TX 77030, USA; Yuanqing.Yan@uth.tmc.edu
3 Department of Physiology, Michigan State University, East Lansing, MI 48824, USA; busik@msu.edu
* Correspondence: meboulton@uabmc.edu

Abstract: Retinal homeostasis is under both diurnal and circadian regulation. We sought to investigate the diurnal expression of autophagy proteins in normal rodent retina and to determine if this is impaired in diabetic retinopathy. C57BL/6J mice and Bio-Breeding Zucker (BBZ) rats were maintained under a 12h/12h light/dark cycle and eyes, enucleated over a 24 h period. Eyes were also collected from diabetic mice with two or nine-months duration of type 1 diabetes (T1D) and Bio-Breeding Zucker diabetic rat (BBZDR/wor rats with 4-months duration of type 2 diabetes (T2D). Immunohistochemistry was performed for the autophagy proteins Atg7, Atg9, LC3 and Beclin1. These autophagy proteins (Atgs) were abundantly expressed in neural retina and endothelial cells in both mice and rats. A differential staining pattern was observed across the retinas which demonstrated a distinctive diurnal rhythmicity. All Atgs showed localization to retinal blood vessels with Atg7 being the most highly expressed. Analysis of the immunostaining demonstrated distinctive diurnal rhythmicity, of which Atg9 and LC3 shared a biphasic expression cycle with the highest level at 8:15 am and 8:15 pm. In contrast, Beclin1 revealed a 24-h cycle with the highest level observed at midnight. Atg7 was also on a 24-h cycle with peak expression at 8:15 am, coinciding with the first peak expression of Atg9 and LC3. In diabetic animals, there was a dramatic reduction in all four Atgs and the distinctive diurnal rhythmicity of these autophagy proteins was significantly impaired and phase shifted in both T1D and T2D animals. Restoration of diurnal rhythmicity and facilitation of autophagy protein expression may provide new treatment strategies for diabetic retinopathy.

Keywords: diurnal rhythm; autophagy; retina; diabetes; diabetic retinopathy

---

1. Introduction

Macroautophagy (hereafter referred to as autophagy) is an evolutionarily conserved cellular catabolic mechanism that facilitates the degradation of damaged cellular organelles and proteins, by targeting them to the lysosomes and recycling the macromolecules for the rebuilding of cellular machinery [? ? ?]. Autophagy undergoes rhythmic variation in accordance with circadian patterns of rest/activity and feeding in adult mammals [?]. Dysregulated autophagy has been implicated in several neurodegenerative disorders, hepatitis, cancer, aging associated diseases and in the general aging process [? ? ? ? ?]. Recently, a growing body of evidence indicates that dysregulated autophagy is also linked to diabetes [? ? ? ?].

The disruption of circadian rhythm has a profound negative impact on health and is associated with elevated risk for several diseases [?]. The physiological relevance of an altered circadian rhythm in diabetes is evidenced by the observation of a high incidence of myocardial dysfunction, acute coronary syndrome, sudden cardiac death, and ischemic stroke in diabetics during the night, compared to a higher frequency during the day in non-diabetics [? ? ? ?]. In diabetic conditions, Bmal1 and Clock are inactivated, causing deregulated glucose homeostasis and suppressed diurnal variation in glucose and triglycerides, along with reduced gluconeogenesis [?]. Streptozotocin (STZ)-induced type 1 diabetes (T1D) in mice exhibits altered phase of the circadian clock in the heart [?] and a significant reduction of circadian sensitivity to low-intensity light in the retina [?]. Furthermore, STZ-mice develop a deficiency in their ability to re-entrain the circadian rhythm when subjected to a phase advance of the 12L/12D cycle [?]. Bio-Breeding Zucker diabetic rat (BBZDR/Wor) and Goto-Kakizaki rat type 2 diabetes (T2D) models also show impairment of the molecular clock, suggesting that the disruption of the circadian clock is a common phenomenon in both T1D and T2D [? ?].

Several hallmarks of diabetic retinopathy can be recapitulated in rodent retina deficient of clock genes [? ?]. Reduced tube formation and increased senescence of endothelial cells coupled with impaired progenitor-mediated repair is observed in Per2 mutant mice, emphasizing the importance of the circadian clock in retinal homeostasis [?]. Recent studies on autophagy in the retina have shed light on the association of key molecules of the autophagic pathway with phagocytosis of photoreceptor outer segments (POS) by the retinal pigmented epithelium (RPE) [? ?]. Photoreceptor disk shedding has been widely reported to exhibit diurnal rhythmicity in the retina [? ?] and the tight coupling of phagocytic ingestion and autophagic degradation of the POS to this diurnal rhythm is a critical aspect of retinal homeostasis [? ?].

The role of the peripheral clock and diurnal variation on the regulation of autophagy in the normal and diabetic rodent retinas and the fate of autophagy in the diabetic retina remain unexplored. Understanding these control mechanisms may help find effective treatments for diabetic retinopathy. In this study, we demonstrate that the spatial distribution and temporal expression of autophagy proteins show a diurnal rhythm and that this is depressed and phase shifted in the diabetic retina.

2. Materials and Methods

2.1. Experimental Animals

All animal procedures were performed in accordance with a) protocols approved by the Institutional Animal Care and Use Committees at University of Florida, Gainesville, FL, USA (#CR-201106001), Michigan State University, Lansing, MI, USA (#Busik09/14-160-00, and Indiana University, Indianapolis, IN, USA (#10574 MD/R), b, the National Institutes of Health Guide for Care and Use of Laboratory Animals and c) the ARVO Statement for the Use of Animals in Ophthalmic and Vision Research. Male C57BL/6J mice were purchased from Jackson Labs at 6 weeks of age and male BBZDR/wor T2D rats and lean heterozygote nondiabetic control littermates were obtained from biomedical research models (BRM, Inc.) Worcester, Massachusetts at 5 months of age. C57BL/6J mice (n = 240) and BBZ rats (n = 75) were maintained on a standard 12/12 h light/dark cycle (6.00 am lights on/6.00 pm lights off). T1D was induced in eight-week-old C57BL/6 mice (n = 120) by five consecutive intraperitoneal injection of freshly prepared streptozotocin (STZ) solution with the concentration of 40mg/kg body weight in 0.1M/citrate buffer, pH 4.5 as previously described [? ?]. The control group received sodium citrate buffer (vehicle) alone. Diabetes was confirmed by two consecutive blood glucose levels >240 mg/dl, using the AlphaTrak® blood glucose monitor and test strip system (Abbot laboratories, Irvine, CA, USA), according to the manufacturer's instruction. No animal used in this study required insulin injections. Eyes from one group were collected at 2 months following establishment of diabetes and the second cohort 9 months after diabetes induction (the age of the animals at these time points being 4 and 11 months, respectively). We also investigated inbred Bio-Breeding Zucker (BBZDR)/wor T2D rats (n = 37) and age-matched controls (n = 38) [?]. BBZDR/wor rats spontaneously became diabetic at ~10 weeks of age and were maintained for 4 months after the onset of diabetes. A second group of C57BL/6J mice (n = 24) were dark adapted for 48 h before sacrifice and referred to as being on the dark/dark cycle. In all groups, animals were euthanized by deep anesthesia with isoflurane followed by cervical dislocation and eyes were immediately enucleated every 2 or 3 h over a 24 h period and prepared for immunofluorescence staining. For animals in the dark cycle, euthanasia and enucleation were performed in a dark room under a red safe light. For each set of experiments, all animals were started at the same time point to clearly identify any phase shift in peak or trough of ATG expression. The number of biological replicates of the enucleated eyes at each time point is n = 10 for mice and n = 3 for rats. Only one eye from each animal was used in the assessment.

2.2. *Immunofluorescence Microscopy*

Eyes were processed for standard paraffin embedding and 4 μm sections were prepared. Rodent Decloaker (Biocare Medical LLC, Concord, CA, USA Catalog# RD913L) was used to unmask antigens and non-specific binding was blocked with 10% normal goat sera and 5% BSA for 1 h at room temperature. Sections received either mouse monoclonal anti-Beclin1 (BD Transduction Lab, San Jose, CA, USA, Cat#612112), or rabbit polyclonal antibodies against Atg7, Atg9 and LC3 (provided by Dr. Dunn, Department of Anatomy and Cell Biology, University of Florida, Gainesville, FL, USA), diluted in phosphate buffered saline (PBS) with 1% normal goat sera plus 1% bovine serum albumin (BSA) (Beclin1 1:20; Atg7- 1:300; Atg9 and LC3 - 1:100). After washing, sections were incubated with an appropriate FITC-conjugated secondary antibody for 1 h. In some sections, colocalization of autophagy proteins within the retinal vasculature was confirmed by dual staining with the endothelial cell marker, TRITC-agglutinin (Vector Labs, Burlingame, CA, USA, Cat#RCA120). Sections were covered with Vectashield mounting medium/DAPI (Vector Labs, Inc.). Sections were viewed using a Zeiss Axioplan 2 Upright Fluorescence Microscope with Qimage/QCapture software Version 8 (QImaging Corporate, Surrey, British Columbia, Canada). Omission of the primary antibody was the baseline control and all the fluorescence photographs were obtained under the same scaled conditions.

2.3. *Grading of Immunostaining*

Three independent masked observers, using a previously described grading system [? ?], graded the intensity of the immunoreactivity for each antibody in transverse retinal sections. The intensity of labeling was graded qualitatively as: 10, strong bright intense immunoreactivity, 9, bright intense; 8, uniformly intense; 7, patchy and intense; 6, uniform and moderate; 5, patchy and moderate; 4, uniform and weak; 3, patchy and weak; 2, uniform and very weak; 1, patchy and very weak; and 0, none. A mean score ±SEM for each group was determined from the scores of all graders for each retina structure.

2.4. *Trypsin Digestion and the Detection of Superoxide*

The retinal vasculature was prepared as previously described [?]. Briefly, mouse eyes were fixed overnight in 4% paraformaldehyde, freshly made in PBS. The retinas were dissected from the eye cups, kept in water overnight, and digested in 3% trypsin (Invitrogen-Gibco, Grand Island, NY, USA) for 3 h at 37 °Celcius. The tissue was mounted carefully on a glass slide under a dissection microscope. The tissue was stained with PAS-H&E (periodic acid Schiff–hematoxylin and eosin; Gill No.3; Sigma-Aldrich), according to the instruction manual. The images were taken using a Zeiss light microscope equipped with a digital camera (AxioCam MRC5, Axiovert 200; Carl Zeiss Meditec, Inc., Dublin, CA, USA), using 20X objective lenses. Eight to ten representative fields from each quadrant of the retina were imaged and the number of acellular capillaries per square millimeter of retina were quantified.

For detecting the reactive oxygen species (ROS), the superoxide indicator, hydroethidine, was used to detect the production of superoxide radicals, as previously described [?]. Superoxide oxidizes hydroethidine to yield a red fluorescent signal at approximately 600 nm. Mice received two intraperitoneal injections, 15 min apart, of freshly prepared hydroethidine (20 mg/kg; Invitrogen) and were euthanized 18 h after injection. The fluorescence intensity was measured in the neural retina using a fluorescent plate reader (BioTek, Winooski, VT, USA) and a spectrofluorometer (FLUOstar Optima; BMG Labtechnologies, Cary, NC, USA). The relative fluorescence intensity was calculated by normalizing to protein concentration.

2.5. Statistical Analysis

The diurnal data are time series data, and single cosine analysis was employed to fit the data. The data was considered as diurnal oscillation by a zero-amplitude test, with a p-value less than 0.05. All experiments were assessed by comparing two groups mean scores from control animals and diabetic animals using a Student's t-test, plus ANOVA for multiple comparisons by using Prism® statistical software ver. 5 (GraphPad, La Jolla, CA, USA) with differences of p value < 0.05 were considered statistically significant. Results are expressed as mean ± SEM.

3. Results

3.1. Autophagy Proteins Exhibit Diurnal Expression/Localization in Normal Mouse Neural Retina

To determine if autophagic protein expression in the neural retina had an intrinsic diurnal rhythm, we assessed the expression and localization of four autophagy proteins, Atg7, LC3, Atg9 and Beclin1 in the normal retinas of young mice (age = 3 months) that were maintained under standard 12 h light/12 h dark conditions. When we examined the tissue at two-hour intervals over a 24 h period, these proteins exhibited not only a distinct diurnal rhythm, but remarkably showed distinct staining patterns across the layers of the neural retina in mice (????). Atg9 and LC3 exhibited a biphasic 12/12 h circadian cycle with zenith at 8:15 AM and 8:15 PM and nadir at 2:15 AM and 2:15 PM ($p < 0.05$) (Figure ??A–D). By contrast, Atg7 and Beclin1 expression showed a monophasic rhythm and the overall expression of these proteins was much lower than either Atg9 or LC3 (Figure ??E–H). The expression of Atg7 started to rise at 4:15 AM, peaked at 8:15 AM and gradually decreased until 10:15 AM ($p < 0.05$) (Figure ??E–G). Beclin1 expression was highest at around midnight and reached lowest levels at midday ($p < 0.05$) (Figure ??F–H). Omission of the primary antibody showed no staining in mouse retina (Figure ??D).

An assessment of the staining pattern of the proteins at zenith revealed that Atg9 and LC3 were localized throughout the retina, predominantly within the retinal ganglion cell (RGC) layer, inner (INL) and outer nuclear layer (ONL) (Figure ??A,B). Atg7 was only weakly localized to the neural retina in both the inner and outer nuclear layers and showed stronger localization in the photoreceptor outer segment. Beclin1 staining was detected throughout the retina, with highest intensity in the inner and outer plexiform layers and in the photoreceptors. Closer observation of the retina revealed that ATG7 and 9 showed remarkably strong association within the inner retinal vasculature (Figure ??C).

Using dual staining for endothelial cells and autophagy proteins, we confirmed that Atg9, LC3, Atg7 and Beclin1 were all expressed in both the inner and outer retinal plexus of the retinal vasculature (Figure ??C).

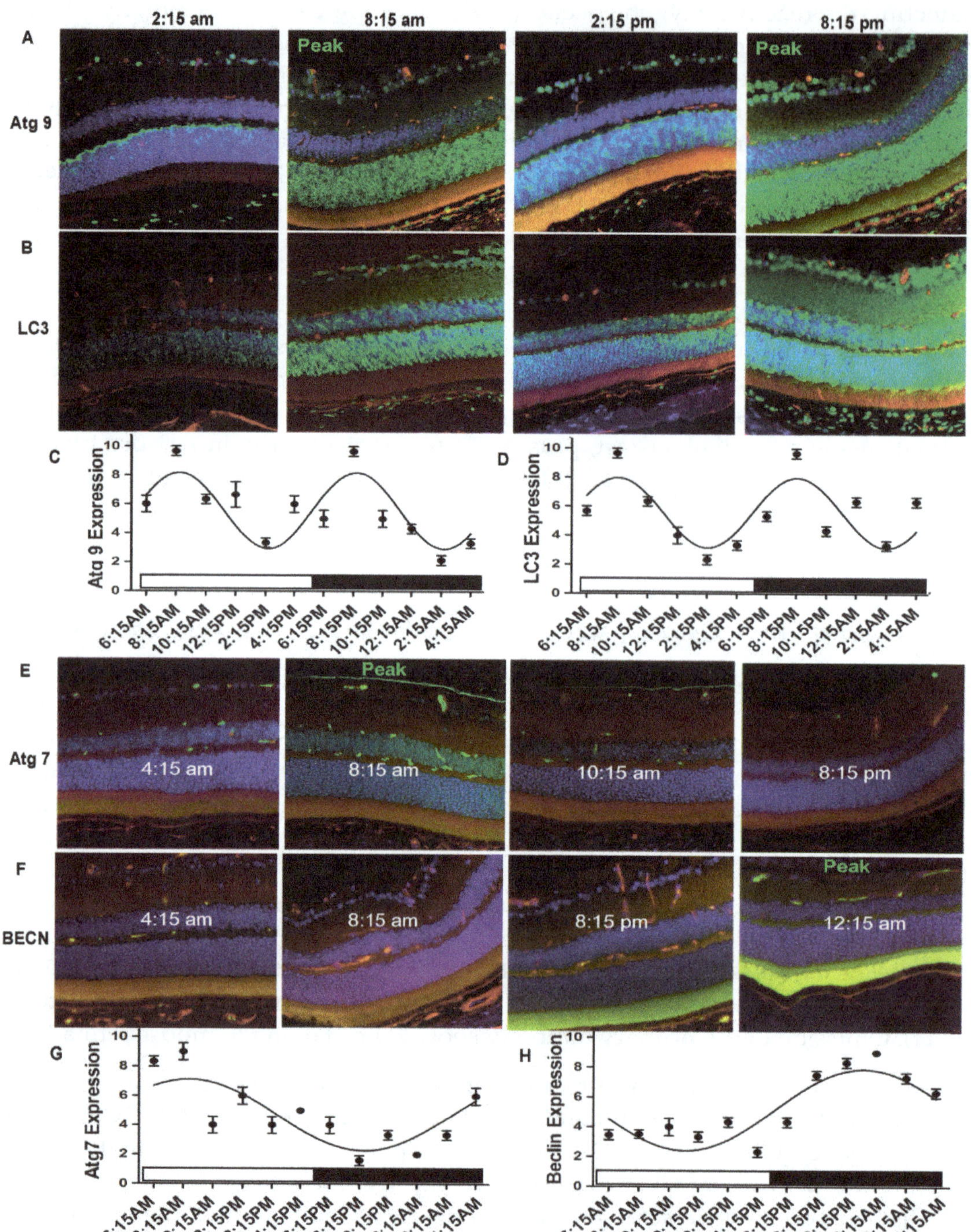

Figure 1. Autophagy proteins exhibited diurnal expression/localization in normal mouse neural retina. Retina were harvested every 2 h over a 24 h time period. Antibodies for autophagy proteins (ATGs) ATG9, Microtubule-associated protein 1A/1B-light chain 3 (LC3), ATG7 and Beclin1 (BECN) were used to detect respective protein expression (green) in the retina, Tetramethylrhodamine (TRITC) agglutinin for vessels (red) and DAPI (blue) shows nuclear staining. Distinct diurnal rhythmic patterns of the autophagic proteins Atg9 and LC3 expressions (**A**,**B**) revealed a biphasic diurnal cycle (12/12 h), with peaks at 8:15 AM and 8:15 PM and lowest levels at 2:15 AM and 2:15 PM (**C**,**D**). Atg7 and Beclin1 (BECN) expressions (**E**,**F**) were on a monophasic 24 h cycle. Atg7 expression peaked at 8:15 AM and lowest levels were at 10:15 AM. The peak of Beclin1 expression was at midnight and lowest levels were observed during the late morning (**H**). All animals were maintained in a standard 12/12 h light/dark phase with lights ON at 6:00 AM and lights OFF at 6:00 PM. The error bars in the diurnal plots represent the mean+SEM and diurnal oscillation had a p-value less than 0.05.

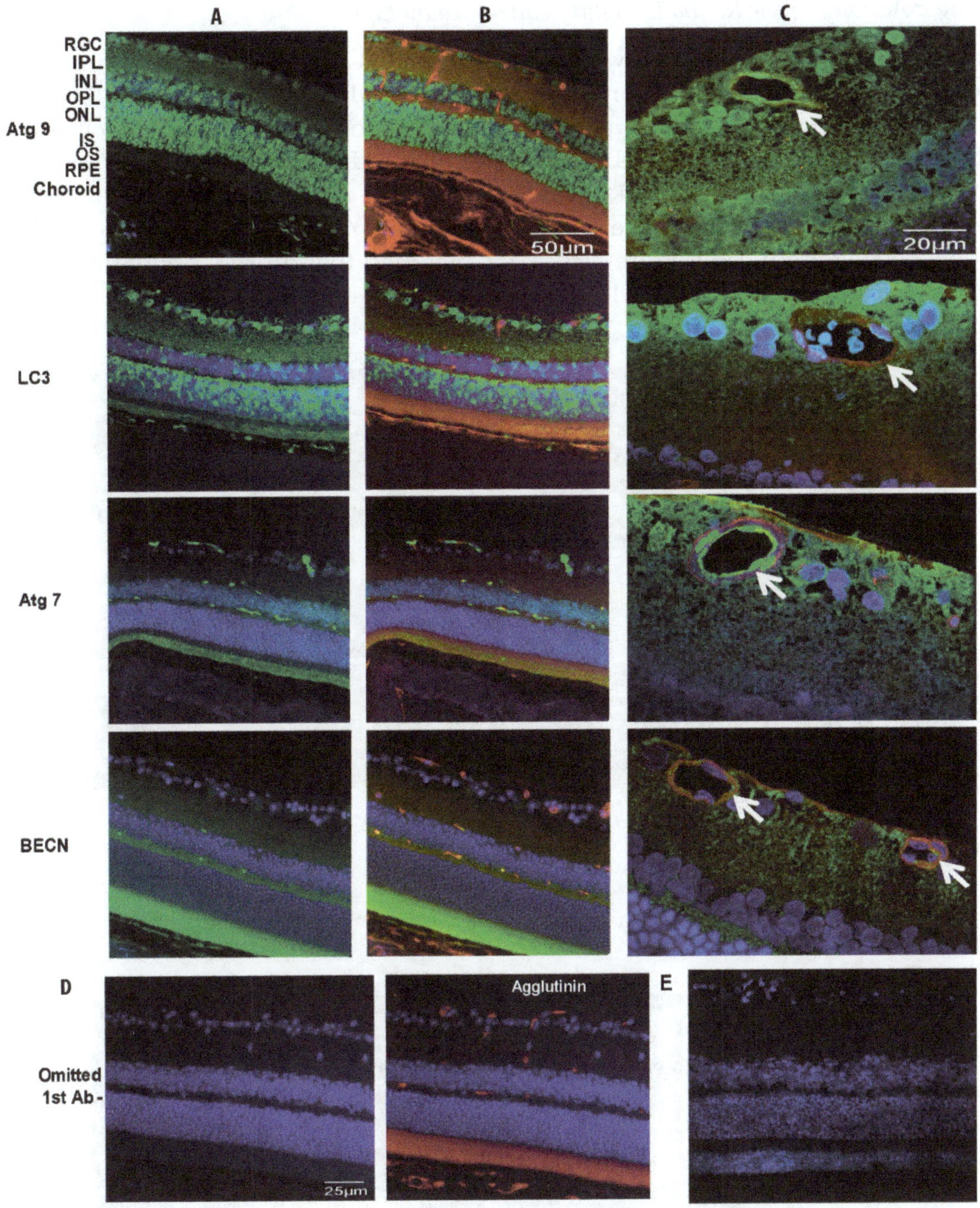

Figure 2. Localization of autophagy proteins in normal mouse retina and vasculature. Animals were kept in tight 12/12-h light/dark cycle before the experiment. Antibodies for ATG9, LC3, ATG7 and Beclin1 (BECN) were used to detect respective protein expression (green) in the retinas with different staining patterns and DAPI was used to stain nuclei (blue) (**A**). Agglutinin, an endothelial cell marker, conjugated with TRITC (red) was used to co-localize with antibodies specific to individual autophagy proteins (FITC) in the retinal vasculature (**B**). High magnification images demonstrated autophagy protein localization to the endothelial cells and pericytes of the retinal vasculature (**C**). No fluorescence was observed with omission of the primary antibody in the mouse retina. Using agglutinin staining, the section displayed retinal vascular patterns with normal architecture (**D**). Omitted autophagy primary antibody in rat retina also was negative (**E**). The arrows indicate autophagy protein localization to retinal vessels. RGC, retina ganglion cell; IPL, inner plexiform layer; INL, inner nuclear layer; OPL, outer plexiform layer; ONL, outer nuclear layer; IS, inner segment; OS, outer segment; RPE, retinal pigment epithelium.

3.2. Autophagic Activity in the Retina Is Tightly Entrained by Light

We repeated immunohistochemistry of ATG9, ATG7, LC3 and Beclin1 in the retina (and the retinal vasculature) of 48 h dark adapted mice and compared the results to those of 12/12 h light/dark adapted mice. The immunohistochemistry data indicated that the periodic oscillations, as well as overall levels of the autophagic proteins ATG9 and LC3, were attenuated in the 48 h dark adapted mice retina when compared to the 12/12 h dark/dark controls, both in the retina and the vasculature (Figure ??A). Similarly, peaks in Atg7 and Beclin1 were phase shifted compared to the light/dark controls and overall expression levels were reduced (Figure ??B). We concluded that diurnal oscillations in autophagic activity in the murine retina depend, at least in part, on light-effected entrainment.

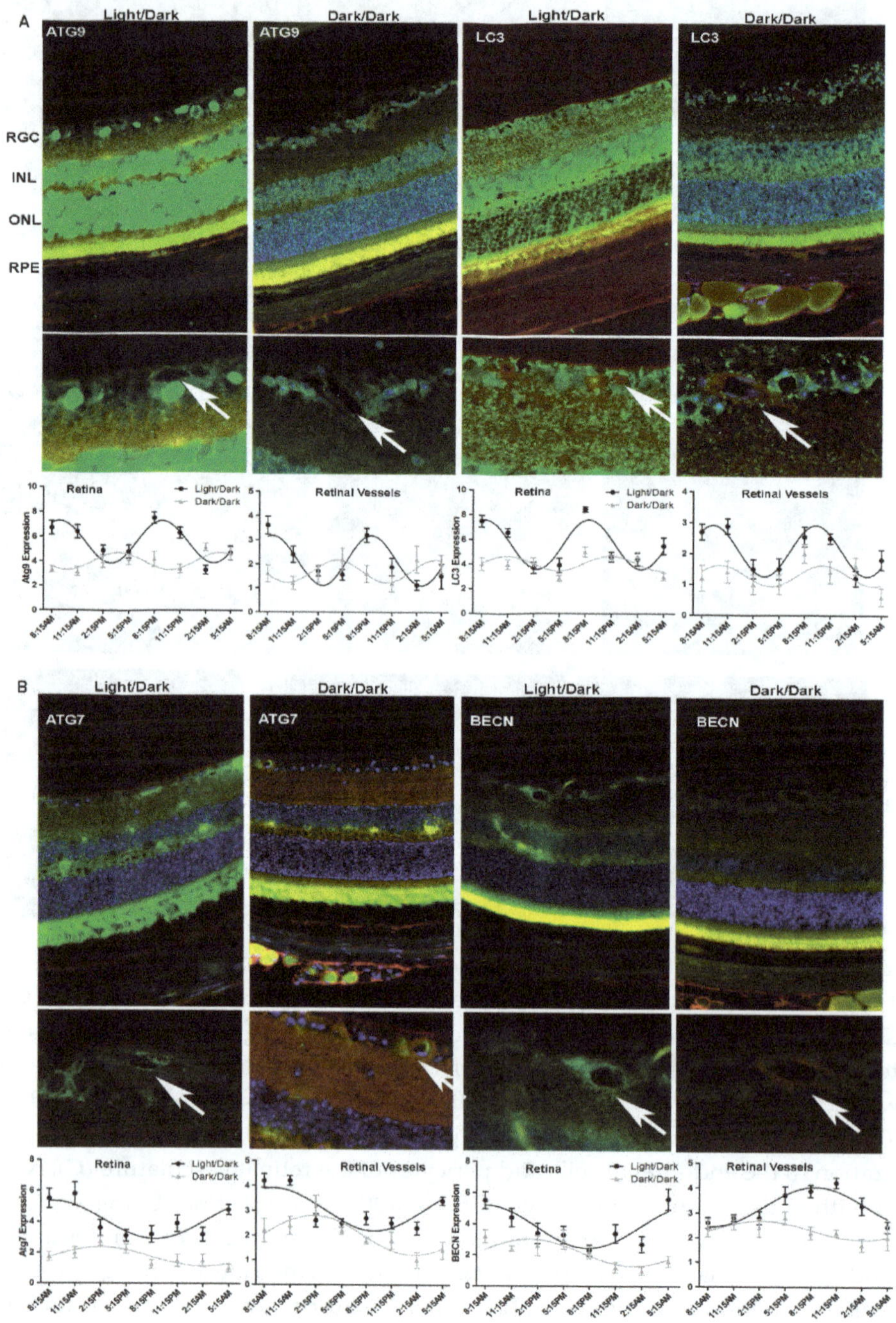

Figure 3. Immunohistochemistry confirmed alterations in diurnal patterns of autophagic gene expression upon light cycle disruption.

Mice were separated into two groups. One group was kept under 12/12-h light/dark cycle and the other group was kept in the dark for 48-h (dark/dark), before being euthanized. Samples were collected every 3 h for 24 h and were analyzed by immunohistochemistry for autophagic markers (**A**) ATG9 (**B**) LC3 (**C**) ATG7 and (**D**) Beclin1 (BECN). Autophagy protein expression is green, TRITC agglutinin for vessels red and DAPI nuclear staining blue. The arrows indicate autophagy protein localization to retinal vessels. RGC, retina ganglion cell; INL, inner nuclear layer; OPL, outer plexiform layer; ONL, outer nuclear layer; RPE, retinal pigment epithelium. The error bars in the circadian plots represent the mean + SEM and diurnal oscillation had a p-value less than 0.05.

3.3. Diurnal Rhythmicity of Expression of Autophagic Proteins Is Dampened in T1D

Having established that autophagy in the retina possesses a diurnal rhythm, we next examined the rhythmicity of autophagy proteins in T1D. We chose mice from 2- and 9-months duration of diabetes to assess the expression of autophagic proteins. To confirm that our T1D mice exhibited the expected retinopathy features [? ?], we performed trypsin-digests of the retina from nondiabetic C57BL/6J (Figure ??A, left) and T1D (Figure ??A, right). T1D mice exhibited an increase in the number of acellular capillaries per unit area. Quantitative measurements of acellular capillaries suggested a dramatic 4-fold increase, in contrast to the age-matched nondiabetic mouse of retinas that showed a normal vascular pattern (Figure ??B). These eyes showed significantly higher levels of superoxide anions in the neural retina, typical of retinopathy in this model (Figure ??C).

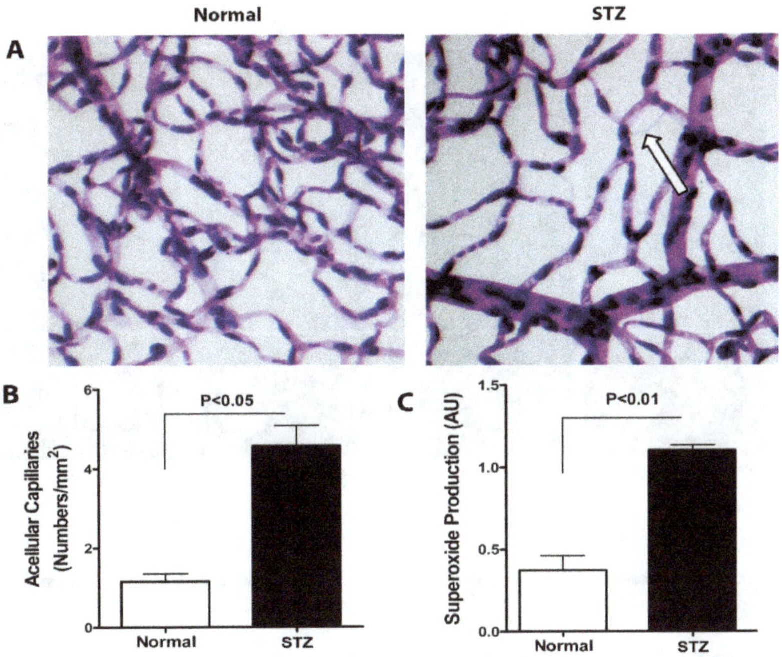

Figure 4. Evaluation of acellular capillary formation and superoxide anion generation in T1D mice. Representative images of trypsin-digested retinal vascular preparations from 4-month old control mice and 4-month old mice with 2-month duration of T1D (**A**) The arrow indicates an acellular capillary. Quantitative measurement of acellular capillaries was significantly increased in diabetic eyes (n = 6). (**B**) STZ-induced diabetic retina showed >1.5 fold increase in superoxide anion levels, $p < 0.01$ (**C**) The errors bars represent SEM.

While immunohistochemistry results from 4-month old normal control mice corresponded with the respective results shown in ????, we observed a dramatic attenuation of diurnal rhythmicity (amplitudes), as well as overall levels of the autophagic proteins in the T1D mice retina (Figure ??). This loss of amplitude was noted for ATG9, LC3 and Beclin1 expression in the diabetic retina, in either duration of diabetes group when compared to the respective age-matched controls (????). ATG7 exhibited a shift in phase in both the retina and the vasculature of mice with 2-month duration of diabetes while in mice with 9-months duration of diabetes the phase-shift was prominent in the retina and there was no significant variation in expression between time-points in the retinal vasculature (Figures ??B and ??B).

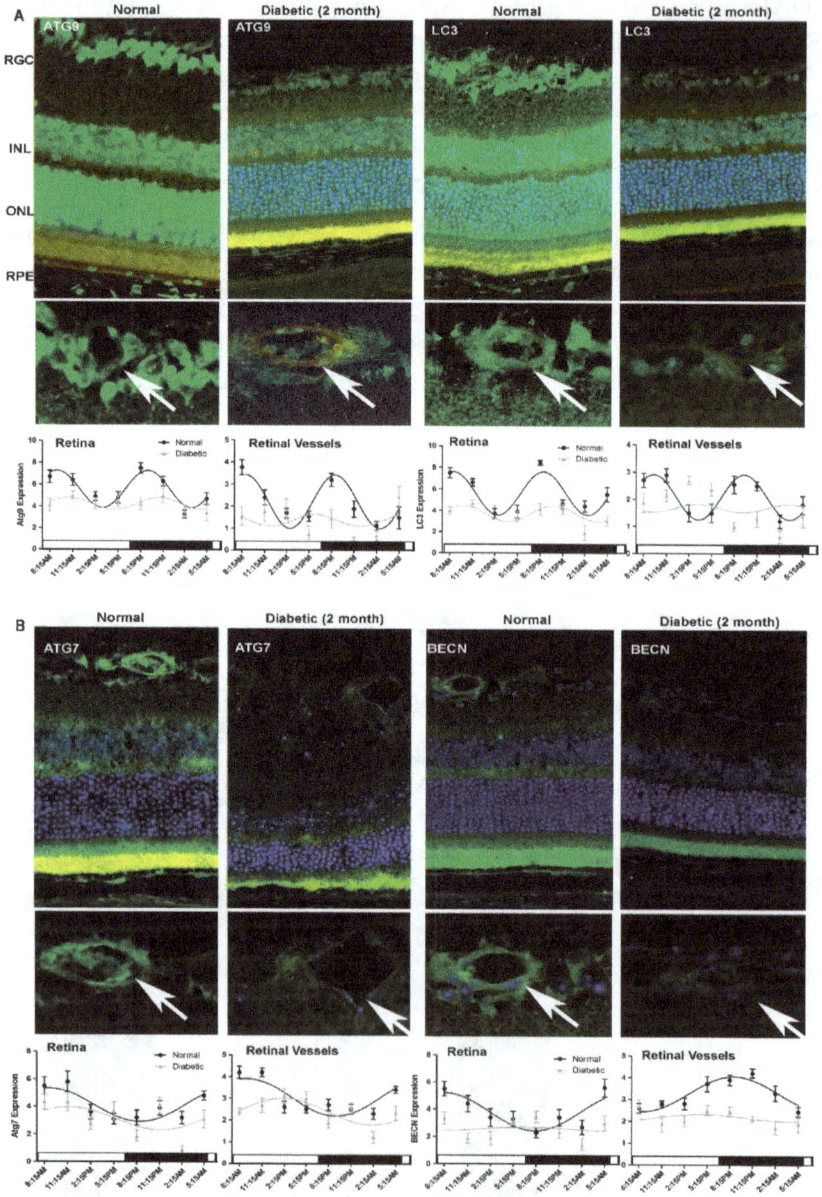

Figure 5. Impairment of diurnal rhythmicity of autophagy in T1D mice with two-months duration of diabetes. Retinas were collected from C57Bl/6J mice with two-months duration of T1D and age-matched control mice. Immunostaining and intensity analyses of retina and retinal vasculature demonstrated a dramatic loss of oscillatory amplitude of autophagic protein expression in the diabetic animals compared to normal mice (**A**,**B**). Autophagy protein expression is green, TRITC agglutinin for vessels red and DAPI nuclear staining blue. The arrows indicate autophagy protein localization to retinal vessels. RGC, retina ganglion cell; INL, inner nuclear layer; OPL, outer plexiform layer; ONL, outer nuclear layer; RPE, retinal pigment epithelium. Loss and phase-shifting of diurnal rhythmicity in diabetic retinopathy is demonstrated in single cosine plots, with ordinary least square fitted ($p < 0.01$, n = 10). All animals were maintained in a standard 12/12-h light/dark phase with lights ON at 6:00 AM and lights OFF at 6:00 PM. The error bars in the circadian plots represent the mean+SEM and diurnal oscillation had a p-value less than 0.05.

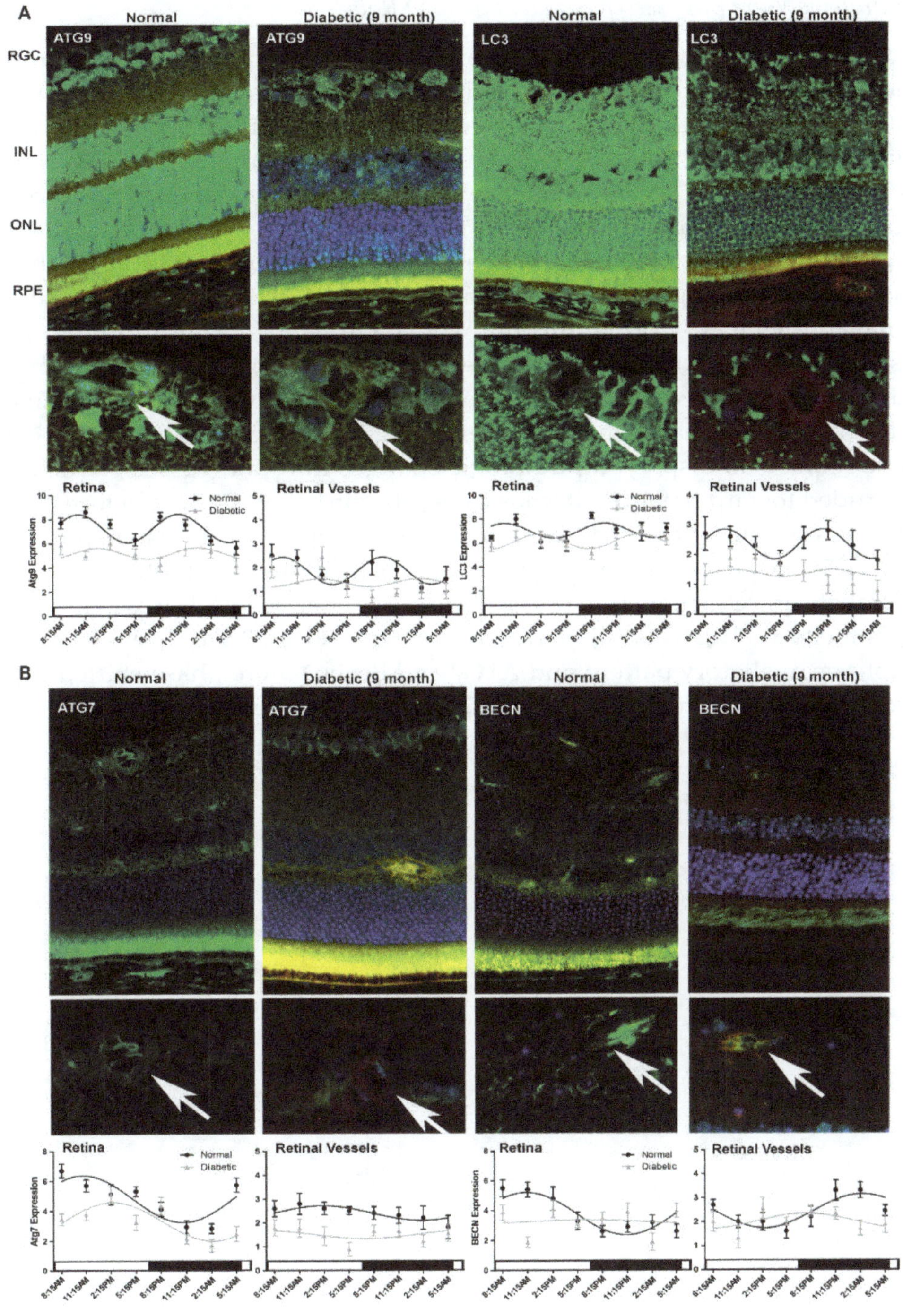

Figure 6. Impairment of diurnal rhythmicity of autophagy in T1D mice with nine-months duration of diabetes. Retinas were collected from C57Bl/6J mice with nine-months duration of T1D and age-matched control mice. Immunostaining and intensity analyses of retina and retinal vasculature demonstrated a dramatic loss of oscillatory amplitude of autophagic protein expression in the diabetic animals compared to normal mice (**A.B**). Autophagy protein expression is green, TRITC agglutinin for vessels red and DAPI nuclear staining blue. The arrows indicate autophagy protein localization to retinal vessels. RGC, retina ganglion cell; INL, inner nuclear layer; OPL, outer plexiform layer; ONL, outer nuclear layer; RPE, retinal pigment epithelium. Loss and phase-shifting of diurnal rhythmicity in diabetic retinopathy is demonstrated in single cosine plot with ordinary least square fitted ($p < 0.01$, n = 10). All animals were maintained in a standard 12/12-h light/dark phase with lights ON at 6:00 AM and lights OFF at 6:00 PM. The error bars in the circadian plots represent the mean+SEM and diurnal oscillation had a p-value less than 0.05.

3.4. Autophagy Proteins Were Suppressed Severely in T2D Rats

We next examined autophagy in the retina of T2D rats following 4-months duration of diabetes (Figure ??). The normal age-matched rats selected as controls demonstrated a similar staining pattern of immunohistochemistry across the retina as were observed in normal mice (Figure ??A–D). Atg9 (Figure ??A) and LC3 (Figure ??B) were mainly present in the ganglion cell layer, inner and outer nuclear layers in the normal rat retina, similar to what was observed in normal mice (Figure ??) but their expression was dramatically decreased in the retinas of the diabetic animals by 49% to 58%, respectively. For better demonstration of changes in autophagic protein levels in the vasculature of diabetic retinas, we showed higher magnification images. Both Atg9 and LC3 clearly distributed within the retinal endothelia of normal rats but were completely absent from the endothelia of the diabetic retinas (Figure ??E,F). Atg7 was strongly expressed in normal retinal vessels near the ganglion cells layer, meanwhile the small vessels in inner and outer plexus layers were also stained (Figure ??C). Semi-quantitative analysis revealed that the level of Atg7 was deceased by 52%, $p < 0.05$ in diabetic retinas. Diabetic retina also displayed pathologic changes in retina vessels, which appeared to be abnormally protruded toward the intravitreous cavity. Beclin1 staining was detected across the retina, including retinal vessels in the plexus and photoreceptors, however, Beclin1 staining was diminished in diabetic retinas by 53%, $p < 0.01$ (Figure ??D). Quantitative analyses of autophagic proteins in the retina of control and diabetic mice demonstrated, not only suppressed levels, but also revealed impairment in diurnal rhythmicity in T2D rats. Expression of Atg9 and LC3 were severely suppressed with insignificant biphasic oscillatory pattern and ATG7 and Beclin1 were phase-shifted by approximately for 4–6 h. We concluded that disruption in autophagy is a characteristic phenomenon of both T1D and T2D.

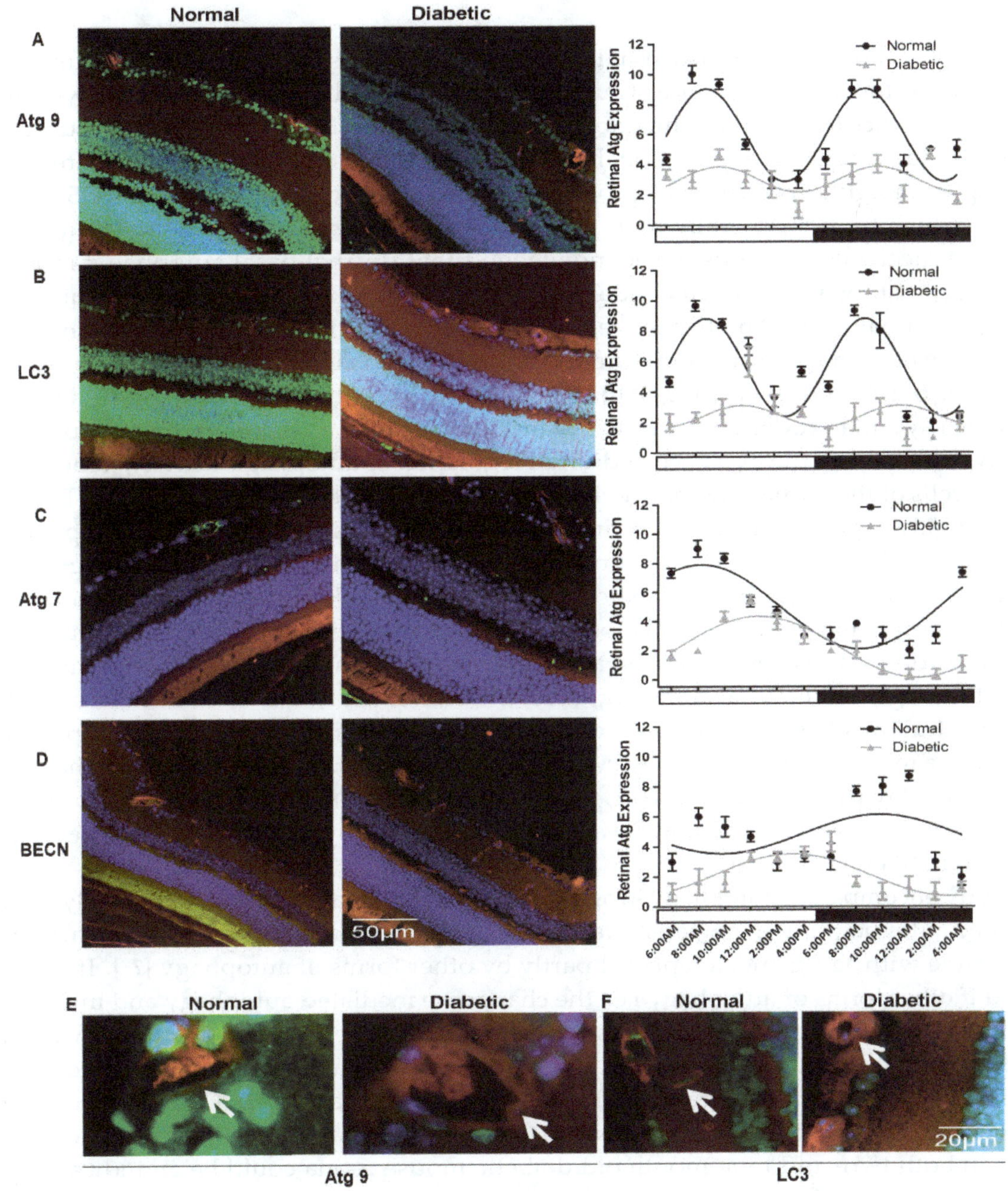

Figure 7. Impairment of diurnal rhythmicity of autophagy in T2D rats. Eyes were collected from 6.5-month old BBZDR/wor type 2 diabetic rats with 4-month duration of diabetes and the normal age-matched rats selected as controls. Immunostaining demonstrated a dramatic decrease in amplitude of diurnal rhythmicity of autophagic protein expression in the retina of the diabetic animals compared to normal rats. Representative micrographs of immunostained sections at 8:15 am are shown for (**A**) ATG9, (**B**) LC3 (**C**) ATG7 (**D**) Beclin1 (BECN). Autophagy protein expression is green, TRITC agglutinin for vessels red and DAPI nuclear staining blue. The arrows indicate autophagy protein localization to retinal vessels. RGC, retina ganglion cell; INL, inner nuclear layer; OPL, outer plexiform layer; ONL, outer nuclear layer; RPE, retinal pigment epithelium. ATG7 and Beclin1 displayed phase-shifting in the diurnal oscillation (**C**) and (**D**) respectively. Loss and phase-shifting of diurnal rhythmicity in diabetic retinopathy is demonstrated in single cosine plot with ordinary least square fitted ($p < 0.01$, n = 10). High magnification images confirmed the loss of autophagy proteins ATG9 and LC3 in the retinal vasculature (**E**). All animals were maintained in a standard 12/12-h light/dark phase with lights ON at 6:00 AM and lights OFF at 6:00 PM. The error bars in the circadian plots represent the mean + SEM and diurnal oscillation had a p-value less than 0.05.

4. Discussion

Autophagy is a critical and indispensable housekeeping process in the cells of the retina. Numerous reports support the functional relevance of autophagy in specific cells of the retina and how dysregulated autophagy contributes to retinal malfunction and degeneration [? ? ? ? ? ?]. While acute short-term noxious stimuli (e.g., nutrient deprivation; hypoxia and endoplasmic reticulum (ER) stress; oxidative stress arising from light, lipofuscin, POS phagocytosis by RPE or mitochondrial ROS generated in retinal cells (which have a generally high metabolic rate)) can stimulate autophagy as a generally cytoprotective mechanism, it must be acknowledged that diurnal basal autophagic modulation is a critical factor in abrogating the unavoidable regular cellular damage that occurs during the basic functioning of retinal cells. An efficient regulatory molecular circuit is required in the retina, that would modulate both the intensity and duration of basal autophagic activity in specific cell types and thus meet their regular housekeeping demands [?]. Previous studies have suggested the existence of autophagic rhythm in rodent heart muscles and liver, as well as kidney proximal tubules [? ? ?]. In this study, we establish the existence of diurnal regulation of autophagic activity, in both the neural and vascular cells of the retina. We show evidence that certain autophagic markers like Beclin1, ATG9 and LC3 are highly expressed across the retina, while ATG7 shows preferential staining patterns and is enriched only in certain layers (**????**). The first report on diurnal rhythmicity in autophagy in the retina recorded increased autophagosome formation following outer disk shedding in rat photoreceptors [?]. Our results regarding the biphasic oscillation of diurnal rhythmicity of LC3 expression agree with the findings in a report by Yao et al. 2014, who also observed two peaks of elevated autophagic activity [?]. Our results in Figure **??** make a strong argument in favor of the influence of external stimuli such as light for the entrainment and maintenance of healthy amplitudes of oscillation of autophagic protein expression in the retina. However, we observed that even in the absence of light entrainment, the retina continued to display rhythmicity in ATG7, ATG9, LC3 and BECN, but were lower in amplitude and out of phase, suggesting that there may be an intrinsic diurnal rhythm of autophagy in the retina not dependent on light entrainment.

Our study encompasses autophagy in aging and diabetic conditions. We successfully demonstrate that perturbed autophagy is a characteristic feature of aging. It has been suggested that macroautophagy suffers a decline with aging and is replaced partly by other forms of autophagy [?]. It remains to be determined if other forms of autophagy i.e., the chaperone mediated autophagy and microautophagy are also under regulation by the circadian system and, if so, whether their rhythmicity is affected in aging and disease. In addition to the above, our study reveals that the level of disruption in T1D and T2D is significant, not only in younger mice, but also in older animals (**????**). Compared to age-matched control mouse retinas, the dramatic deviations in the oscillatory patterns or the overall levels of one or more Atgs in both two- and nine-month old diabetic mouse retina could be an indication of faulty housekeeping and pathological outcomes, such as the accumulation of damaged mitochondria and ROS production [? ? ? ?].

A limitation of this study is that it relies on immunohistochemistry to determine changes in the expression of autophagy proteins throughout the neural retina. We did not attempt to confirm our findings by assessing gene expression or protein levels using Western blot. Neither did we assess autophagic flux by determining the LC3II:LC3I ratio. The reasons for this were a combination of the large number of animals needed; regional/cell-specific changes would be masked in whole retinal preps and the non-canonical role of LC3 in retinal and immune cell phagocytosis [?] could complicate the analysis of the autophagic flux. Furthermore, based on our data, there is a need to determine the mechanistic link between diurnal changes and autophagy in the neural retina. There is considerable evidence that diurnal/circadian rhythm is associated with the induction of autophagy [? ?], a key regulator of autophagy; the mechanistic target of rapamycin (mTOR) is regulated by the circadian clock [?] and the circadian regulation of metabolism is mediated through reciprocal signaling between the clock and metabolic regulatory networks such as autophagy [?]. Recently, Ryzhikov and colleagues reported that diurnal rhythms spatially and temporarily organize autophagy [?]. They reported that basal autophagy rhythms could be resolved into two antiphase clusters that were distinguished by the subcellular location of targeted proteins. Daytime autophagy was directed towards cytosolic proteins and proteosomal degradation, while nighttime autophagy was directed towards ER and mitochondrial removal. There is now a need to better understand the mechanistic control of these processes.

As mentioned above, autophagy in diabetes and related diseases has become an area of intense research, with focus on how this pathway may be targeted in synergy, with other therapeutic approaches to encourage a better clinical outcome. Our study, along with other recent reports, adds a novel extension to the mammalian diurnal rhythmicity in its relevance in regulation of biological processes. It provides a novel link between dysregulated autophagy and disrupted diurnal rhythm in the aging and diabetic retina and suggests that our analyses of myriad biological processes in the retina should be reconsidered from a diurnal perspective, in order to better comprehend age-related vision loss and disease pathology.

Author Contributions: Conceptualization, M.E.B., M.B.G. and J.V.B; Data curation, X.Q., S.K.M; Formal analysis, X.Q., Y.Y.; Investigation, X.Q., S.K.M., M.E.B. Resources, M.E.B., J.V.B., M.B.G.; Project administration: M.E.B., J.V.B., M.B.G. Writing—original draft preparation, X.Q., M.E.B.; Writing—review and editing, X.Q., S.K.M., Y.Y., J.V.B., M.B.G., M.E.B. All authors have read and agreed to the published version of the manuscript.

Acknowledgments: The animal experiments were performed over a period of time when MEB, MBG, XQ and SKM were at University of Florida and then Indiana University, before moving to UAB. All data were analyzed at UAB.

References

1. Choi, A.M.; Ryter, S.W.; Levine, B. Autophagy in human health and disease. *N. Engl. J. Med.* **2013**, *368*, 651–662. [CrossRef]
2. Mitter, S.K.; Boulton, M.E. Autophagy in ocular physiology. In *Autophagy in Current Trends in Cellular Physiology and Pathology*; Gorbunov, N.V., Schneider, M., Eds.; InTech: Open Access: London, UK, 2016; pp. 287–327.
3. Sridhar, S.; Botbol, Y.; Macian, F.; Cuervo, A.M. Autophagy and disease: Always two sides to a problem. *J. Pathol.* **2012**, *226*, 255–273. [CrossRef]
4. Sachdeva, U.M.; Thompson, C.B. Diurnal rhythms of autophagy: Implications for cell biology and human disease. *Autophagy* **2008**, *4*, 581–589. [CrossRef]
5. Boya, P.; Esteban-Martinez, L.; Serrano-Puebla, A.; Gomez-Sintes, R.; Villarejo-Zori, B. Autophagy in the eye: Development, degeneration, and aging. *Prog. Retin. Eye Res.* **2016**, *55*, 206–245. [CrossRef]
6. Czaja, M.J.; Ding, W.X.; Donohue, T.M., Jr.; Friedman, S.L.; Kim, J.S.; Komatsu, M.; Lemasters, J.J.; Lemoine, A.; Lin, J.D.; Ou, J.H.; et al. Functions of autophagy in normal and diseased liver. *Autophagy* **2013**, *9*, 1131–1158. [CrossRef]
7. Kiriyama, Y.; Nochi, H. The Function of Autophagy in Neurodegenerative Diseases. *Int. J. Mol. Sci.* **2015**, *16*, 26797–26812. [CrossRef]
8. Mancias, J.D.; Kimmelman, A.C. Mechanisms of Selective Autophagy in Normal Physiology and Cancer. *J. Mol. Biol.* **2016**, *428*, 1659–1680. [CrossRef]
9. Yin, Y.; Sun, G.; Li, E.; Kiselyov, K.; Sun, D. ER stress and impaired autophagy flux in neuronal degeneration and brain injury. *Ageing Res. Rev.* **2016**. [CrossRef]
10. Ebato, C.; Uchida, T.; Arakawa, M.; Komatsu, M.; Ueno, T.; Komiya, K.; Azuma, K.; Hirose, T.; Tanaka, K.; Kominami, E.; et al. Autophagy is important in islet homeostasis and compensatory increase of beta cell mass in response to high-fat diet. *Cell Metab.* **2008**, *8*, 325–332. [CrossRef]
11. Fujitani, Y.; Kawamori, R.; Watada, H. The role of autophagy in pancreatic beta-cell and diabetes. *Autophagy* **2009**, *5*, 280–282. [CrossRef]
12. Goldman, S.; Zhang, Y.; Jin, S. Autophagy and adipogenesis: Implications in obesity and type II diabetes. *Autophagy* **2010**, *6*, 179–181. [CrossRef] [PubMed]

13. Graham, T.E.; Abel, E.D. Autophagy in diabetes and the metabolic syndrome. In *Autophagy in Health and Disease*; Gottlieb, R.A., Ed.; Academic Press: London, UK, 2013; pp. 117–140.
14. Shi, S.Q.; Ansari, T.S.; McGuinness, O.P.; Wasserman, D.H.; Johnson, C.H. Circadian disruption leads to insulin resistance and obesity. *Curr. Biol. Cb* **2013**, *23*, 372–381. [CrossRef] [PubMed]
15. Busik, J.V.; Tikhonenko, M.; Bhatwadekar, A.; Opreanu, M.; Yakubova, N.; Caballero, S.; Player, D.; Nakagawa, T.; Afzal, A.; Kielczewski, J.; et al. Diabetic retinopathy is associated with bone marrow neuropathy and a depressed peripheral clock. *J. Exp. Med.* **2009**, *206*, 2897–2906. [CrossRef] [PubMed]
16. Ikeda, H.; Yong, Q.; Kurose, T.; Todo, T.; Mizunoya, W.; Fushiki, T.; Seino, Y.; Yamada, Y. Clock gene defect disrupts light-dependency of autonomic nerve activity. *Biochem. Biophys. Res. Commun.* **2007**, *364*, 457–463. [CrossRef] [PubMed]
17. Ruiter, M.; Buijs, R.M.; Kalsbeek, A. Hormones and the autonomic nervous system are involved in suprachiasmatic nucleus modulation of glucose homeostasis. *Curr. Diabetes Rev.* **2006**, *2*, 213–226. [CrossRef] [PubMed]
18. Thomas, H.E.; Redgrave, R.; Cunnington, M.S.; Avery, P.; Keavney, B.D.; Arthur, H.M. Circulating endothelial progenitor cells exhibit diurnal variation. *Arterioscler. Thromb. Vasc. Biol.* **2008**, *28*, e21–e22. [CrossRef]
19. Kohsaka, A.; Laposky, A.D.; Ramsey, K.M.; Estrada, C.; Joshu, C.; Kobayashi, Y.; Turek, F.W.; Bass, J. High-fat diet disrupts behavioral and molecular circadian rhythms in mice. *Cell Metab.* **2007**, *6*, 414–421. [CrossRef]
20. Young, M.E.; Razeghi, P.; Taegtmeyer, H. Clock genes in the heart: Characterization and attenuation with hypertrophy. *Circ. Res.* **2001**, *88*, 1142–1150. [CrossRef]
21. Lahouaoui, H.; Coutanson, C.; Cooper, H.M.; Bennis, M.; Dkhissi-Benyahya, O. Clock genes and behavioral responses to light are altered in a mouse model of diabetic retinopathy. *PLoS ONE* **2014**, *9*, e101584. [CrossRef]
22. Ando, H.; Ushijima, K.; Yanagihara, H.; Hayashi, Y.; Takamura, T.; Kaneko, S.; Fujimura, A. Clock gene expression in the liver and adipose tissues of non-obese type 2 diabetic Goto-Kakizaki rats. *Clin. Exp. Hypertens.* **2009**, *31*, 201–207. [CrossRef]
23. Bhatwadekar, A.D.; Yan, Y.; Qi, X.; Thinschmidt, J.S.; Neu, M.B.; Li Calzi, S.; Shaw, L.C.; Dominiguez, J.M.; Busik, J.V.; Lee, C.; et al. Per2 mutation recapitulates the vascular phenotype of diabetes in the retina and bone marrow. *Diabetes* **2013**, *62*, 273–282. [CrossRef]
24. Frost, L.S.; Lopes, V.S.; Bragin, A.; Reyes-Reveles, J.; Brancato, J.; Cohen, A.; Mitchell, C.H.; Williams, D.S.; Boesze-Battaglia, K. The Contribution of Melanoregulin to Microtubule-Associated Protein 1 Light Chain 3 (LC3) Associated Phagocytosis in Retinal Pigment Epithelium. *Mol. Neurobiol.* **2015**, *52*, 1135–1151. [CrossRef] [PubMed]
25. Kim, J.Y.; Zhao, H.; Martinez, J.; Doggett, T.A.; Kolesnikov, A.V.; Tang, P.H.; Ablonczy, Z.; Chan, C.C.; Zhou, Z.; Green, D.R.; et al. Noncanonical autophagy promotes the visual cycle. *Cell* **2013**, *154*, 365–376. [CrossRef] [PubMed]
26. Bosch, E.; Horwitz, J.; Bok, D. Phagocytosis of outer segments by retinal pigment epithelium: Phagosome-lysosome interaction. *J. Histochem. Cytochem. Off. J. Histochem. Soc.* **1993**, *41*, 253–263. [CrossRef] [PubMed]
27. Young, R.W. The daily rhythm of shedding and degradation of cone outer segment membranes in the lizard retina. *J. Ultrastruct. Res.* **1977**, *61*, 172–185. [CrossRef]
28. Rodriguez-Muela, N.; Koga, H.; Garcia-Ledo, L.; de la Villa, P.; de la Rosa, E.J.; Cuervo, A.M.; Boya, P. Balance between autophagic pathways preserves retinal homeostasis. *Aging Cell* **2013**, *12*, 478–488. [CrossRef]
29. Yao, J.; Jia, L.; Shelby, S.J.; Ganios, A.M.; Feathers, K.; Thompson, D.A.; Zacks, D.N. Circadian and noncircadian modulation of autophagy in photoreceptors and retinal pigment epithelium. *Investig. Ophthalmol. Vis. Sci.* **2014**, *55*, 3237–3246. [CrossRef]
30. Feit-Leichman, R.A.; Kinouchi, R.; Takeda, M.; Fan, Z.; Mohr, S.; Kern, T.S.; Chen, D.F. Vascular damage in a mouse model of diabetic retinopathy: Relation to neuronal and glial changes. *Investig. Ophthalmol. Vis. Sci.* **2005**, *46*, 4281–4287. [CrossRef]
31. Hazra, S.; Rasheed, A.; Bhatwadekar, A.; Wang, X.; Shaw, L.C.; Patel, M.; Caballero, S.; Magomedova, L.; Solis, N.; Yan, Y.; et al. Liver X receptor modulates diabetic retinopathy outcome in a mouse model of streptozotocin-induced diabetes. *Diabetes* **2012**, *61*, 3270–3279. [CrossRef]
32. Bhutto, I.A.; McLeod, D.S.; Hasegawa, T.; Kim, S.Y.; Merges, C.; Tong, P.; Lutty, G.A. Pigment epithelium-derived factor (PEDF) and vascular endothelial growth factor (VEGF) in aged human choroid and eyes with age-related macular degeneration. *Exp. Eye Res.* **2006**, *82*, 99–110. [CrossRef]

33. McLeod, D.S.; Lefer, D.J.; Merges, C.; Lutty, G.A. Enhanced expression of intracellular adhesion molecule-1 and P-selectin in the diabetic human retina and choroid. *Am. J. Pathol.* **1995**, *147*, 642–653. [PubMed]
34. Kuwabara, T.; Cogan, D.G. Studies of retinal vascular patterns. I. Normal architecture. *Arch. Ophthalmol.* **1960**, *64*, 904–911. [CrossRef] [PubMed]
35. Komeina, K.; Usui, S.; Shen, J.; Rogers, B.S.; Campochiaro, P.A. Blockade of neuronal nitric oxide synthase reduces cone cell death in a model of retinitis pigmentosa. *Free Radic. Biol. Med.* **2008**, *45*, 905–912. [CrossRef] [PubMed]
36. Hammes, H.P.; Lin, J.; Renner, O.; Shani, M.; Lundqvist, A.; Betsholtz, C.; Brownlee, M.; Deutsch, U. Pericytes and the pathogenesis of diabetic retinopathy. *Diabetes* **2002**, *51*, 3107–3112. [CrossRef] [PubMed]
37. Toda, N.; Nakanishi-Toda, M. Nitric oxide: Ocular blood flow, glaucoma, and diabetic retinopathy. *Prog. Retin. Eye Res.* **2007**, *26*, 205–238. [CrossRef] [PubMed]
38. Krohne, T.U.; Kaemmerer, E.; Holz, F.G.; Kopitz, J. Lipid peroxidation products reduce lysosomal protease activities in human retinal pigment epithelial cells via two different mechanisms of action. *Exp. Eye Res.* **2010**, *90*, 261–266. [CrossRef]
39. Viiri, J.; Amadio, M.; Marchesi, N.; Hyttinen, J.M.; Kivinen, N.; Sironen, R.; Rilla, K.; Akhtar, S.; Provenzani, A.; D'Agostino, V.G.; et al. Autophagy activation clears ELAVL1/HuR-mediated accumulation of SQSTM1/p62 during proteasomal inhibition in human retinal pigment epithelial cells. *PLoS ONE* **2013**, *8*, e69563. [CrossRef]
40. Chu, Y.K.; Lee, S.C.; Byeon, S.H. VEGF rescues cigarette smoking-induced human RPE cell death by increasing autophagic flux: Implications of the role of autophagy in advanced age-related macular degeneration. *Investig. Ophthalmol. Vis. Sci.* **2013**, *54*, 7329–7337. [CrossRef]
41. Mohlin, C.; Taylor, L.; Ghosh, F.; Johansson, K. Autophagy and ER-stress contribute to photoreceptor degeneration in cultured adult porcine retina. *Brain Res.* **2014**, *1585*, 167–183. [CrossRef]
42. Rodriguez-Muela, N.; Hernandez-Pinto, A.M.; Serrano-Puebla, A.; Garcia-Ledo, L.; Latorre, S.H.; de la Rosa, E.J.; Boya, P. Lysosomal membrane permeabilization and autophagy blockade contribute to photoreceptor cell death in a mouse model of retinitis pigmentosa. *Cell Death Differ.* **2015**, *22*, 476–487. [CrossRef]
43. Mitter, S.K.; Song, C.; Qi, X.; Mao, H.; Rao, H.; Akin, D.; Lewin, A.; Grant, M.; Dunn, W., Jr.; Ding, J.; et al. Dysregulated autophagy in the RPE is associated with increased susceptibility to oxidative stress and AMD. *Autophagy* **2014**, *10*, 1989–2005. [CrossRef] [PubMed]
44. Ma, D.; Li, S.; Molusky, M.M.; Lin, J.D. Circadian autophagy rhythm: A link between clock and metabolism? *Trends Endocrinol. Metab. Tem.* **2012**, *23*, 319–325. [CrossRef]
45. Ma, D.; Panda, S.; Lin, J.D. Temporal orchestration of circadian autophagy rhythm by C/EBPbeta. *Embo J.* **2011**, *30*, 4642–4651. [CrossRef] [PubMed]
46. Pfeifer, U.; Scheller, H.; Ormanns, W. Diurnal rhythm of lysosomal organelle decomposition in liver, kidney and pancreas. *Acta Histochemica Suppl.* **1976**, *16*, 205–210.
47. Pfeifer, U.; Strauss, P. Autophagic vacuoles in heart muscle and liver. A comparative morphometric study including circadian variations in meal-fed rats. *J. Mol. Cell. Cardiol.* **1981**, *13*, 37–49.
48. Reme, C.E.; Sulser, M. Diurnal variation of autophagy in rod visual cells in the rat. *Graefes Arch. Clin. Exp. Ophthalmol.* **1977**, *203*, 261–270. [CrossRef]
49. Kanwar, M.; Chan, P.S.; Kern, T.S.; Kowluru, R.A. Oxidative damage in the retinal mitochondria of diabetic mice: Possible protection by superoxide dismutase. *Investig. Ophthalmol. Vis. Sci.* **2007**, *48*, 3805–3811. [CrossRef]
50. Kowluru, R.A.; Chan, P.S. Oxidative stress and diabetic retinopathy. *Exp. Diabetes Res.* **2007**, *2007*, 43603. [CrossRef]
51. Wu, Y.; Tang, L.; Chen, B. Oxidative stress: Implications for the development of diabetic retinopathy and antioxidant therapeutic perspectives. *Oxid. Med. Cell. Longev.* **2014**, *2014*, 752387. [CrossRef]
52. Zhong, Q.; Kowluru, R.A. Diabetic retinopathy and damage to mitochondrial structure and transport machinery. *Investig. Ophthalmol. Vis. Sci.* **2011**, *52*, 8739–8746. [CrossRef]
53. Maiese, K. Moving to the Rhythm with Clock (Circadian) Genes, Autophagy, mTOR, and SIRT1 in Degenerative Disease and Cancer. *Curr. Neurovasc. Res.* **2017**, *14*, 299–304. [CrossRef]

54. Cao, R. mTOR Signaling, Translational Control, and the Circadian Clock. *Front. Genet.* **2018**, *9*, 367. [CrossRef]
55. Ryzhikov, M.; Ehlers, A.; Steinberg, D.; Xie, W.; Oberlander, E.; Brown, S.; Gilmore, P.E.; Townsend, R.R.; Lane, W.S.; Dolinay, T.; et al. Diurnal Rhythms Spatially and Temporally Organize Autophagy. *Cell Rep.* **2019**, *26*, 1880–1892.e6. [CrossRef] [PubMed]

10

Role of FGF and Hyaluronan in Choroidal Neovascularization in Sorsby Fundus Dystrophy

Alyson Wolk [1,2], Dilara Hatipoglu [1], Alecia Cutler [1], Mariya Ali [1], Lestella Bell [1,3], Jian Hua Qi [1], Rupesh Singh [1], Julia Batoki [1], Laura Karle [1], Vera L. Bonilha [1,2,3], Oliver Wessely [2,4], Heidi Stoehr [5], Vincent Hascall [6] and Bela Anand-Apte [1,2,3,*]

1 Cole Eye Institute & Lerner Research Institute, Cleveland Clinic Foundation, Cleveland, OH 44195, USA; wolka@ccf.org (A.W.); Hatipod@ccf.org (D.H.); cutlera@ccf.org (A.C.); alim2@ccf.org (M.A.); belll3@ccf.org (L.B.); qij@ccf.org (J.H.Q.); Singhr4@ccf.org (R.S.); Batokij@ccf.org (J.B.); lauraikarle@gmail.com (L.K.); bonilhav@ccf.org (V.L.B.)

2 Cleveland Clinic Lerner College of Medicine, Department of Molecular Medicine, Case Western Reserve University, Cleveland, OH 44195, USA; Wesselo@ccf.org

3 Cleveland Clinic Lerner College of Medicine at Case Western Reserve University, Department of Ophthalmology, Cleveland, OH 44195, USA

4 Department of Cardiovascular and Metabolic Sciences, Lerner Research Institute, Cleveland Clinic Foundation, Cleveland, OH 44195, USA

5 Institute of Human Genetics, University of Regensburg, 93053 Regensburg, Germany; Heidi.Stoehr@klinik.uni-regensburg.de

6 Department of Biomedical Engineering, Lerner Research Institute, Cleveland Clinic Foundation, Cleveland, OH 44195, USA; Hascalv@ccf.org

* Correspondence: anandab@ccf.org

Abstract: Sorsby's fundus dystrophy (SFD) is an inherited blinding disorder caused by mutations in the tissue inhibitor of metalloproteinase-3 (*TIMP3*) gene. The SFD pathology of macular degeneration with subretinal deposits and choroidal neovascularization (CNV) closely resembles that of the more common age-related macular degeneration (AMD). The objective of this study was to gain further insight into the molecular mechanism(s) by which mutant TIMP3 induces CNV. In this study we demonstrate that hyaluronan (HA), a large glycosaminoglycan, is elevated in the plasma and retinal pigment epithelium (RPE)/choroid of patients with AMD. Mice carrying the S179C-TIMP3 mutation also showed increased plasma levels of HA as well as accumulation of HA around the RPE in the retina. Human RPE cells expressing the *S179C-TIMP3* mutation accumulated HA apically, intracellularly and basally when cultured long-term compared with cells expressing wildtype *TIMP3*. We recently reported that RPE cells carrying the *S179C-TIMP3* mutation have the propensity to induce angiogenesis via basic fibroblast growth factor (FGF-2). We now demonstrate that FGF-2 induces accumulation of HA in RPE cells. These results suggest that the TIMP3-MMP-FGF-2-HA axis may have an important role in the pathogenesis of CNV in SFD and possibly AMD.

Keywords: sorsby's fundus dystrophy; hyaluronan; neovascularization; retina

---

1. Introduction

Sorsby's fundus dystrophy (SFD) is a dominantly inherited, degenerative disease of the macula that is characterized by bilateral loss of central vision as a consequence of choroidal neovascularization (CNV) [1–6]. Specific mutations in the tissue inhibitor of metalloproteinase 3 (*TIMP3*) gene involving exon 5, exon 1 or the intron 4-exon 5 boundary have been shown to be causative [7–14]. In comparative studies using TIMP3 deficient mice, S179C-TIMP3 transgenic mice and in vitro culture experiments we have determined that TIMP3 partially inhibits angiogenesis by blocking the binding of vascular endothelial growth factor (VEGF) to VEGF Receptor 2 (VEGFR2). We have also demonstrated that the S179C-TIMP3 mutant protein induces angiogenesis via VEGF and fibroblast growth factor 2 (FGF-2) [15–21].

TIMP3 is produced constitutively by the retinal pigment epithelium (RPE) and choroidal endothelial cells [2,20]. It is a normal component of Bruch's membrane [22] and binds to sulfated glycosaminoglycans of the extracellular matrix (ECM) [23,24]. Hyaluronan (HA) is a large glycosaminoglycan that is a significant component of peri-cellular and extracellular matrices. HA is essential for numerous physiological functions that are dependent on its chain size and its interactions with various effector proteins and receptors [25]. HA has been implicated in the regulation of neovascularization and endothelial barrier function [26]. While studies have demonstrated that signaling via HA and its cell surface receptor CD44 accentuates CNV in mice using a laser-induced model [27], the exact molecular mechanism by which HA regulates tissue remodeling and neovascularization is unknown.

We have recently reported that RPE cells expressing mutant TIMP3 secrete increased amounts of FGF-2 [28] and that this contributes to increased angiogenesis. FGF-2 has been shown to be important in tumor angiogenesis, but its role in CNV has been less well studied. The most direct evidence for a role of FGF-2 in CNV comes from studies in which Flk1-Cre or Tie2-Cre mediated deletions of FGF receptor 1 (FGFR1) and FGF receptor 2 (FGFR2) in endothelial cells resulted in reduced laser-induced CNV in mice [29]. Extracellular matrix components such as heparan sulfate proteoglycans (HSPGs) bind and regulate the activity of growth factors such as FGF-2 [30] and have a critical role in the regulation of neovascularization [31]. In addition, the observation that activation of the FGFR-STAT3 pathway can induce a hyaluronan-rich microenvironment that can affect tumor growth [32] led us to test the hypothesis that in addition to VEGF, FGF-2 and hyaluronan also have critical roles in the increased neovascularization induced by mutant TIMP3 in Sorsby's fundus dystrophy.

2. Materials and Methods

2.1. Human Samples

Patients with AMD and controls (without AMD or any other retinal disease) were recruited from the eye clinics at Cole Eye Institute under Cleveland Clinic Foundation approved IRB protocols. Plasma samples were prepared and stored at −80 °C. Samples from patients (n = 49, with 26 males and 23 females) given a clinical diagnosis of geographic atrophy or CNV and age-matched controls (n = 59 with 28 males and 31 females) were included in this pilot study to evaluate HA in the plasma. Normal and/or AMD post-mortem eyes were obtained from the Cleveland Eye Bank, the National Disease Research Interchange (Philadelphia, PA, USA) or from the Cole Eye Institute Eye Tissue Repository through the Foundation Fighting Blindness (FFB) Eye Donor Program (Columbia, MD, USA). All post-mortem tissue were obtained in accordance with the policies of the Eye Bank Association of America and the Institutional Review Board of the Cleveland Clinic Foundation (IRB#14-057). Eye bank records accompanying the donor eyes indicated whether the donor had AMD or no known eye diseases. The analyzed tissue included FFB donations #714 (82 y.o.), #781 (80 y.o.), #711 (83 y.o.), #722 (90 y.o.), #716 (80 y.o.) and #739 (90 y.o.), identified as AMD. Postmortem eyes from a 95 (#784), 92 (#979) and a 91 year-old donor without a history of retinal disease were used as controls. Eyes were enucleated 4 to 22 h postmortem and fixed in 4% paraformaldehyde and 0.5% glutaraldehyde in phosphate buffer. The globes were stored in 2% paraformaldehyde in D-PBS.

2.2. Mice

All mice utilized in this study were housed in the Cole Eye Institute vivarium under approved Institutional Animal Care and Use Committee (IACUC) protocols. All procedures on the mice were in accordance with ARVO statement for the Use of Animals in Ophthalmic and Vision Research and conformed to the National Institutes of Health Guide for the Care and Use of Animals in Research and to the ARVO statement for the use of animals in ophthalmic and vision research. $Timp3^{+/S179C}$ mice were generated in the laboratory of Dr. Bernhard Weber using site-directed mutagenesis and homologous recombination in embryonic stem (ES) cells to generate mutant ES cells carrying the $Timp3^{S179C}$ allele. Heterozygous breeding of $Timp3^{+/S179C}$ [33] produced homozygous $Timp3^{S179C/S179C}$ mice and age-matched littermate controls in a C57BL6 background. Similarly, heterozygous $Timp3^{+/-}$ mice [34] were bred to generate $Timp3^{-/-}$ knockouts and $TIMP3^{+/+}$ littermate controls. Eyes were enucleated following euthanasia and fresh frozen in tissue-plus optical cutting temperature embedding medium (Scigen, #4583) for sectioning and histology. Blood samples were collected via cardiac puncture and plasma prepared via standard protocols.

2.3. *Hyaluronan Enzyme-Linked Immunosorbent Assay (ELISA)*

Plasma from human patients with and without AMD and from SFD mouse models were measured for HA contents by solid-phase sandwich ELISA in 96-well plates (Costar, #9018) using the Hyaluronan Duo-Set ELISA kit (R&D Systems, #DY3614-05).

2.4. *Immunofluorescence*

Retina sections and flat-mounted ARPE-19 cells grown on polyester trans-wells were fixed for 5 min in 4% paraformaldehyde and blocked in 1% bovine serum albumin with 0.1% Triton X-100 in phosphate-buffered saline. Human sections were processed with melanin bleaching kit to remove autofluorescence (Polysciences, Inc., Warrington, PA, USA, #24883A-B). Samples were incubated overnight with biotinylated HA binding protein, (Millipore Sigma, #385911) or primary antibodies (anti-ezrin, clone 3C12, Invitrogen, Carlsbad, CA, USA #MA5-13862) in humidified chambers at 4 °C. Subsequently, secondary antibodies (anti-mouse AlexaFluor 594, streptavidin-AlexaFluor 488, streptavidin-AlexaFluor 647, all from ThermoFisher Scientific, Waltham, MA, USA) were incubated with samples at room temperature for one hour in the dark. Rhodamine-phalloidin (Thermo Fisher Scientific, R415) was incubated together with secondary antibodies. Then, 4′,6-diamidino-2-phenylindole (DAPI) was used to stain nuclei of murine sections and cell culture mounts and SYTOX green (ThermoFisher Scientific, #S7020) was used to stain nuclei in human sections. Imaging by confocal microscopy was performed (Leica TCS-SP8, Exton, PA, USA). The localization of Bruch's membrane was determined by its autofluorescence at 405 nm.

2.5. *Hyaluronidase Treatment of Retina Sections*

Hyaluronidase from *Streptomyces hyalurolyticus* (Millipore Sigma, Burlington, MA USA, #H1136) was used to treat retina sections as described previously [35]. Streptomyces hyaluronidase was resuspended in 0.1 M sodium acetate buffer, pH 5.0, at 100 U/mL. To prevent any nonspecific digestion, the following protease inhibitors were added to the sodium acetate buffer: 1 mM iodoacetic acid, 1 mM phenylmethyl sulfonylfluoride, 1 mM EDTA, 1 μg/mL pepstatin A, 250 μg/mL ovomucoid. Hyaluronidase solution (100 mU/mL of hyaluronidase in PBS with $CaCl_2$ (0.1 g/L) and $MgCl_2$ (0.1 g/L)) was applied onto the sections for 3 h at 37 °C. Slides were subsequently fixed in 4% paraformaldehyde and examined by fluorescence microscopy.

2.6. *Cells and Reagents*

ARPE-19 cells stably expressing S179C-TIMP3, wild-type-TIMP3 (WT), or vector alone were reported previously [19]. Cells were expanded in DMEM-F12 with 10% FBS before transfer to polyester inserts coated with mouse laminin (Corning Inc., Corning, NY, USA, #23017). 720,000 cells and 100,000 cells were plated per well in each well of a 12-well plate or 24-well plate, respectively using a previously published protocol [36]. Essentially, ARPE-19 cells were cultured for at least 2 weeks in nicotinamide-supplemented media with 1% FBS. Media were replaced twice per week. Cells were serum-starved for 24 h before treatment with the FGF Receptor inhibitor BGJ-398 (Selleckchem, Houston, TX, USA, #S2183) for 48 h. Similarly, cells were treated with FGF-2 (Gibco from Thermo

Fisher Scientific, #13256-029) with the required cofactor heparin sodium salt (1 μg/mL, Sigma Aldrich, #H3149) for 48 h after serum starving for 24 h.

2.7. *Quantitation of Immunofluorescence by Integrated Density Analysis*

Fluorescence intensity of HABP staining was quantified using integrated density analysis as previously described [37,38]. For all the RPE cell culture confocal microscopy images, fluorescence was quantitated using a standard measure of integrated density, which is the product of area and mean gray value. A custom written automated image analysis code was developed using Matlab (MATLAB 2019a, The MathWorks, Inc., Natick, MA, USA) for separating the desired color channel from the image, thereby obtaining the total area (in pixels), the mean gray value, and the integrated density.

2.8. *In Vivo Imaging and Laser Injury Model*

Laser mediated CNV was induced as described previously [28]. Briefly, mice were anesthetized with 65–68 mg/kg sodium pentobarbital delivered intra-peritoneally. Topical 0.5% procaine solution was applied for cornea anesthesia. Following anesthesia, pupils were dilated with 0.5% topical tropicamide/phenylephrine combination drops (Santen Pharmaceuticals, Osaka, Japan).

Four laser spots were placed in the superior, superior-temporal, or superior-nasal quadrants of the fundus using a green solid-state laser (Oculight by Iridex Corp., Mountain View, CA, USA) (532 nm; 2500 mW; 0.50 s pulse duration; 50 μm spot size) using a slit lamp delivery system and a microscope coverslip placed and affixed to the cornea with a drop of Systane Ultra artificial tears (Alcon, Ft Worth, TX, USA). All animals were scanned immediately after laser injury with optical coherence tomography (Envisu R2210 UHR Leica Microsystems Inc., Wetzlar, Germany) to confirm successful RPE-Bruch's membrane rupture, an endpoint in laser-induced CNV models.

2.9. *Statistical Analysis*

All parameters in the study were distributed normally. Data are expressed as mean ± SEM. Differences were tested by unpaired t-test (Figure 1, Figure 2 and Figure 3) or by using multiple t-tests employing two-stage linear step-up procedure of Benjamini, Krieger and Yekutieli, with a false discovery rate set to 1% (Figure 4 and Figure 5). Each group was analyzed separately without the assumption of consistent standard deviation. $p < 0.05$ values were considered statistically significant. Statistical analysis was performed with GraphPad Prism 7.03 (GraphPad Software, Inc., San Diego, CA, USA).

3. Results

3.1. *Hyaluronan is Elevated in Plasma and RPE/Choroid of Patients with AMD*

Age-related macular degeneration (AMD) is usually seen as two main types. "Dry" AMD where deposits called drusen develop in the macular region that ultimately progress to a late stage in which there is atrophy of the macula (geographic atrophy). "Wet" AMD describes AMD in which patients develop abnormal growth and leakage of the choroid vessels beneath and into the retina, termed choroidal neovascularization (CNV). HA contents were measured in plasma from patients with late stage AMD (geographic atrophy or choroidal neovascularization) and from age-matched controls without the disease. ELISA analysis (Figure 1A) indicates that HA contents were significantly increased in the plasma of patients with late-stage AMD (mean ± SEM: 111.8 ± 5.78 ng/mL) compared with plasma of controls without AMD (32.91 ± 5.75).

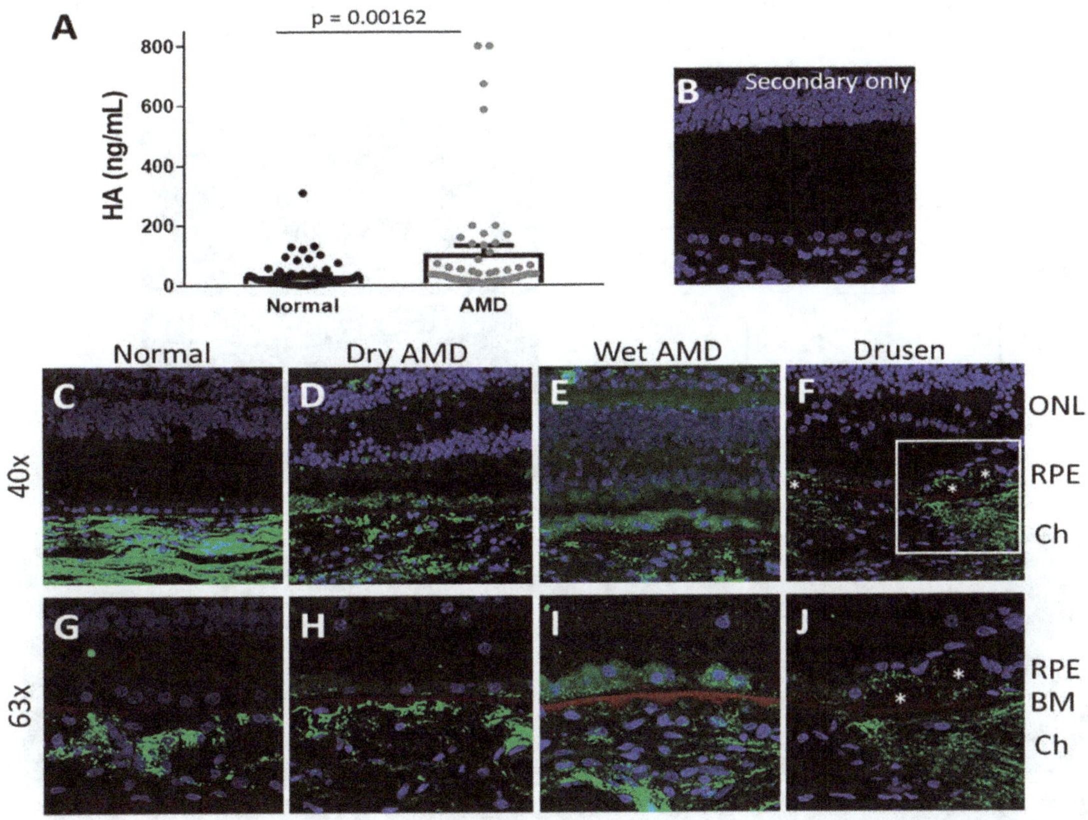

Figure 1. Hyaluronan HA is increased in circulation and in the RPE of age-related macular degeneration (AMD) patients. (**A**) HA was increased in plasma from patients with late-stage AMD (GA or CNV) compared to age-matched, normal controls. Data are presented as mean ± SEM (**B–J**) Representative human retina sections stained with HA binding protein (HABP) (**B**) Human retina section stained with streptavidin-AlexaFluor 647 in the absence of HA binding protein serves as a specificity control. (**C–J**) Human retina sections stained with streptavidin-AlexaFluor 647 in the presence of HA binding protein. HA is increased in the RPE in patients with dry AMD (**D**,**H**), wet AMD (**E**,**I**), and around drusen (**F**,**J**) compared to the RPE from an aged-match normal control (**C**,**G**). 40× images (**B–F**), 63× images (**G–J**). Green: HA; red: Bruch's membrane determined by its autofluorescence at 405 nm; blue: DAPI. Asterisks indicate drusen (**F**,**J**). GA—geographic atrophy; CNV—choroidal neovascularization; ONL—outer nuclear layer; RPE—retinal pigment epithelium; Ch—choroid; DAPI—4′,6-diamidino-2-phenylindole.

To evaluate the distribution of HA in the retina under physiological and pathological conditions, sections from post-mortem human donor eyes from 3 controls and 6 AMD (4 dry and 2 wet AMD) patients were stained for HA using biotinylated HA binding protein (HABP). HA was found to be localized predominantly in the choroid of normal eyes (Figure 1C) as described previously [39,40]. Increased deposition of HA was seen around the RPE in AMD eyes (both in the dry (Figure 1D,H) and wet AMD specimens (Figure 1E,I)). HA was particularly enhanced in drusen and in areas of atrophy (Figure 1F,J) in AMD specimens. The sections stained with secondary antibody alone serves as a specificity control and shows minimal staining compared with sections stained with HABP (Figure 1B).

3.2. Increased Plasma HA and Accumulation of HA in the RPE of SFD Mice

We utilized two mouse models to study the potential role of TIMP3 in the regulation of HA in the retina: mice lacking TIMP3 [34] and mice carrying the S179C-TIMP3 SFD mutation [33]. Plasma from S179C-TIMP3 and TIMP3-KO mice at 4–6 weeks of age was collected and HA contents were analyzed by ELISA. HA content of plasma was significantly increased in mice lacking TIMP3 as well as in mice carrying the S179C-TIMP3 mutation (Figure 2A), suggesting that TIMP3 may be important in regulating HA.

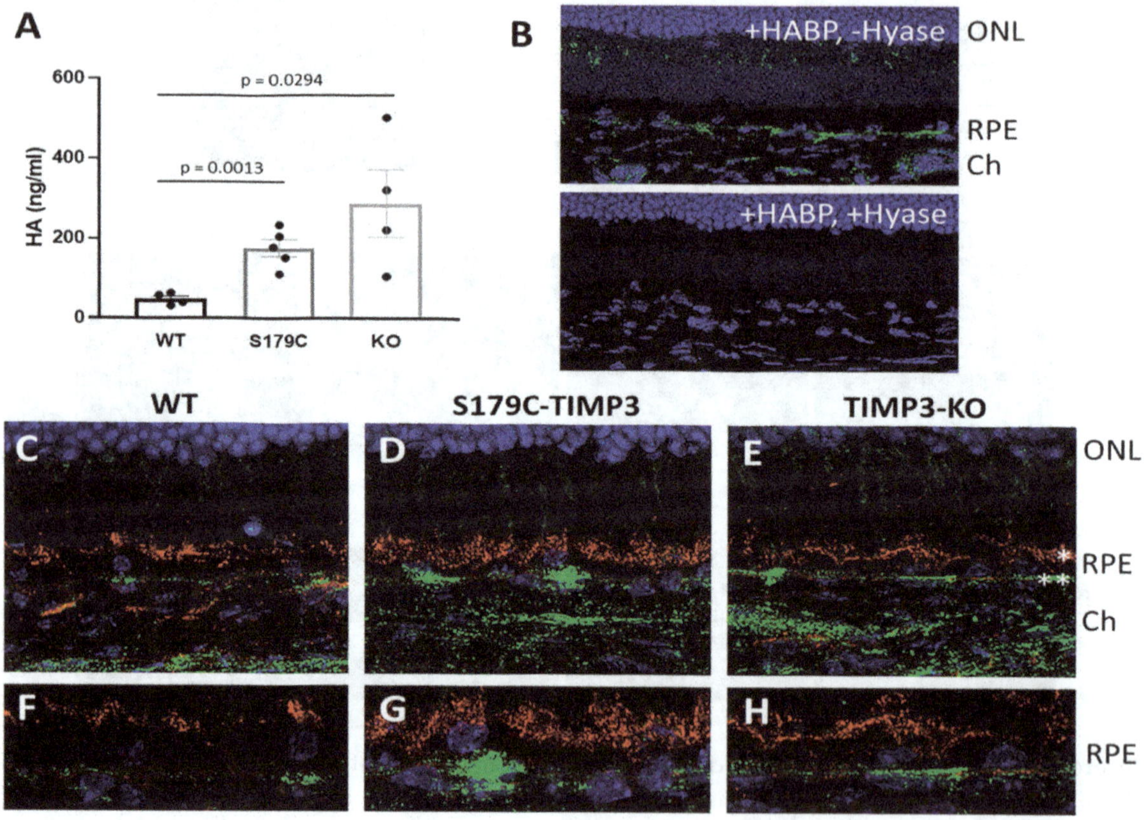

Figure 2. HA is increased in circulation and in the RPE and choroid in mouse models of Sorsby's fundus dystrophy. (**A**) HA was increased in plasma from S179C-TIMP3 knockin mice ($Timp3^{S179C6/S179C}$) and TIMP3-KO ($Timp3^{-/-}$) mice compared to wild-type (WT) littermates. ($n \geq 5$). Data are presented as mean ± SEM. (**B**) Mouse retina sections stained with biotinylated HA binding protein (HABP) in the absence (upper panel) or presence (lower panel) of hyaluronidase to detect HA. HABP staining is specific for HA as shown by the absence of staining in sections treated with hyaluronidase (lower panel). Green: HA; blue: DAPI. (**C–H**) Representative images of HA staining of mouse sections from wild-type (WT) mice (**C**,**F**), S179C-TIMP3 mutant mice (**D**,**G**) and TIMP3-KO mice (**E**,**H**). HA is increased in the RPE and choroid of S179C-TIMP3 (**D**) and TIMP3-KO (**E**) mice compared to wild-type (WT) littermate controls (**C**). HA (green) is predominantly localized to the basal surface of the RPE (**) (**F–H**) and not to the apical surface (*) as shown by co-staining with ezrin, a marker for the apical microvilli of RPE (red). 40× images (**C–E**); 63× images (**F–H**). $n \geq 3$ for all immunohistochemistry data.

To determine if there was a similar correlation between the plasma HA levels and the accumulation of HA in the RPE as observed in human sections with AMD, we evaluated accrual of HA in the retinas of mice (8 weeks of age) lacking TIMP3 or carrying the SFD mutation. Cryosections of retina from mice of each specific genotype and wild-type littermates were stained for HA content with HABP. To ascertain that HABP binds HA specifically, sections were treated with hyaluronidase prior to staining with HABP. Indeed, pre-treatment with hyaluronidase resulted in absence of staining with HABP (Figure 2B, lower panel). S179C-TIMP3 mice (Figure 2D) and TIMP3-KO mice (Figure 2E) show increased accumulation of HA beneath the RPE and in the choroid compared to that seen in wildtype littermates (Figure 2C). Staining with antibodies to ezrin served as a marker for RPE apical microvilli (Figure 2C–H), and the higher magnification images (Figure 2F–H) confirmed the RPE localization of HA to the basal surface of the cells.

To identify the potential mechanism by which S179C-TIMP3 regulates HA we utilized stable human RPE lines (ARPE-19) expressing S179C-TIMP3 [20]. ARPE-19 cells (expressing S179C-TIMP3, wildtype TIMP3 (WT-TIMP3) and empty vector (Vector)) were cultured for 2–6 weeks in 1% serum on trans-well inserts and stained for HA. Increased accumulation of HA was observed in RPE cells expressing S179C-TIMP3 (Figure 3C,G) compared with cells transfected with empty vector (Figure 3A,G) or expressing wildtype TIMP3 (Figure 3B,G). The accumulation was predominantly intracellular and apical in the RPE (Figure 3D–F). There appear to be multiple layers of S179C-TIMP3 RPE cells on the transwell compared with a single monolayer for WT-TIMP3 and vector cells, which might suggest epithelial-mesenchymal transition.

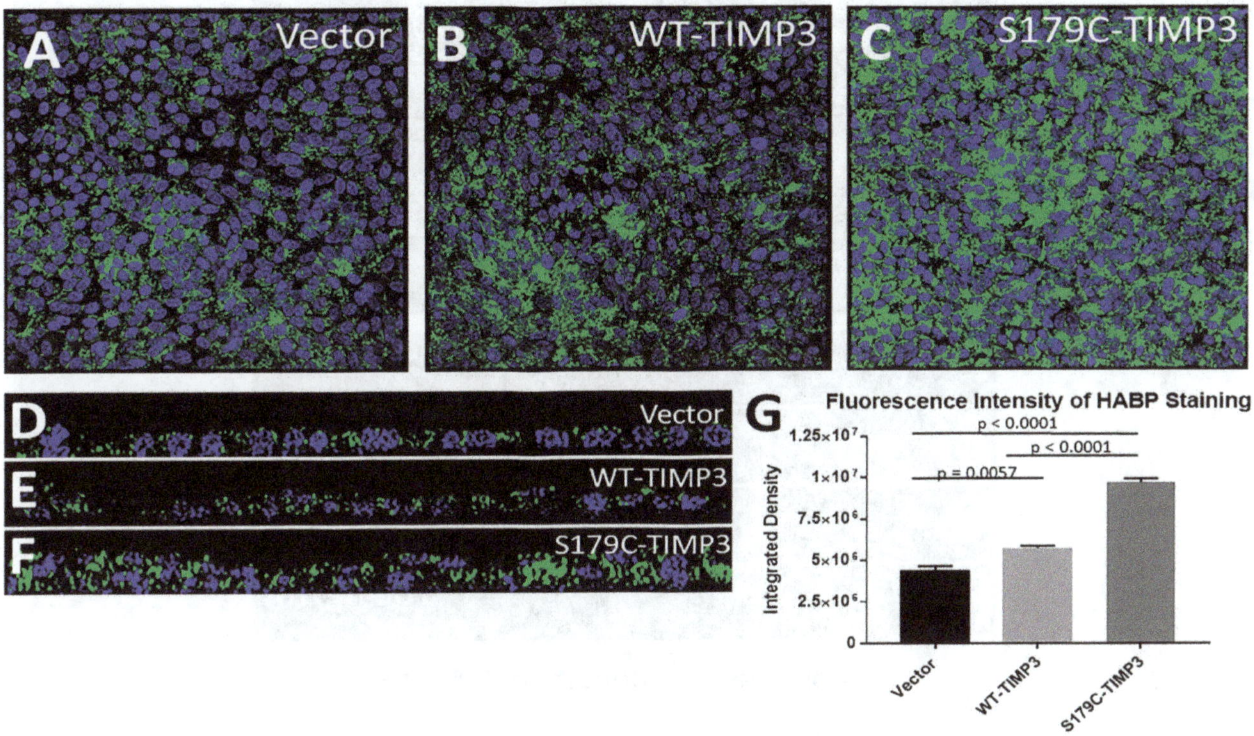

Figure 3. HA is increased in S179C-TIMP3 RPE cells in culture. (**A–C**) ARPE-19 cells expressing S179C-TIMP3 grown in culture for at least 2 weeks on trans-well inserts have increased HA (**C**) compared to WT-TIMP3 expressing cells (**B**) or vector only controls (**A**).(**D–F**) Z-plane images of HA in RPE monolayers grown on trans-well inserts show increased intracellular HA in S179C-TIMP3 cells. Green: HA; blue: DAPI. (**G**) Fluorescence intensity was quantitated by integrated density measurement ($n \geq 4$, for each cell line). Data are presented as mean ± SEM.

3.3. FGF-2 Contributes to HA Accumulation in the RPE

We have recently reported that RPE cells expressing S179C-TIMP3 secrete higher amounts of FGF-2 compared with control cells [28]. Previous studies have suggested that FGF signaling has the propensity to increase HA accumulation [32]. To experimentally test this hypothesis in RPE cells, we evaluated the ability of FGF-2 to induce HA accumulation in primary porcine RPE cells. Cells cultured for 3 weeks on trans-well inserts in 1% serum were treated with 0 ng/mL, 10 ng/mL, 25 ng/mL, or 100 ng/mL of FGF-2 in the presence of 1 µg/mL heparin, a cofactor for FGF receptor signaling. FGF-2 induced HA accumulation in a dose-dependent manner (Figure 4A–I) with maximum HA deposits being observed with a dose of 25 and 100 ng/mL (Figure 4D,H). This was confirmed by quantitation of fluorescence by integrated density measurements (Figure 4I). The FGF-2 induced accumulation of HA was seen predominantly on the apical surface of the RPE with increased basal and peri-cellular accumulation at higher doses (Figure 4E–H).

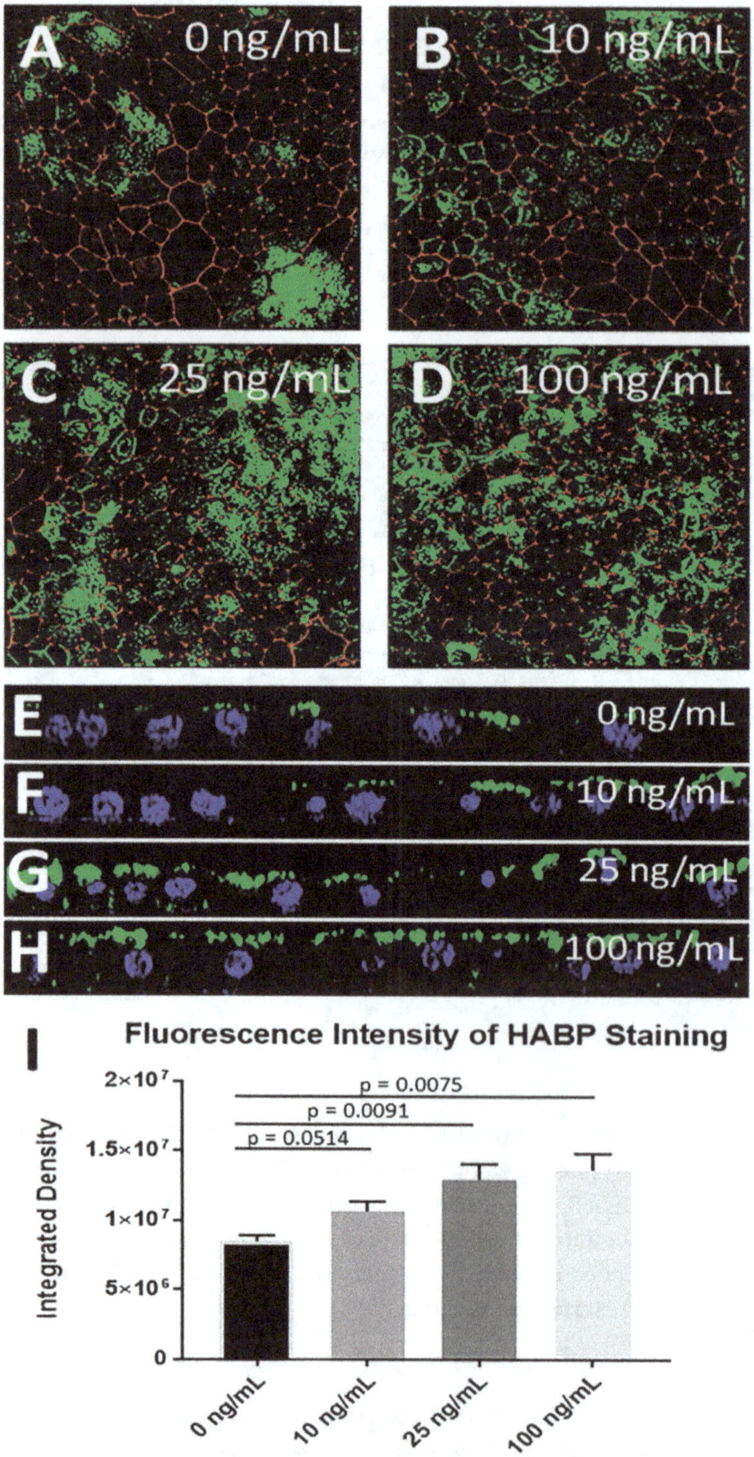

Figure 4. FGF-2 induces HA accumulation in primary RPE cells. (**A–D**) FGF-2 induced HA accumulation in primary porcine RPE cells in a dose-dependent manner (**A**) 0 ng/mL, (**B**) 10 ng/mL, (**C**) 25 ng/mL, (**D**) 100 ng/mL. Fluorescence intensity was quantitated by integrated density measurement (**I**) ($n \geq 4$, for each cell line). Data are presented as mean ± SEM (**E–H**) Z-plane images show that increased concentrations of FGF-2 induce increased apical accumulation of HA in addition to some peri-cellular and basal deposits of HA at high doses of FGF-2. Green: HA, red: phalloidin; blue: DAPI.

To determine if the accumulation of HA seen in RPE cells expressing S179C-TIMP3 was a consequence of increased FGF signaling, cells (RPE cells expressing S179C-TIMP3, wildtype TIMP3 or empty vector) were treated with BGJ-398, an FGF receptor inhibitor. 10 μM BGJ-398 decreased HA content in RPE cells expressing S179C-TIMP3 (Figure 5C,F,H,I) and WT-TIMP3 (Figure 5B,E,I) but not vector only transfected cells (Figure 5A,D,I) when compared with their respective untreated cells that served as controls (Figure 5A: vector, 5B: WT-TIMP3 and 5C,G: S179C-TIMP3). Quantitation of fluorescence by integrated density analysis revealed that 10 μM BGJ-398 decreased HA accumulation in S179C-TIMP3 cells 63.1% (SD = 0.241) and only 43.4% (SD = 0.291) in wildtype cells (Figure 5I). Quantitation confirmed that BGJ-398 had no significant effect on vector only cells (Figure 5I), suggesting an FGF-specific mechanism for HA accumulation in S179C-TIMP3 cells.

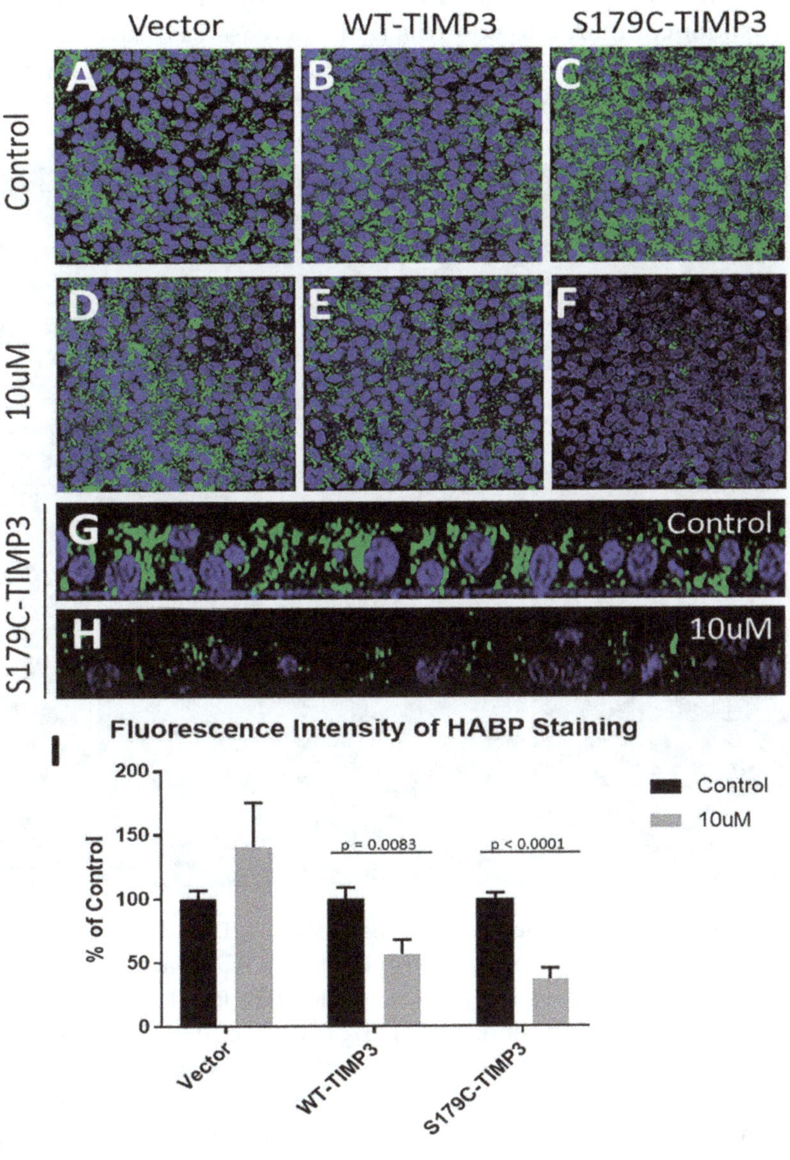

Figure 5. Inhibition of FGF signaling decreases HA accumulation in S179C-TIMP3 RPE cells. Vector only (**A**), WT-TIMP3 (**B**), and S179C-TIMP3 (**C**) expressing ARPE-19 cells were grown on trans-well inserts for 4 weeks before treatment with FGF receptor inhibitor BGJ-398. Treatment with BGJ-398 decreased HA accumulation in S179C-TIMP3 expressing RPE cells (**F**,**H**,**I**) and to a lesser extent in WT-TIMP3 expressing cells (**E**,**I**) but has no effect on control vector RPE cells (**A**,**D**,**I**). (**I**) Control (Black Bar) indicates respective untreated cells compared with BGJ-398 treated cells (Grey bar). (**G**,**H**) Z-plane images of S179C-TIMP3 cells in the absence (**G**) and presence (**H**) of 10 μM BGJ-398 S179C-TIMP3 cells show an overall reduction in HA accumulation, including intracellular HA, after treatment with BGJ-398. Green: HA; blue: DAPI. (**I**) data are presented as mean ± SEM (n ≥ 6).

3.4. Increased HA is Associated with CNV in AMD and SFD

Sections of post-mortem eyes from a patient with CNV showed significant HA deposition around the RPE (Figure 6C,D) when compared with control eyes (Figure 6A,B). While S179C-TIMP3 mice do not demonstrate a florid SFD phenotype as seen in humans, they do have increased susceptibility to experimental laser-induced CNV [28] as do the TIMP3-KO mice [41]. We have previously shown that FGF-2 from S179C-TIMP3 RPE cells can stimulate angiogenesis [28]. Since FGF-2 contributes to HA accumulation in the RPE and to angiogenesis, we evaluated if HA content and distribution was altered in laser-induced CNV lesions in S179C-TIMP3 mice. As described previously lesions in S179C-TIMP3 mice were larger and leakier compared to controls [28]. Increased HA accumulation was observed in CNV in S179C-TIMP3 mice (Figure 6H–J) when compared to lesions in control mice (Figure 6E–G) which appears to be a consequence of altered distribution to the CNV lesions in S179C-TIMP3 mice.

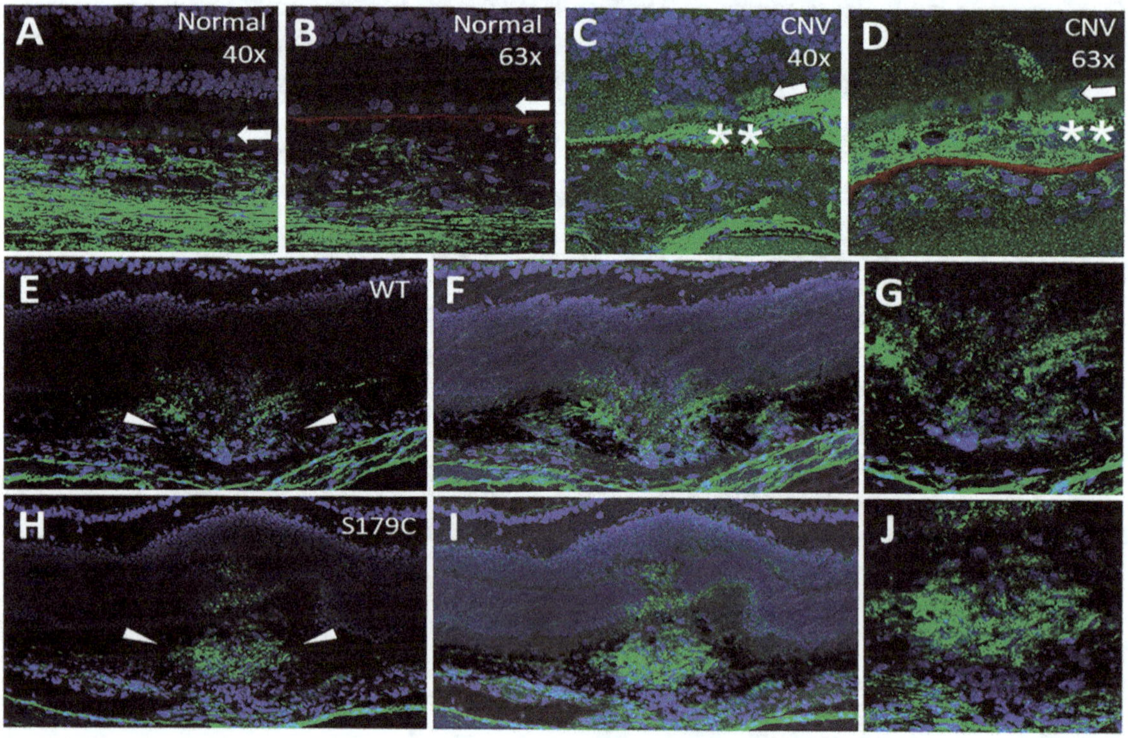

Figure 6. HA is increased in choroidal neovascular lesions in AMD patients and in S179C-TIMP3 mice. (**A–D**) HA is increased in the RPE in a patient with CNV (**C,D**) and in the CNV lesion compared to the RPE of a normal patient (**A,B**). Green: HA; blue: nuclei; red: Bruch's membrane. Arrows indicate RPE, double asterisks indicate CNV lesion. (**E–G**) HA is increased in laser-induced CNV lesions in S179C-TIMP3 mice compared to wild-type (WT) littermates 5 days post injury. (**E,H**) Arrows indicate CNV lesion. (**F,I**) Brightfield image overlaid on fluorescent image shows disruption of RPE and Bruch's membrane. (**G,J**) HA accumulation is diffuse and appears predominantly in the borders of the lesion in WT (**E–G**) compared to dense mass within the lesions of S179C-TIMP3 mice (**H–J**). Green: HA; blue: nuclei.

4. Discussion

Sorsby's fundus dystrophy (SFD) is a rare macular dystrophy characterized by vision loss due to persistent choroidal neovascularization [1–6]. SFD is an autosomal dominant, fully penetrant degenerative disease of the macula and is notable for its similarity in histopathological features to AMD [3–6]. The majority of SFD patients develop CNV, as well as confluent, 20–30 µm thick, amorphous deposits between the basement membrane of the RPE and Bruch's membrane. TIMP3 and/or its downstream substrates have been postulated to have a role in the pathogenesis of both SFD and AMD, because accumulation of TIMP3 has been observed in subretinal deposits in SFD [42] as well as in AMD drusen [43–45]. In this study, we show that hyaluronan accumulates around the RPE in AMD as well as in CNV lesions of mice expressing S179C-TIMP3.

One interesting observation from our studies was the increase in HA in the plasma of patients with AMD as well as in mice lacking TIMP3 or carrying the S179C-TIMP3 mutation. Although we observe significant differences in the plasma levels of HA in patients with advanced AMD (GA and CNV), the number of patients analyzed (n = 49 controls) and n = 59 (AMD) is not sufficient to determine if this is of prognostic value. In addition, we did not have access to samples from patients at different degrees of severity to be able to draw conclusions with this or the rate of progression of the disease. Future studies are warranted to address this question. While patients with SFD generally demonstrate disease localized to the retina, our results may be a consequence of ubiquitous expression of TIMP3 in a variety of tissues in the body [46] which could potentially explain the systemic increase in HA. Whether there is accumulation of HA in other tissues in S179C TIMP3 mice has not been evaluated.

Our studies with RPE cells suggest that the increase in HA in these cells is likely a consequence of increased FGF. A recent study [47] suggests that TIMP proteins can control FGF-2 bioavailability in skeletal tissue and the same might be true of multiple tissues leading to systemic increase in HA in the plasma. The exact mechanism by which TIMP3 regulates FGF bioavailability in the RPE is currently unknown, but it is highly likely that the TIMP-metalloproteinase axis likely has a key role. The extracellular matrix (ECM) serves as a high capacity reservoir for FGF-2 and early studies have demonstrated that matrix metalloproteases (MMPs) have the ability to mobilize FGF-2 to a soluble phase that results in receptor activation [48]. Additional studies identifying the molecular mechanisms by which TIMP3 regulates FGF-2 bioavailability will provide insight into the pathophysiology of the disease.

FGF-2 is sufficient to increase HA accumulation and distribution in the RPE, and blocking FGF signaling in S179C-TIMP3 RPE cells brings HA levels back to normal. The mechanism by which FGF-2 increases HA accumulation is not understood. HA is endogenously synthesized by a family of membrane-integrated glycosyltransferases, called hyaluronan synthases (HAS 1-3) and is exported directly into the ECM [49,50]. Hyaluronidases (HYAL1-2) are a class of enzymes that degrade HA [51]. A balance between HA synthesizing and degrading activity keeps HA at physiological levels. In order to determine the mechanism of accumulation of HA in the RPE in SFD, we performed quantitative PCR analysis of HAS1-3 and HYAL1-2 from RPE isolated from S179C-TIMP3, TIMP3-KO mice and wildtype littermate controls. Interestingly, we observed no changes in gene expression of any of these enzymes in the mutant mice (Supplementary Figure S1). Therefore, at least in the RPE in SFD mice, the differences in HA content are not due to increased expression of the synthases nor decreased expression of canonical degradation enzymes. However, there are other possibilities that need to be explored in the future. HA production could be modulated by decreasing enzyme recycling from endosomes back to the cell surface as seen in keratocytes [52]. Additionally, there is a possibility that other non-canonical hyaluronidases such as KIAA1199 [53] and Tmem2 [54] could be involved. Alternatively, as previously reported degradation might be prevented by increased binding proteins on HA and leading to net accumulation [55].

HA has been shown to exhibit a diverse array of biological functions including a role in the response to tissue damage and inflammation [56]. Our studies demonstrating accumulation of HA in laser-induced CNV lesions corroborates previous studies [27]. This study also reported an increase in *CD44* and *HAS2* mRNA following laser injury [27]. It is possible that the increased accumulation of HA in laser-induced CNV lesions in S179C-TIMP3 mice might result from similar increases in mRNA transcription.

Chronic low-grade inflammation has been suggested to contribute to age-related macular degeneration [57]. In the laser-induced mouse model of CNV, inflammatory processes have been shown to play a role in the development and regression of the lesions. A number of reports link HA remodeling to the modulation of neuroinflammation with low-molecular weight HA being pro-inflammatory and high molecular weight HA being anti-inflammatory [58–60]. While we see increased deposition of HA in and around the RPE, we have not determined its physical properties such as size and molecular weight distribution in the tissue.

The receptor engagement of HA in the retina or it's downstream signaling under physiological or pathological conditions has not yet been identified and will be important as we determine its exact role in the pathology of macular degenerative disease. In our study we demonstrate that primary porcine RPE cells deposited HA predominantly on the apical surface under physiological conditions similar to what had been previously reported for human RPE cells [61]. Our data revealed that FGF-2 induced HA accumulation apically as well as between cells and on the basal surface, suggesting that in addition to increased total HA content, the distribution of HA may be important for disease pathogenesis and warrants further investigation. We have recently reported that the secretion of FGF-2 by RPE cells expressing S179C-TIMP3 led to increased angiogenesis [28]. Whether HA is modified in the endothelial glycocalyx as a consequence of FGF-2 has not been studied and might provide further insight into the pathogenesis of CNV in AMD and SFD leading to the identification of novel therapeutic approaches.

Author Contributions: Conceptualization, A.W., O.W., V.H. and B.A.-A.; data curation, A.W.; formal analysis, B.A.-A.; funding acquisition, B.A.-A.; methodology, A.W., D.H., A.C., M.A., L.B., J.H.Q., R.S., J.B. and L.K.; project administration, B.A.-A.; resources, V.L.B., O.W. and H.S.; software, R.S.; supervision, B.A.-A.; validation, A.W.; writing—original draft, A.W.; writing—review and editing, A.W., H.S., V.H. and B.A.-A. All authors have read and agreed to the published version of the manuscript.

Acknowledgments: The authors thank the retina specialists at Cole Eye Institute from whose clinics patients with or without AMD were recruited. The authors are grateful for the generous gift of TIMP-3 null mice from Rama Khokha at the Princess Margaret Cancer Centre-Ontario Cancer Institute, Toronto, Canada and to Emma Lessieur who served as the research coordinator at the time the blood samples were collected from patients The authors also acknowledge the support of Foundation Fighting Blindness in setting up the Eye Tissue Repository. We wish to extend a sincere apology to colleagues whose work was not cited due to space limitations.

References

1. Sorsby, A.; Mason, M.E.; Gardener, N. A fundus dystrophy with unusual features (late onset and dominant inheritance of a central retinal lesion showing oedema, haemorrhage and exudates developing into generalised choroidal atrophy with massive pigment proliferation). *Br. J. Ophthalmol.* **1949**, *33*, 67–97. [CrossRef] [PubMed]
2. Della, N.G.; Campochiaro, P.A.; Zack, D.J. Localization of timp-3 mRNA expression to the retinal pigment epithelium. *Investig. Ophthalmol. Vis. Sci.* **1996**, *37*, 1921–1924.
3. Holz, F.G.; Haimovici, R.; Wagner, D.G.; Bird, A.C. Recurrent choroidal neovascularization after laser photocoagulation in sorsby's fundus dystrophy. *Retina* **1994**, *14*, 329–334. [CrossRef] [PubMed]
4. Jacobson, S.G.; Cideciyan, A.V.; Regunath, G.; Rodriguez, F.J.; Vandenburgh, K.; Sheffield, V.C.; Stone, E.M. Night blindness in sorsby's fundus dystrophy reversed by vitamin a. *Nat. Genet.* **1995**, *11*, 27–32. [CrossRef]
5. Kalmus, H.; Seedburgh, D. Probable common origin of a hereditary fundus dystrophy (sorsby's familial pseudoinflammatory macular dystrophy) in an english and australian family. *J. Med. Genet.* **1976**, *13*, 271–276. [CrossRef]

6. Polkinghorne, P.J.; Capon, M.R.; Berninger, T.; Lyness, A.L.; Sehmi, K.; Bird, A.C. Sorsby's fundus dystrophy. A clinical study. *Ophthalmology* **1989**, *96*, 1763–1768. [CrossRef]
7. Barbazetto, I.A.; Hayashi, M.; Klais, C.M.; Yannuzzi, L.A.; Allikmets, R. A novel timp3 mutation associated with sorsby fundus dystrophy. *Arch. Ophthalmol.* **2005**, *123*, 542–543. [CrossRef]
8. Felbor, U.; Benkwitz, C.; Klein, M.L.; Greenberg, J.; Gregory, C.Y.; Weber, B.H. Sorsby fundus dystrophy: Reevaluation of variable expressivity in patients carrying a timp3 founder mutation. *Arch. Ophthalmol.* **1997**, *115*, 1569–1571. [CrossRef]
9. Felbor, U.; Stohr, H.; Amann, T.; Schonherr, U.; Weber, B.H. A novel ser156cys mutation in the tissue inhibitor of metalloproteinases-3 (timp3) in sorsby's fundus dystrophy with unusual clinical features. *Hum. Mol. Genet.* **1995**, *4*, 2415–2416. [CrossRef]
10. Langton, K.P.; Barker, M.D.; McKie, N. Localization of the functional domains of human tissue inhibitor of metalloproteinases-3 and the effects of a sorsby's fundus dystrophy mutation. *J. Biol. Chem.* **1998**, *273*, 16778–16781. [CrossRef]
11. Langton, K.P.; McKie, N.; Curtis, A.; Goodship, J.A.; Bond, P.M.; Barker, M.D.; Clarke, M. A novel tissue inhibitor of metalloproteinases-3 mutation reveals a common molecular phenotype in sorsby's fundus dystrophy. *J. Biol. Chem.* **2000**, *275*, 27027–27031. [PubMed]
12. Lin, R.J.; Blumenkranz, M.S.; Binkley, J.; Wu, K.; Vollrath, D. A novel his158arg mutation in timp3 causes a late-onset form of sorsby fundus dystrophy. *Am. J. Ophthalmol.* **2006**, *142*, 839–848. [CrossRef] [PubMed]
13. Tabata, Y.; Isashiki, Y.; Kamimura, K.; Nakao, K.; Ohba, N. A novel splice site mutation in the tissue inhibitor of the metalloproteinases-3 gene in sorsby's fundus dystrophy with unusual clinical features. *Hum. Genet.* **1998**, *103*, 179–182. [PubMed]
14. Weber, B.H.; Vogt, G.; Pruett, R.C.; Stohr, H.; Felbor, U. Mutations in the tissue inhibitor of metalloproteinase-3 (timp-3) in patients with sorsby's fundus dystrophy. *Nat. Genet.* **1994**, *8*, 352–356. [CrossRef]
15. Qi, J.H.; Anand-Apte, B. Tissue inhibitor of metalloproteinase-3 (timp3) promotes endothelial apoptosis via a caspase-independent mechanism. *Apoptosis* **2015**, *20*, 523–534. [CrossRef]
16. Qi, J.H.; Dai, G.; Luthert, P.; Chaurasia, S.; Hollyfield, J.; Weber, B.H.; Stohr, H.; Anand-Apte, B. S156c mutation in tissue inhibitor of metalloproteinases-3 induces increased angiogenesis. *J. Biol. Chem.* **2009**, *284*, 19927–19936. [CrossRef]
17. Qi, J.H.; Ebrahem, Q.; Ali, M.; Cutler, A.; Bell, B.; Prayson, N.; Sears, J.; Knauper, V.; Murphy, G.; Anand-Apte, B. Tissue inhibitor of metalloproteinases-3 peptides inhibit angiogenesis and choroidal neovascularization in mice. *PLoS ONE* **2013**, *8*, e55667. [CrossRef]
18. Qi, J.H.; Ebrahem, Q.; Anand-Apte, B. Tissue inhibitor of metalloproteinases-3 and sorsby fundus dystrophy. *Adv. Exp. Med. Biol.* **2003**, *533*, 97–105.
19. Qi, J.H.; Ebrahem, Q.; Moore, N.; Murphy, G.; Claesson-Welsh, L.; Bond, M.; Baker, A.; Anand-Apte, B. A novel function for tissue inhibitor of metalloproteinases-3 (timp3): Inhibition of angiogenesis by blockage of VEGF binding to vegf receptor-2. *Nat. Med.* **2003**, *9*, 407–415. [CrossRef]
20. Qi, J.H.; Ebrahem, Q.; Yeow, K.; Edwards, D.R.; Fox, P.L.; Anand-Apte, B. Expression of sorsby's fundus dystrophy mutations in human retinal pigment epithelial cells reduces matrix metalloproteinase inhibition and may promote angiogenesis. *J. Biol. Chem.* **2002**, *30*, 30. [CrossRef]
21. Stohr, H.; Anand-Apte, B. A review and update on the molecular basis of pathogenesis of sorsby fundus dystrophy. *Adv. Exp. Med. Biol.* **2012**, *723*, 261–267. [PubMed]
22. Fariss, R.N.; Apte, S.S.; Olsen, B.R.; Iwata, K.; Milam, A.H. Tissue inhibitor of metalloproteinases-3 is a component of bruch's membrane of the eye. *Am. J. Pathol.* **1997**, *150*, 323–328. [PubMed]
23. Troeberg, L.; Lazenbatt, C.; Anower, E.K.M.F.; Freeman, C.; Federov, O.; Habuchi, H.; Habuchi, O.; Kimata, K.; Nagase, H. Sulfated glycosaminoglycans control the extracellular trafficking and the activity of the metalloprotease inhibitor timp-3. *Chem. Biol.* **2014**, *21*, 1300–1309. [CrossRef] [PubMed]
24. Yu, W.H.; Yu, S.; Meng, Q.; Brew, K.; Woessner, J.F., Jr. Timp-3 binds to sulfated glycosaminoglycans of the extracellular matrix. *J. Biol. Chem.* **2000**, *275*, 31226–31232. [CrossRef] [PubMed]
25. Itano, N.; Kimata, K. Altered hyaluronan biosynthesis in cancer progression. *Semin. Cancer Biol.* **2008**, *18*, 268–274. [CrossRef] [PubMed]
26. Singleton, P.A. Hyaluronan regulation of endothelial barrier function in cancer. *Adv. Cancer Res.* **2014**, *123*, 191–209.

27. Mochimaru, H.; Takahashi, E.; Tsukamoto, N.; Miyazaki, J.; Yaguchi, T.; Koto, T.; Kurihara, T.; Noda, K.; Ozawa, Y.; Ishimoto, T.; et al. Involvement of hyaluronan and its receptor cd44 with choroidal neovascularization. *Investig. Ophthalmol. Vis. Sci.* **2009**, *50*, 4410–4415. [CrossRef]
28. Qi, J.H.; Bell, B.; Singh, R.; Batoki, J.; Wolk, A.; Cutler, A.; Prayson, N.; Ali, M.; Stoehr, H.; Anand-Apte, B. Sorsby fundus dystrophy mutation in tissue inhibitor of metalloproteinase 3 (timp3) promotes choroidal neovascularization via a fibroblast growth factor-dependent mechanism. *Sci. Rep.* **2019**, *9*, 17429. [CrossRef]
29. Oladipupo, S.S.; Smith, C.; Santeford, A.; Park, C.; Sene, A.; Wiley, L.A.; Osei-Owusu, P.; Hsu, J.; Zapata, N.; Liu, F.; et al. Endothelial cell fgf signaling is required for injury response but not for vascular homeostasis. *Proc. Natl. Acad. Sci. USA* **2014**, *111*, 13379–13384. [CrossRef]
30. Sarrazin, S.; Lamanna, W.C.; Esko, J.D. Heparan sulfate proteoglycans. *Cold Spring Harb. Perspect. Biol.* **2011**, *3*, a004952. [CrossRef]
31. Weis, S.M.; Cheresh, D.A. Tumor angiogenesis: Molecular pathways and therapeutic targets. *Nat. Med.* **2011**, *17*, 1359–1370. [CrossRef] [PubMed]
32. Bohrer, L.R.; Chuntova, P.; Bade, L.K.; Beadnell, T.C.; Leon, R.P.; Brady, N.J.; Ryu, Y.; Goldberg, J.E.; Schmechel, S.C.; Koopmeiners, J.S.; et al. Activation of the fgfr-stat3 pathway in breast cancer cells induces a hyaluronan-rich microenvironment that licenses tumor formation. *Cancer Res.* **2014**, *74*, 374–386. [CrossRef] [PubMed]
33. Weber, B.H.; Lin, B.; White, K.; Kohler, K.; Soboleva, G.; Herterich, S.; Seeliger, M.W.; Jaissle, G.B.; Grimm, C.; Reme, C.; et al. A mouse model for sorsby fundus dystrophy. *Investig. Ophthalmol. Vis. Sci.* **2002**, *43*, 2732–2740.
34. Leco, K.J.; Waterhouse, P.; Sanchez, O.H.; Gowing, K.L.; Poole, A.R.; Wakeham, A.; Mak, T.W.; Khokha, R. Spontaneous air space enlargement in the lungs of mice lacking tissue inhibitor of metalloproteinases-3 (timp-3). *J. Clin. Investig.* **2001**, *108*, 817–829. [CrossRef]
35. Tammi, R.; Ripellino, J.A.; Margolis, R.U.; Maibach, H.I.; Tammi, M. Hyaluronate accumulation in human epidermis treated with retinoic acid in skin organ culture. *J. Investig. Dermatol.* **1989**, *92*, 326–332. [CrossRef]
36. Hazim, R.A.; Volland, S.; Yen, A.; Burgess, B.L.; Williams, D.S. Rapid differentiation of the human rpe cell line, arpe-19, induced by nicotinamide. *Exp. Eye Res.* **2019**, *179*, 18–24. [CrossRef]
37. Venkatareddy, M.; Verma, R.; Kalinowski, A.; Patel, S.R.; Shisheva, A.; Garg, P. Distinct requirements for vacuolar protein sorting 34 downstream effector phosphatidylinositol 3-phosphate 5-kinase in podocytes versus proximal tubular cells. *J. Am. Soc. Nephrol.* **2016**, *27*, 2702–2719. [CrossRef]
38. Scheuring, D.; Lofke, C.; Kruger, F.; Kittelmann, M.; Eisa, A.; Hughes, L.; Smith, R.S.; Hawes, C.; Schumacher, K.; Kleine-Vehn, J. Actin-dependent vacuolar occupancy of the cell determines auxin-induced growth repression. *Proc. Natl. Acad. Sci. USA* **2016**, *113*, 452–457. [CrossRef]
39. Hollyfield, J.G. Hyaluronan and the functional organization of the interphotoreceptor matrix. *Investig. Ophthalmol. Vis. Sci.* **1999**, *40*, 2767–2769.
40. Hollyfield, J.G.; Rayborn, M.E.; Tammi, R. Hyaluronan localization in tissues of the mouse posterior eye wall: Absence in the interphotoreceptor matrix. *Exp. Eye Res.* **1997**, *65*, 603–608. [CrossRef]
41. Ebrahem, Q.; Qi, J.H.; Sugimoto, M.; Ali, M.; Sears, J.E.; Cutler, A.; Khokha, R.; Vasanji, A.; Anand-Apte, B. Increased neovascularization in mice lacking tissue inhibitor of metalloproteinases-3. *Investig. Ophthalmol. Vis. Sci.* **2011**, *52*, 6117–6123. [CrossRef] [PubMed]
42. Fariss, R.N.; Apte, S.S.; Luthert, P.J.; Bird, A.C.; Milam, A.H. Accumulation of tissue inhibitor of metalloproteinases-3 in human eyes with sorsby's fundus dystrophy or retinitis pigmentosa. *Br. J. Ophthalmol.* **1998**, *82*, 1329–1334. [CrossRef] [PubMed]
43. Crabb, J.W.; Miyagi, M.; Gu, X.; Shadrach, K.; West, K.A.; Sakaguchi, H.; Kamei, M.; Hasan, A.; Yan, L.; Rayborn, M.E.; et al. Drusen proteome analysis: An approach to the etiology of age-related macular degeneration. *Proc. Natl. Acad. Sci. USA* **2002**, *99*, 14682–14687. [CrossRef] [PubMed]
44. Kamei, M.; Apte, S.S.; Rayborn, M.E.; Lewis, H.; Hollyfield, J.G. Timp-3 accumulation in drusen and bruch's membrane in eyes from donors with age-related macular degeneration (1997). In *Degenerative Diseases of the Retina*; Luvail, M.M., Anderson, R.E., Hollyfield, J.G., Eds.; Plenum Press: New York, NY, USA, 1997; pp. 11–15.
45. Kamei, M.; Hollyfield, J. Timp-3 in bruch's membrane: Changes during aging and in age-related macular degeneration. *Investig. Ophthalmol. Vis. Sci.* **1999**, *40*, p2367–p2375.

46. Apte, S.S.; Mattei, M.-G.; Olsen, B.R. Cloning of the cdna encoding human tissue inhibitor of metalloproteinase-3 (timp-3) and mapping of the timp-3 gene to chromosome 22. *Genomics* **1994**, *19*, 86–90. [CrossRef]
47. Saw, S.; Aiken, A.; Fang, H.; McKee, T.D.; Bregant, S.; Sanchez, O.; Chen, Y.; Weiss, A.; Dickson, B.C.; Czarny, B.; et al. Metalloprotease inhibitor timp proteins control fgf-2 bioavailability and regulate skeletal growth. *J. Cell Biol.* **2019**, *218*, 3134–3152. [CrossRef]
48. Rifkin, D.B.; Moscatelli, D.; Bizik, J.; Quarto, N.; Blei, F.; Dennis, P.; Flaumenhaft, R.; Mignatti, P. Growth factor control of extracellular proteolysis. *Cell Differ. Dev.* **1990**, *32*, 313–318. [CrossRef]
49. DeAngelis, P.L. Hyaluronan synthases: Fascinating glycosyltransferases from vertebrates, bacterial pathogens, and algal viruses. *Cell Mol. Life Sci.* **1999**, *56*, 670–682. [CrossRef]
50. Tien, J.Y.; Spicer, A.P. Three vertebrate hyaluronan synthases are expressed during mouse development in distinct spatial and temporal patterns. *Dev. Dyn.* **2005**, *233*, 130–141. [CrossRef]
51. Stern, R.; Kogan, G.; Jedrzejas, M.J.; Soltes, L. The many ways to cleave hyaluronan. *Biotechnol. Adv.* **2007**, *25*, 537–557. [CrossRef]
52. Tammi, R.; Rilla, K.; Pienimaki, J.P.; MacCallum, D.K.; Hogg, M.; Luukkonen, M.; Hascall, V.C.; Tammi, M. Hyaluronan enters keratinocytes by a novel endocytic route for catabolism. *J. Biol. Chem.* **2001**, *276*, 35111–35122. [CrossRef] [PubMed]
53. Marella, M.; Jadin, L.; Keller, G.A.; Sugarman, B.J.; Frost, G.I.; Shepard, H.M. Kiaa1199 expression and hyaluronan degradation colocalize in multiple sclerosis lesions. *Glycobiology* **2018**, *28*, 958–967. [CrossRef] [PubMed]
54. De Angelis, J.E.; Lagendijk, A.K.; Chen, H.; Tromp, A.; Bower, N.I.; Tunny, K.A.; Brooks, A.J.; Bakkers, J.; Francois, M.; Yap, A.S.; et al. Tmem2 regulates embryonic VEGF signaling by controlling hyaluronic acid turnover. *Dev. Cell* **2017**, *40*, 123–136. [CrossRef] [PubMed]
55. Nagaoka, A.; Yoshida, H.; Nakamura, S.; Morikawa, T.; Kawabata, K.; Kobayashi, M.; Sakai, S.; Takahashi, Y.; Okada, Y.; Inoue, S. Regulation of hyaluronan (ha) metabolism mediated by hybid (hyaluronan-binding protein involved in ha depolymerization, kiaa1199) and ha synthases in growth factor-stimulated fibroblasts. *J. Biol. Chem.* **2015**, *290*, 30910–30923. [CrossRef]
56. Garantziotis, S.; Savani, R.C. Hyaluronan biology: A complex balancing act of structure, function, location and context. *Matrix Biol.* **2019**, *78–79*, 1–10. [CrossRef]
57. Nita, M.; Grzybowski, A.; Ascaso, F.J.; Huerva, V. Age-related macular degeneration in the aspect of chronic low-grade inflammation (pathophysiological parainflammation). *Mediators Inflamm.* **2014**, *2014*, 930671. [CrossRef]
58. Avenoso, A.; Bruschetta, G.; D'Ascola, A.; Scuruchi, M.; Mandraffino, G.; Saitta, A.; Campo, S.; Campo, G.M. Hyaluronan fragmentation during inflammatory pathologies: A signal that empowers tissue damage. *Mini Rev. Med. Chem.* **2020**, *20*, 54–65. [CrossRef]
59. Mueller, A.M.; Yoon, B.H.; Sadiq, S.A. Inhibition of hyaluronan synthesis protects against central nervous system (cns) autoimmunity and increases cxcl12 expression in the inflamed cns. *J. Biol. Chem.* **2014**, *289*, 22888–22899. [CrossRef]
60. Scuruchi, M.; D'Ascola, A.; Avenoso, A.; Campana, S.; Abusamra, Y.A.; Spina, E.; Calatroni, A.; Campo, G.M.; Campo, S. 6-mer hyaluronan oligosaccharides modulate neuroinflammation and alpha-synuclein expression in neuron-like sh-sy5y cells. *J. Cell Biochem.* **2016**, *117*, 2835–2843. [CrossRef]
61. deS Senanayake, P.; Calabro, A.; Nishiyama, K.; Hu, J.G.; Bok, D.; Hollyfield, J.G. Glycosaminoglycan synthesis and secretion by the retinal pigment epithelium: Polarized delivery of hyaluronan from the apical surface. *J. Cell Sci.* **2001**, *114*, 199–205.

11

Molecular Therapies for Inherited Retinal Diseases—Current Standing, Opportunities and Challenges

Irene Vázquez-Domínguez, Alejandro Garanto *,† and Rob W. J. Collin *,†

Department of Human Genetics and Donders Institute for Brain, Cognition and Behaviour, Radboud University Medical Center, 6525GA Nijmegen, The Netherlands

* Correspondence: alex.garanto@radboudumc.nl (A.G.); rob.collin@radboudumc.nl (R.W.J.C.);

† Both senior authors contributed equally.

Abstract: Inherited retinal diseases (IRDs) are both genetically and clinically highly heterogeneous and have long been considered incurable. Following the successful development of a gene augmentation therapy for biallelic *RPE65*-associated IRD, this view has changed. As a result, many different therapeutic approaches are currently being developed, in particular a large variety of molecular therapies. These are depending on the severity of the retinal degeneration, knowledge of the pathophysiological mechanism underlying each subtype of IRD, and the therapeutic target molecule. DNA therapies include approaches such as gene augmentation therapy, genome editing and optogenetics. For some genetic subtypes of IRD, RNA therapies and compound therapies have also shown considerable therapeutic potential. In this review, we summarize the current state-of-the-art of various therapeutic approaches, including the pros and cons of each strategy, and outline the future challenges that lie ahead in the combat against IRDs.

Keywords: inherited retinal diseases; IRD; DNA therapies; RNA therapies; compound therapies; clinical trials

---

1. Introduction

1.1. Inherited Retinal Diseases (IRDs)

Inherited retinal diseases (IRDs) are a rare and heterogeneous group of neurodegenerative disorders that collectively result in progressive visual impairment. IRDs are estimated to affect around 1 in 2000 people worldwide [1]. Over 250 causative genes have been identified in which mutations can cause one or more of the clinical subtypes of IRD (https://sph.uth.edu/retnet/). IRDs can be familial or sporadic, isolated (non-syndromic) or syndromic and stationary or progressive. In terms of geographic distribution, they could be diffused or localized. Most forms of IRD mainly affect photoreceptors but other forms can also primarily affect the retinal pigment epithelium (RPE) or the inner retina. IRDs can propagate through all modes of inheritance—autosomal dominant (AD), autosomal recessive (AR), X-linked (XL) or mitochondrial, whilst digenic cases or uniparental disomy have also been described occasionally [2].

1.2. Present Treatment of IRD

The eye is an ideal target for molecular therapies, for various reasons. First, the tight junctions of the blood-retina barrier (BRB) define the retina to be a relatively immune-privileged tissue [3]. In other words, the introduction of a foreign antigen (like a viral vector) is generally well tolerated without evoking severe inflammatory responses [4,5]. The risk of widespread dissemination of the locally administered vector is low, preventing unwanted systemic effects. Furthermore, relatively small amounts of the vector are needed to achieve a therapeutic response [6,7]. The eye is easily accessible by surgery [8], which allows intravitreal and subretinal administration of vectors to the affected tissue. As retinal cells are differentiated and non-dividing, there is no loss of the transgene even with the use of non-integrating vectors [9]. Finally, there are many different non-invasive approaches that are able to monitor disease progression [10]. Examples include fundus autofluorescence that provides a topographical map of lipofuscin changes in the RPE cells, spectral domain OCT to assess retinal thickness and photoreceptor layer architecture, as well as other known tests like visual acuity and biomicroscopy [11–13].

Currently, there are various (overlapping) approaches to treat IRDs under development, including molecular therapies but also stem cell-based therapies and retinal prostheses [14–18] (Figure 1). Despite the promising results obtained with some of these approaches, there are still many challenges that must be overcome in order to reach a broad implementation of treatment modalities for IRDs. The great heterogeneity of these diseases [19] hampers the development of a common treatment for a large number of patients [20]. In addition, a significant proportion of genes involved in IRDs has a cDNA size that exceeds the cargo capacity of adeno-associated viral (AAV) vectors, generally considered the most preferred viral vector for retinal delivery of therapeutic molecules [21]. Finally, the costs of developing gene or even mutation-specific approaches are substantial, while often having only a limited number of individuals that could potentially benefit from a given therapeutic molecule.

In this review, we summarize the current state-of-the-art of the therapeutic approaches for IRDs, with a strong emphasis on molecular therapies.

2. Molecular therapies

Due to the severity and heterogeneity of IRDs, avid research is ongoing to identify therapeutic strategies that could ameliorate symptoms and/or disease progression, including many that focus on resolving the consequences of a particular genetic defect [22]. However, a good candidate for molecular therapies requires—(i) a substantial disease burden and a favourable risk/benefit ratio compared to another therapy, if any; (ii) the relevant gene/locus involved in the disease has already been identified and there is ample knowledge of the molecular mechanism of disease and its progression; (iii) the right target cell(s) can be reached, with or without using a therapeutic vehicle; (iv) phenotypic improvement can preferably be achieved with limited expression levels of the therapeutic gene, while its overexpression does not exert any toxic effect [23].

We can subdivide the molecular strategies into different groups—DNA, RNA and compound therapies, as graphically depicted in Figures 1 and 2. Ongoing clinical trials for genetic subtypes of IRDs are summarized in Table 1 (DNA therapies), Table 2 (RNA therapies) and Table 3 (Compound therapies).

2.1. DNA Therapies

2.1.1. Gene Augmentation

In gene augmentation therapy (also known as gene replacement therapy), a normal copy of the mutated gene is inserted into the host cells using therapeutic vectors (for details on the various types of vectors, see Section 3). To enable this, the gene of interest could be delivered as DNA, as messenger RNA (mRNA) or as mRNA analogue. The big advantage of the mRNA platform is that it does not require delivery into the nucleus and the risk of integration into the host genome is reduced [24,25]. Two of the main challenges of mRNA delivery however are immunogenicity and stability of the RNA molecule [24,26]. Thus, since sustained production of the protein of interest is required for continued improvement of visual function, the DNA platform is the preferred strategy for ocular gene augmentation therapy [25]. With this, the gene of interest is introduced to the cell nucleus, where it often remains in an episomal state while promoters and enhancers can facilitate its expression [25,27].

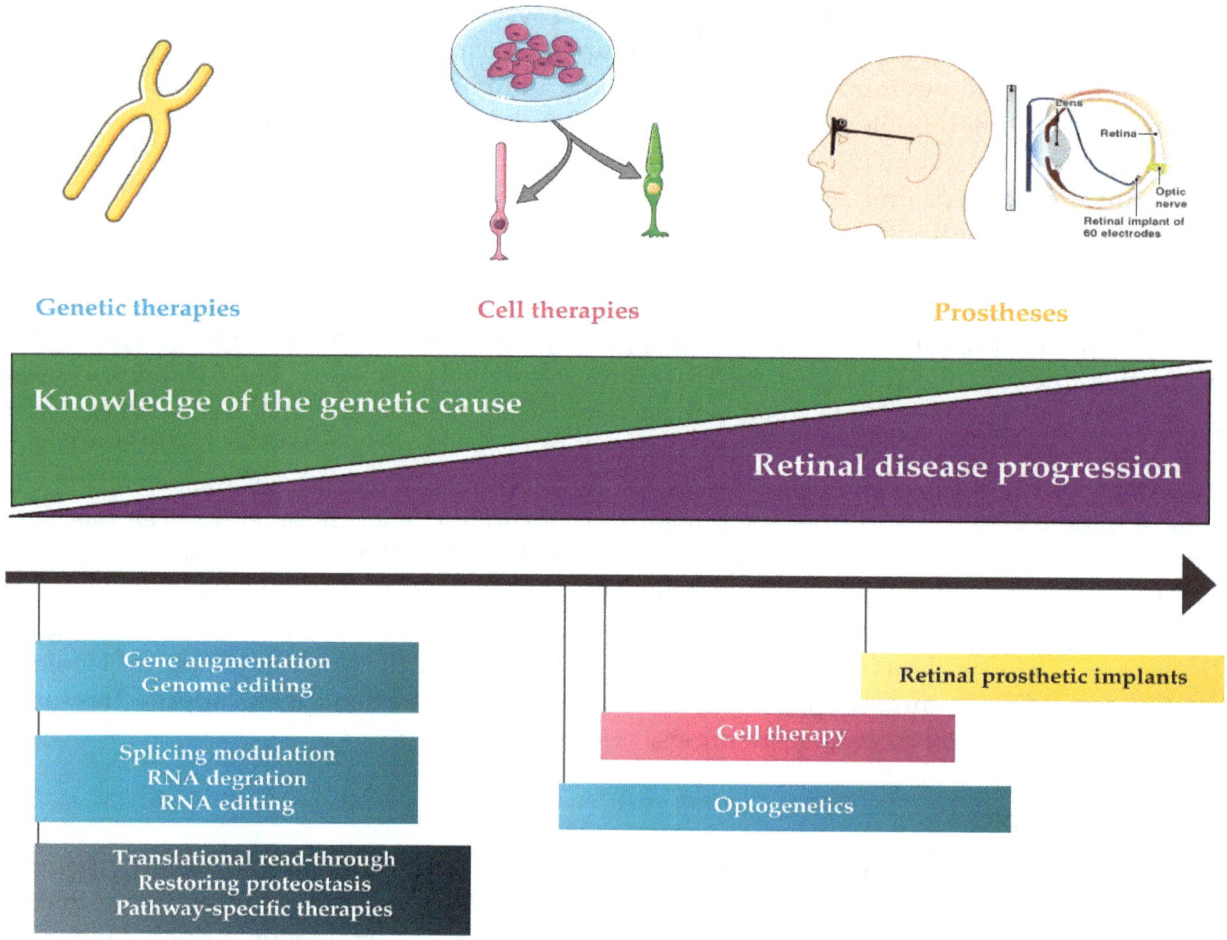

Figure 1. Schematic representation of potential therapeutic approaches according to the retinal disease progression and the knowledge of the genetic cause of the retinal disease. Genetic therapies (blue boxes) are preferred in the first steps of the disease progression (retinal cells are still alive) and when knowledge of the genetic causes of the diseases is present. As the disease progresses and the knowledge of the pathogenesis decreases, other approaches such as cell therapies (pink box) or retinal prosthetic implants (yellow box) can be used. Compound therapies (black box), based on pharmacological treatments, could be used as an alternative approach when the genetic cause of the disease or the pathway involved are either known or unknown. For late-stage diseases, optogenetics or retinal prostheses may be the only option. Image sources—smart.servier.com and Doheny Retina Institute (new.bbc.co.uk/2/hi/science/nature/6368089).

DNA can be delivered using one of several different vectors but in particular for IRDs, adeno-associated viruses (AAVs) have been most commonly used due to their high tropism for certain retinal cells and their low immunogenicity [14]. Other vectors under study are lentiviruses and nanoparticles, which have larger cargo capacities [28].

Advanced stages of retinal degeneration are not compatible with the use of gene augmentation therapy, since this approach requires the target cells to be alive [29]. Moreover, reaching substantial levels of gene expression is crucial for a significant and strong rescue of the phenotype [30]. This requirement can for instance be improved by varying the serotypes of AAVs that are used to deliver the transgene [31–33], by varying the promoter sequence [30] or by producing codon-optimized cDNA versions of a given gene [34,35].

For IRDs, gene augmentation is currently the most advanced therapeutic strategy, with market approval for one gene (*RPE65*, Luxturna™), several ongoing clinical studies for other genes (Table 1) and preclinical development for a plethora of genes mutated in these diseases [36]. Despite these promising results, gene augmentation strategies may not be the best approach when treating dominant conditions [37], as the mutated allele underlying the disease most often first needs to be inactivated such that it does not interfere with the normal allele [38]. Such an allele-specific inhibition of expression can be achieved either at the DNA level (Section 2.1.2) or at the RNA level (Section 2.2) and, if needed, can be combined with gene augmentation [39]. In addition, the cargo capacity of AAV remains a challenge, since several of the recurrently mutated genes (e.g., *USH2A*, *EYS*, etc.) are by far exceeding it. Several studies using dual or even triple AAVs [40–43], or microgenes (smaller versions of the gene) [44] are ongoing.

2.1.2. Genome Editing

In addition to gene augmentation, precise editing of genomic DNA has gained an enormous attention over the last five years. Currently, there are two main approaches in genome editing—an in vivo approach, in which the disease-causing mutations are corrected inside the retina and an *ex vivo* approach to first correct the mutation in patient-derived cells, which can be followed by cell transplantation [45]. The editing itself can be achieved by different classes of molecules, as outlined below.

ZFNs and TALENs: Zinc-finger nucleases (ZFNs) and transcription activator like effector nucleases (TALENs) are molecules that pioneered genome editing. Both can induce a wide range of genetic modifications by generating double-strand breaks (DSBs) in the DNA that subsequently stimulate one of the DNA repair pathways of the cell—non-homologous end-joining (NHEJ), homology-directed repair (HDR) or microhomology-mediated end joining [46,47]. To induce DSBs, either nuclease needs to be guided to its target sequence by a DNA-binding protein domain. These approaches are thus depending on the engineering of new proteins for each target, making them laborious and challenging [48]. Nevertheless, ZFNs have been used as a proof-of-concept treatment in IRD. Human embryonic cells carrying the c.68C>A; p.P23H mutation in *RHO* were targeted using ZFNs, which led to an increase in homologous recombination events when the ZFNs were transfected with a homologous donor template, compared to delivery in the absence of this template [49].

TALENs have been used in the correction of the *Crbrd8* allele in C57BL/6N mice. HDR triggered by a combination of TALEN and a single-stranded donor oligonucleotide repair template was observed in 27% of the treated mouse embryos and resulted in an improvement of retinal function [50].

CRISPR/Cas system: The CRISPR/Cas system is considered a more advanced genome editing tool compared to ZFNs and TALENs, as it presents many advantages including the simple design of the target, its higher efficacy and its ability to introduce mutations in multiple genes at the same time by using a combination of guide RNAs (gRNAs) [25]. The CRISPR/Cas system has been improved to a simpler version, CRISPR/Cas9, which nowadays is commonly used for mammalian genome editing [51–53]. The Cas9 endonuclease is delivered into a cell in conjunction with a gRNA, after which it can cut the genome specifically at any desired location [52,54].

As for other genome-editing tools, its major limitation is the possibility of off-target effects [46]. To overcome this aspect, researchers have developed different strategies—(i) using ribonucleoproteins (RNPs) as a form of delivery [55]; (ii) titrating the concentration of gRNA and Cas9 or using two gRNAs flanking the target region [56]; (iii) adding two additional guanine bases at the 5′ end of the gRNA sequence for Cas9 derived from *Streptococcus pyogenes* (SpCas9); interestingly, this modification in the design did not reduce the on-target ratio both in vivo and *in vitro* [57]; (iv) selecting unique DNA target sites with no homology to any other gene sequence [58]; (v) using paired Cas9 nickases, modified Cas9 nucleases that cut only one strand of DNA and thus can produce DSBs with two times more specificity [52,57,59], (vi) employing a high-fidelity version of Cas9 (SpCas9-HF1) [59] or (vii) using the 'enhanced specificity' SpCas9, which is reported to not only decrease the off-target events but also to obtain a higher on-target efficacy [60]. All these strategies have allowed researchers to yield relatively high editing rates *in vitro* but these rates are generally lower in vivo, for instance in treated retinas [52,61–72]. The first challenge is the delivery of the CRISPR system directly into the cells or tissue of interest. As it was previously mentioned, AAV vectors are currently considered the most potent therapeutic vector for retinal delivery. However, its limited cargo capacity hampers an efficient delivery of the complete CRISPR/Cas9 system [73]. One solution for this problem is the delivery of the SpCas9 and gRNA separated into two vectors, with which Hung and colleagues obtained an editing efficacy of 84% in the mouse retina [52]. Other studies using two AAV vectors have also obtained good results over the last years, although it should be mentioned that these in vivo studies only used CRISPR/Cas9 technology to activate NHEJ, resulting in indels and subsequent gene inactivation [55,74–77]. A major concern that remains to be solved is how to increase the efficacy of genome correction in the retina, since photoreceptors are post-mitotic cells that to a large extent lack HDR mechanisms. Suzuki and colleagues developed a strategy coined homology-independent targeted integration which allows for targeted knock-in in non-dividing cells like photoreceptors [45,77]. This appears as a promising approach, as it is based on the NHEJ mechanism, as opposed to HDR, for specific integration of a desired DNA sequence [45,77].

Besides precise editing, the CRISPR/Cas9-system can also be used in other ways, such as the invalidation of mutant alleles that underlie autosomal dominant IRD (reviewed by Diakatou et al.) [78], or the removal of intronic sequences harbouring pathogenic pseudoexons. For the latter, Maeder and colleagues recently developed a CRISPR/Cas9-based approach (EDIT-101) for the splice mutation c.2991+1655A>G in *CEP290*. EDIT-101 promotes the deletion of part of intron 26 where the deep-intronic variant is located. It was tested in a humanized *Cep290* mouse model carrying the c.2991+1655A>G variant [79] and a comparable surrogate non-human primate (NHP) vector also showed efficient editing in photoreceptor and somatic primate cells [80].

Although several hurdles still need to be overcome, the development of the CRISPR/Cas9 system has opened new avenues for the future treatment of various genetic subtypes of IRD.

2.1.3. Optogenetics

Although gene-specific augmentation therapy is a very attractive approach in patients with a known genotype and at a relative early stage of the disease, it is not suitable for patients who present a more advanced stage of the disease in which many of the photoreceptors have been lost (Figure 1).

Optogenetics is a technique used to monitor or control neural activity with light, which can be achieved by the genetic introduction of light-sensitive proteins into retinal cells. This strategy is often used to convert secondary or tertiary neurons into "photoreceptors" or, less often, to restore sensitivity of degenerating photoreceptor cells [81–83]. One advantage of optogenetics is that it may more precisely excite the neural pathway compared to for example, electronic retinal implants [82,84]. In addition, optogenetics can be used independent of the primary genetic defect.

Opsins represent the major optogenetic tool [85]. They function as sensory receptors or light-responsive ion channels. Two types of opsin have been described—microbial opsins (type I) and animal opsins (type II) [81,82]. Type-I opsins (channelrhodopsins, halorhodopsins and archaerhodopsins), following light capture, result in a passive flow of ions across the cell membrane. When they are introduced into non-light sensitive cells, microbial opsins can induce rapid optical control of specific cellular processes. Type-I opsins allow high-speed neural activation and silencing, without requiring any additional chemicals [86]. Type-II opsins (rhodopsin and melanopsin) are part of the large family of naturally occurring light-sensitive G protein-coupled receptors (GPCRs). In contrast to microbial opsins, animal opsins present a much higher light sensitivity, as the light signal is amplified by G-protein-coupled signalling cascades [87]. Both types of opsins are small enough to be encapsidated in AAVs [81,82].

Experiments in animal models (mouse, rat and dog) revealed that expression of type-II opsins resulted in increased light sensitivity, within 1–2 log units of the threshold for normal cone vision, although this sensitivity may come at the cost of slower kinetics [88]. In contrast, the use of type-I opsins is superior in terms of kinetics, yet its sensitivity is lower. Both types however are limited in their operational range of light levels and will likely require modification of the incoming light signal [89]. Moreover, many questions still need to be addressed such as the identification of the best vector and surgical approach for delivery. Although a wide range of ubiquitous, photoreceptor-, bipolar- or ganglion-cell specific promoters have been used, the ideal condition so far remains unclear [82].

Currently, there are two clinical trials ongoing that use optogenetics for vision restoration. One comprises a phase I/II clinical trial (NCT02556736; Table 1) and a second trial is still in a recruiting state (NCT03326336; Table 1), without any results reported yet for both trials.

2.2. RNA Therapies

2.2.1. Splicing Modulation

Antisense oligonucleotides (AONs): Around 15% of all IRD-causing mutations affect the splicing process [90]. Currently, the most widely used genetic therapy to correct aberrant splicing employs antisense oligonucleotides (AONs) [91], small DNA or RNA molecules that bind to their target pre-mRNA in a complementary way [91,92]. Their ability to modulate splicing in fact offers several advantages over gene replacement approaches, especially for IRDs [93]. Initially, AONs were simple antisense RNA molecules but found to be rapidly degraded by nucleases [91]. Therefore, multiple chemical modifications for the backbone or sugar groups were added to improve their target affinity and resistance to nuclease activity [91,94]. These new AONs were classified as first or second generation AONs, depending on their chemical modifications [94]. A third generation class of AONs consists of analogues of nucleic acids. Due to their relatively small size, it has been shown that AONs can be delivered to the eye either as naked molecules or in an AAV using a modified U7-snRNA system [95,96].

The first approved AON-based drug was Formivirsen, also known as Vitravene [97]. Vitravene was used to treat cytomegalovirus retinitis in patients whose immune system was compromised [97,98]. In the last years, the number of IRD-causing mutations that affect pre-mRNA splicing has rapidly increased. An example is a recurrent deep-intronic mutation in *CEP290* (c.2991+1665A>G) underlying congenital blindness [99]. For this mutation, the potential of AON-based therapy was demonstrated first in *in vitro* and in vivo models [96,100–104] and later on, in a phase I/II clinical trial [105]. Promising proof-of-concept studies employing AONs have also been developed for other mutations in *CEP290* [106], and for other genes mutated in IRD such as *OPA1* [107], *CHM* [108], *USH2A* [109] and *ABCA4* [110–113].

Besides the clinical trial for *CEP290* (NCT03140969) there is also an ongoing clinical trial for *USH2A* (Table 2). The results obtained so far indicate that AON-based therapy is a promising therapeutic strategy, albeit only for a selected group of IRD-causing mutations. However, the use of whole genome sequencing or targeted full-gene sequencing will likely identify more mutations amenable for this type of therapy in the near future. Overall, the remaining challenges for AON-based splicing modulation are mainly related to delivery, longevity and potential off-target effects.

U1 spliceosomal RNA: Many exonic splice donor site (SD) mutations have been identified in the last nucleotide of an exon and over 95% of these are predicted to result in aberrant splicing [114]. The splicing process needs the recognition of splice sites and subsequent assembly of the spliceosome. The latter is started by formation of stable complexes consisting of U1 small nuclear RNA (U1 snRNA), pre-mRNA and splice factor proteins. Splice donor sites are recognized directly by the U1 complex and are crucial for a proper splicing of exons. In case nucleotides within the splice donor site of an exon are mutated, an attractive therapeutic approach is to use a modified U1 snRNA. Tanner and colleagues demonstrated that a mutation that induces exon skipping in *RHO* (c.936G>A; p.Q311Q) can be rescued by adapting the U1 snRNA to the mutation [114]. In the last years, this approach has also been successfully employed *in vitro*, to rescue a mutation in exon 5 of the *BBS1* gene that underlies Bardet-Biedl syndrome [115], or a mutation in intron 10 causing *RPGR*-associated X-linked RP [116]. Thus, the U1 snRNA system definitely holds some therapeutic potential for mutations affecting the splice donor site. However, possible off-target effects caused by the delivery of an exogenous modified U1 snRNA are still poorly studied [117,118].

Table 1. Summary of clinical trials for inherited retinal diseases (IRDs) using DNA therapies.

Gene/Condition	Therapeutic Molecule	Clinical Trial Identifier	Status
Gene Augmentation			
ABCA4	SAR422459	NCT01367444	Recruiting
	SAR422459	NCT01736592	Enrolling by invitation
CHM	AAV2-hCHM	NCT02341807	Active, not recruiting
	AAV2-REP1	NCT03496012	Recruiting
	AAV2-REP1	NCT03507686	Recruiting
	AAV2-REP1	NCT02407678	Active, not recruiting
	rAAV2.REP1	NCT02671539	Active, not recruiting
	rAAV2.REP1	NCT02077361	**Completed**
	rAAV2.REP1	NCT01461213	**Completed**
	AAV2-REP1	NCT03584165	Enrolling by invitation
	AAV2-REP1	NCT02553135	**Completed**
CNGA3	AGTC-402	NCT02935517	Recruiting
	AAV2/8-hG1.7p.coCNGA3	NCT03758404	Recruiting
	rAAV.hCNGA3	NCT02610582	Active, not recruiting
CNGB3	rAAV2tYF-PR1.7-hCNGB3	NCT02599922	Recruiting
	AAV2/8-hCARp.hCNGB3	NCT03001310	Recruiting
	AAV-CNGB3	NCT03278873	Recruiting
MERTK	rAAV2-VMD2-hMERTK	NCT01482195	Recruiting
MYO7A	UshStat	NCT02065011	Enrolling by invitation
PDE6B	AAV2/5-hPDE6B	NCT03328130	Recruiting
RPE65	AAV OPTIREP	NCT02946879	Recruiting
	rAAV2-CBSB-hRPE65	NCT00481546	Active, not recruiting
	AAV2-hRPE65v2-	NCT00516477	Active, not recruiting
	AAV2-hRPE65v2	NCT00999609	Active, not recruiting
	AAV2-hRPE65v2	NCT01208389	Active, not recruiting
	AAV2-hRPE65v2	NCT03602820	Active, not recruiting
	tgAAG76 (rAAV 2/2.hRPE65p.hRPE65)	NCT00643747	**Completed**
	rAAV2-CB-hRPE65	NCT00749957	**Completed**
	rAAV2-hRPE65	NCT00821340	**Completed**
	rAAV2/4.hRPE65	NCT01496040	**Completed**
	AAV RPE65	NCT02781480	**Completed**
RLBP1	CPK850	NCT03374657	Recruiting
RPGR	AAV8-RPGR	NCT03116113	Recruiting
	AAV2/5-hRKp.RPGR	NCT03252847	Recruiting
	rAAV2tYF-GRK1-RPGR	NCT03316560	Recruiting
RS1	AAV8-scRS/IRBPhRS	NCT02317887	Recruiting
	rAAV2tYF-CB-hRS1	NCT02416622	Active, not recruiting
Genome editing			
CEP290	EDIT-101 (AGN-151587)	NCT03872479	Recruiting
Optogenetics			
Advanced RP	RST-001	NCT02556736	Recruiting
Non-syndromic RP Retinitis Pigmentosa	GS030-DP	NCT03326336	Recruiting

Black and gray are just used to indicate the different sectiond and can be considered as headers. Gene or disease condition (first column), therapeutic molecule (second column), clinical trial identifier (third column) and the current status of the trial (last column) are indicated. Completed trials are highlighted in bold. Data obtained from https://clinicaltrials.gov/. RP: retinitis pigmentosa.

Trans-splicing: Trans-splicing is a naturally occurring process that results in an alternative processing of the pre-mRNA and was first reported in plants and bacteria [119,120]. Unlike in cis-splicing, trans-splicing takes place between two independent RNA molecules [93,119,120]. In vertebrates, these trans-splicing events occur in some key physiological processes, for example, the regulation of gene expression [121–123]. In humans, trans-splicing has also been reported in some diseases such as cancer [120].

Therapeutic trans-splicing offers an intriguing strategy to remove mutations from the mRNA. Only the introduction of an exogenous RNA molecule can be sufficient to activate the trans-splicing process. This exogenous RNA, also called PTM (pre-mRNA trans-splicing molecule), is constituted by a binding domain that specifically targets the molecule towards a specific region within the endogenous pre-mRNA, an artificial intron sequence harbouring all the elements required for splicing and the sequence that needs to be replaced [93,119]. For a 5′ PTM, the partial coding sequence has to end at the 3′ end of an exon to allow for a 5′ splice site and vice versa for a 3′ splice site [124]. In the last years, trans-splicing has revealed promising results for the correction of mutations in *RHO* and *CEP290*. In the first example, Berger and collaborators were able to correct *RHO* mutations located in exons 2 through 5 by delivering the correct sequence of those exons in an AAV. This led to successful trans-splicing events, both in vivo and *in vitro* [119]. Dooley and colleagues delivered a part of the *CEP290* gene in an AAV and thereby could successfully replace the aforementioned c.2991+1655A>G mutation using the trans-splicing approach [124]. These data support the usefulness of trans-splicing as a therapeutic tool in IRDs.

2.2.2. Post-transcriptional Gene Silencing

iRNA and Ribozymes: Both Hammerhead ribozymes (hhRz) and (short) interference RNA ((s)iRNA) catalyse the sequence-specific cleavage of target mRNAs. iRNA molecules are double-stranded RNAs that are able to inhibit gene expression by binding to specific mRNAs (cellular or viral) [93,125]. Despite their affordability and speed, the effect of iRNA is often incomplete and temporary, with potential off-target effects [126]. In addition, variations between experiments and laboratories often occur. These variations limit the broad application of iRNA technology in many diseases including IRDs [46], although promising results have been obtained in age-related macular degeneration, a multifactorial subtype of retinal disease. Specifically, Ryoo and colleagues used a novel siRNA-based anti-VEGF nanoball that, upon intravitreal administration in mice, showed therapeutic effects for at least two weeks [127].

HhRzs are small RNA molecules causing enzymatic cleavage of polyribonucleotides [128]. The hhRz consists of three helixes surrounding an evolutionary conserved catalytic core. This gives rise to an antisense complementary region that provides the unimolecular RNA the capacity to recognize and subsequently enzymatically cleave its target mRNA [128].

Both types of molecules (iRNA and hhRz) have been successfully used to degrade an incorrect *RHO* transcript responsible for dominant retinitis pigmentosa, a common subtype of IRD [128]. Another alternative is employing microRNAs (miRNAs), which act at the post-transcriptional level to regulate gene expression in the retina. miRNAs generally bind to mRNA and cause a reduction of translated products. Some miRNAs are commonly expressed in all retinal cell types while others are specifically expressed in one or the other [5,129], suggesting that there are possibilities to employ these molecules therapeutically. However, more studies are needed before miRNAs can actually be used [130]. Overall, post-transcriptional gene silencing mediated by iRNA and ribozymes are believed to be a promising strategy for treating dominant-negative mutations.

RNAse H-dependent AONs: Besides redirecting splicing, AONs can also be used to specifically degrade transcripts, even in an allele-specific manner. Some oligonucleotide modifications combine AON segments with conformationally restricted residues that affect cleavage of their intended targets [131]. With this, catalytic activation of RNase H, a ubiquitous enzyme cleaving the RNA part of DNA/RNA hybrid duplexes, can be induced. The big advantage of these hybrid duplexes is that only a low amount of AON is sufficient to induce catalytic turnover. Furthermore, this catalytic turnover provides enough time for AONs to act as a potential drug due to their stability in blood serum, that is, a few days [132]. Murray and colleagues used rodent models genetically modified for *RHO* (p.P23H) to test RNAse H-activating AONs in vivo. They observed that the AON-mediated knockdown of mutant p.P23H rhodopsin expression reduced photoreceptor degradation, thereby preserving the function of photoreceptors in the transgenic rats [133]. Recently, AON-mediated transcript downregulation has also been assessed *in vitro* for a *NR2E3* variant underlying autosomal dominant RP [134], underscoring the usefulness of this approach for some (dominant) mutations.

Cas13: The editing system based on Cas13 can reduce off-target effect rates shown by other systems as explained previously [135]. RNA-guided RNA-targeting CRISPR-Cas effector Cas13 (previously named C2c2) can be engineered to bind and subsequently knockdown mammalian RNA [136]. Abudayyeh and colleagues verified that, for endogenous genes, the knockdown efficiency is transcript-dependent. Despite, the efficacy was comparable to that shown by iRNA, thus the substantially lower off-target ratio makes this approach well-suited for therapeutic applications [137].

2.2.3. RNA Editing (dCas13 and ADAR)

The ADAR (adenosine deaminase acting on RNA) family of proteins can mediate endogenous editing of transcripts via the deamination of adenosine to inosine, a nucleobase that is functionally equivalent to guanosine both in splicing and in translation [135]. Cox and colleagues designed a catalytically inactivated Cas13 (dCas13) that is able to retain its RNA-binding capacity, to direct an ADAR towards the RNA transcript of interest and to perform its adenosine-to-inosine deaminase function [135]. This demonstrated the flexibility of Cas13 to be adapted as a tool for nucleic acid modification. The system that was created is called REPAIRv2 and generates a higher specificity compared to other RNA-editing platforms reported so far [138,139] with high levels of on-target activity. Other advantages include—(i) Cas13 has no targeting sequence constraints and does not present any preferential motif surrounding the target adenosine, allowing any adenosine in the transcriptome to be potentially targeted; (ii) the REPAIRv2 system directly deaminates target adenosines to inosines and does not depend on endogenous repair pathways, thereby enabling RNA editing in post-mitotic cells like neurons and photoreceptors and, (iii) RNA editing, contrary to DNA editing, is transient and thus can be more readily reversed, allowing temporal control over editing events [135]. These features make RNA editing an interesting strategy to be used in future therapeutic studies in IRDs.

Table 2. List of clinical trials for IRDs using RNA therapies.

Gene	Therapeutic Molecule	Clinical Trial Identifier	Status
CEP290	QR-110	NCT03140969	Active, not recruiting
	QR-110	NCT03913130	Recruiting
	QR-110	NCT03913143	Recruiting
USH2A	QR-421a	NCT03780257	Recruiting

Black is just used to indicate the different sectiond and can be considered as headers. Gene (first column), therapeutic molecule (second column), clinical trial identifier (third column) and current status of the trial (last column) are indicated. Data obtained from https://clinicaltrials.gov/.

2.3. *Compound Therapies*

As happens in other types of diseases, pharmacological development can offer an entirely different approach to the treatment of IRD. However, the great heterogeneity observed in IRDs and the access-limiting BRB present major challenges towards an effective compound therapy [140]. In this section, we focus our attention on some promising drugs for the treatment of IRDs.

2.3.1. Translational Read-Through

Translational read-through (TR) therapy is based on small molecules, also known as TR-inducing drugs (TRIDs), that allow the translation machinery to bypass a premature termination codon (PTC) during translation [141]. In addition, PTCs can induce mRNA degradation through nonsense-mediated decay and thereby also inhibit full-length protein expression [141,142]. The incorporation of an amino acid at the site of the premature stop codon can increase the expression of the full-length protein as well as the reduction of nonsense-mediated decay [142]. Until now, the detailed mechanisms by which TRIDs induce their therapeutic effect are not completely understood. However, it is known that TR efficiency depends on the competition between decoding of the stop codon by a near-cognate tRNA and stop codon recognition by eRF1 [141]. There are two main classes of TRIDs—aminoglycoside and non-aminoglycoside TRIDs. From the first group, gentamicin has been most widely used to analyse TR in different disease models, including those affected with IRD. The efficacy of gentamicin was studied in different rat and mouse models—(i) the S334ter rat model that carries a nonsense mutation (c.1002T>A; p.S334*) in the gene encoding the visual pigment rhodopsin (*Rho*) and (ii) the *rd12* mouse, a model for retinal degeneration caused by a nonsense mutation in *Rpe65*. Systematic gentamicin treatment showed different results between the two models. In S334ter rats, a partial rescue of photoreceptor survival was noticed however, no rescue was observed in *rd12* mice [143]. Studies on genes mutated in Usher syndrome (a syndromic form of IRD accompanied by hearing impairment) demonstrated that aminoglycosides and derivatives thereof can mediate TR of different disease-causing PTCs in the *PCDH15* and *USH1C* genes, in *in vitro* translation assays as well as in cell culture experiments [144–149].

The non-aminoglycoside TRID PTC124 (also known as Ataluren) is used in a wide range of diseases including Duchenne muscular dystrophy and cystic fibrosis [150–153], with several clinical studies having been performed or ongoing. For IRDs, promising results using PTC124 have been reported by the restoration of full-length RP2 protein, the encoding gene of which is mutated in X-linked RP, as well as for the REP1 protein, encoded by the *CHM* gene that is mutated in choroideremia. In X-linked RP, rod photoreceptors mainly suffer from the loss of RP2, although the effect on cone photoreceptors and RPE cells should not be neglected. Schwarz and colleagues used TRIDs (both the aminoglycoside G418 as well as PTC124) to successfully increase full-length RP2 protein levels in the presence of the p.R120ter (c.358C>T; p.R120 *) mutation. In choroideremia, many nonsense mutations in *CHM* have been described. Several studies attempted to use TRIDs, including PTC124 or its analogue PTC-414, to increase REP1 protein levels, either in cellular (human fibroblasts, iPSC-derived RPE) or animal (zebrafish) models [154–156]. The efficacy of read-through was found to be considerably variable, not only depending on the type of nonsense codon and its surrounding sequence but also on the remaining transcript levels that can differ significantly between patients [142]. Another study, based on topical administration of PTC124 to the eye, demonstrated functional restoration of the harmonin protein in a mouse model for Usher syndrome type 1c (USH1C) [141,145].

One of the disadvantages of the systemic use of TRIDs is that for many diseases, drugs need to go through physical barriers (such as the blood-brain barrier or BRB). These barriers can reduce compound availability in the targeted organ after treatment, illustrating the need to increment the dosage administered to the patients or to change the delivery method of TRIDs (commonly intraperitoneal) towards local administration [141]. One strategy to overcome this is the encapsulation of drugs into tissue-specific liposomes [157]. In particular for IRDs, topical applications or intraocular injections should be considered in the future.

2.3.2. Restoring Proteostasis (Protein Therapies)

Photoreceptor cells require a rigorous regulation of proteostasis (maintaining a healthy protein balance) to ensure their correct function and viability. As a result, certain genetic changes in specific genes with an essential function in the photoreceptor cell can have dramatic effects. One example is the dominant-negative effect of mutations in *RHO*, which leads to the disruption of outer segments in the photoreceptor cell [158]. The manipulation of proteostasis mechanisms such as the heat-shock response (HSR) or unfolded protein response could be a good therapeutic target in order to alleviate misfolding diseases (e.g., targeted up-regulation of these pathways to reduce aggregation of proteins such as rhodopsin) [159]. This could be achieved either by the administration of drugs that restore proteostasis (e.g., pharmacological chaperones, kosmotropes, molecular chaperones or autophagy inducers) or by targeting key molecules in the photoreceptor proteostasis network [160,161].

So far, "proteostasis" therapies are mainly focused on rhodopsin, as *RHO* is one of the most frequently mutated genes in autosomal dominant RP. One of the most common mutations in this gene is the p.P23H mutation, which acts in a dominant-negative fashion on wild-type rhodopsin by inducing misfolding [160]. Intriguingly, it was reported that misfolded proteins could be rescued by a ligand that works as a chaperone [161].

Pharmacological chaperones are small, substrate-specific molecules that are able to directly target the protein structure and shift the protein folding equilibrium towards its native state [158,162]. Studies using this kind of chaperones suggested that correction of mutant rhodopsin folding, without improving its stability, could further compromise the outer segments and increase rod cell death. Thus, these data underscore the necessity to ensure opsin stability using parallel treatment strategies [163,164].

Kosmotropes are small, low molecular weight compounds that can enhance the stability of proteins in their native conformation and decrease aggregation. Kosmotropes bind to proteins non-specifically and thus have the potential to be used in a wide range of protein-misfolding diseases [161]. The chemical chaperone tauroursodeoxycholic acid (TUDCA) has been studied in several retinal degeneration models [165–167], although its efficacy was found to vary between different studies, even in the presence of the same IRD-causing mutation, namely p.P23H, in the gene encoding rhodopsin. It has been hypothesized that activation of PERK, one of the receptors responsible for UPR [168] differs between models, thereby explaining the ineffectiveness of TUDCA in some of them [161,165].

Finally, another alternative to restore proteostasis is through the control of the adaptative machinery that is responsible for its maintenance via HSR and UPR [158]. Inhibition of molecular chaperones can activate the HSR by releasing HSF1 and inducing cell stress, which triggers the production of molecular chaperones. The Hsp90 inhibitors and HSR inducers geldanamycin, radicicol and 17-AAG reduced P23H aggregation and cell death *in vitro* [162]. Hsp90 works as a crucial chaperone in the maturation of many proteins. Targeting Hsp90 directly however could affect normal vision, suggesting that an alternative therapeutic approach could include the stimulation of both the HSR and UPR pathways with arimoclomol (a heat shock protein inducer). In rat models carrying the p.P23H rhodopsin mutation, it has been demonstrated that administering arimoclonol via intraperitoneal injection reduced mutant rhodopsin aggregation and ameliorated photoreceptor degeneration [160,161].

2.3.3. Pathway-Specific Therapies

Cyclic guanosine-monophosphate (cGMP) is a crucial molecule for photoreceptor signal transduction and has two main cellular effectors—cyclic nucleotide gated ion channels (CNGCs) and cGMP-dependent protein kinase G (PKG) [169]. It has been reported that over-activation of PKG can be enough to cause photoreceptor cell death and that its activation levels are higher in mutant photoreceptors. Knowing that CNGCs play an important role in driving phototransduction, some interesting observations have been made. The deletion of CNGC beta subunits protects photoreceptors in *rd1* mice that harbour a defect in the *Pde6b* gene, which encodes the phosphodiesterase protein involved in the phototransduction cascade. Therefore, either PKG or CNGCs can be considered as critical disease drivers; consequently, both of them are therapeutic targets for prevention of (further) retinal degeneration [140]. As mentioned above, the BRB can prevent the access of therapeutic agents to the retina. Vighi and colleagues overcame this problem using a liposomal drug delivery method, the liposomal cGMP analogue formulation LP-CN03, and demonstrated improved visual function as well as reduced photoreceptor degeneration in mouse models harbouring mutations in different IRD gene orthologues [140]. Together, these data suggest that cGMP signalling could be a common pathway to target for the treatment of genetically and phenotypically divergent kinds of retinal degeneration [140,169].

Another drug previously tested in clinical trials is an orally delivered synthetic cis-retinoid also known as QLT091001. This drug triggered visual restoration in transgenic and naturally occurring mouse and dog models mutant for *Rpe65* [170]. The results of the clinical trial NCT01014052 (Table 3) showed that QLT091001 did improve visual function in subjects with IRD due to *LRAT* or *RPE65* mutations. Mutations in these genes can cause different subtypes of IRD, usually classified as LCA or RP. Despite this, the exact genetic defect apparently did not affect the drug response in both LCA and RP patients [171]. Upon oral administration of QLT091001, patients showed beneficial effects in the remaining photoreceptors of the retina in both eyes, although it did not stop the progression of photoreceptor degradation completely. The safety profile of this drug showed transient adverse effects such as headaches or nausea [171]. In theory, QLT091001 could be combined with gene augmentation therapy, although the combination of treatments, in particular for orphan diseases, poses additional challenges on drug development.

Table 3. Summary of clinical trials for IRDs using compound therapies.

Gene	Therapeutic Molecule	Clinical Trial Identifier	Status
ABCA4	ALK-001	NCT02402660	Recruiting
	Zimura	NCT03364153	Active, not recruiting
	Emuxustat	NCT03772665	Recruiting
	Emuxustat	NCT03033108	**Completed**
RPE65	QLT091001	NCT01014052	**Completed**
	QLT091001	NCT01521793	**Completed**
	QLT091001	NCT01543906 *	**Completed**
RS1	Dorzolamide 2% TID or brinzolamide 1% TID	NCT02331173	**Completed**

Black is just used to indicate the different sectiond and can be considered as headers. Gene (first column), therapeutic molecule (second column), clinical trial identifier (third column) and current status of the trial (last column) are indicated. Completed trials are highlighted in bold. Data obtained from https://clinicaltrials.gov/. * Of note, Trial NCT01543906 describes the use of QLT091001 in patients with a dominant *RPE65* mutation (unlike most *RPE65* mutations inherited in an autosomal recessive manner).

3. Delivery of Therapeutic Molecules

3.1. Methods of Ocular Delivery

Despite its small size, the eye contains several cell and tissue types that can be targeted by therapeutic agents [172]. Local tolerability of vector administration in IRDs has been reported in various studies and no serious systemic problems have been indicated so far [23]. Commonly, we can identify two main potential delivery methods—subretinal and intravitreal injections. Subretinal injections are considered to be more prone towards complications (e.g., retinal detachment), especially in patients with affected retinal integrity, compared to intravitreal injection. Despite, the vector is delivered much closer to its target cells/region, allowing an efficient vector transduction in RPE cells and/or photoreceptors [173]. In contrast, intravitreal injections allow an easier targeting of the optic nerve, lens or inner retina and less often the outer retina or the anterior chamber. It also shows fewer procedure-related complications but the transduction of the viral vector into photoreceptors and RPE cells is less efficient when compared with subretinal injections [23,174]. Apart from these two methods, there is an alternative system—Suprachoroidal delivery. With this, therapeutic agents are delivered directly to the suprachoroidal space located between the sclera and choroid [175,176]. Preclinical animal studies showed that suprachoroidal drug delivery has the same safety profile as intravitreal injections [177–179]. Results from completed clinical trials (e.g., NCT01789320) have also showed encouraging safety profiles [180], although potential spreading of therapeutic vectors into the systemic circulation needs to be considered.

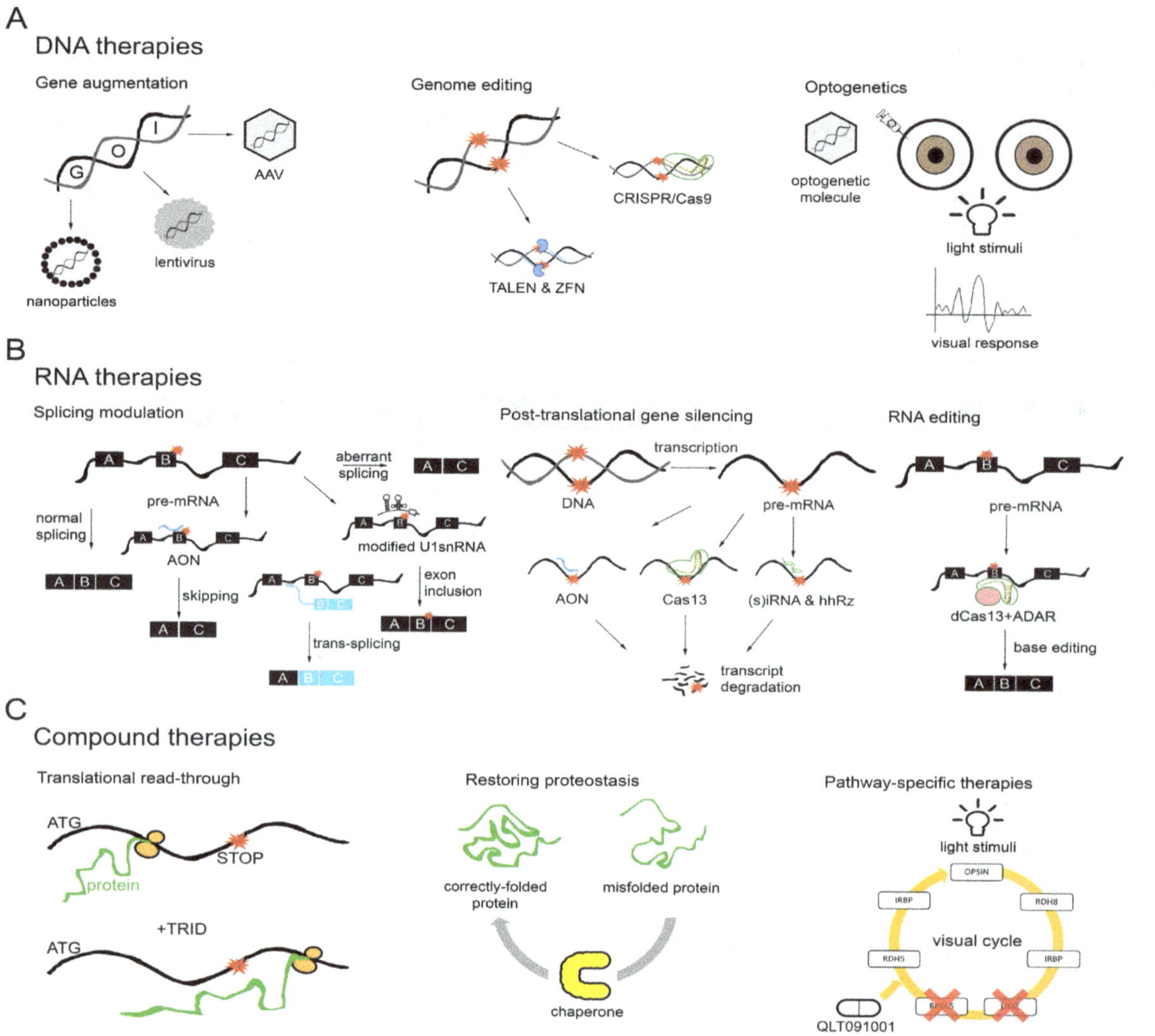

Figure 2. Schematic and simplified representation of the several types of molecular therapies. (**A**) DNA therapies are represented by gene augmentation, genome editing and optogenetics. In gene augmentation, the entire coding sequence of the gene of interest (GOI) is delivered using different vectors. Genome editing employs nucleases able to edit the DNA at a specific position; CRISPR/Cas9 is depicted in green, guide RNA in dark yellow and ZFN and TALEN in blue. Mutations are depicted in red. In optogenetics, a light-sensitive molecule is delivered to the eye to give photosensitive properties to remaining retinal neurons. (**B**) RNA therapies; splicing modulation can be achieved using AONs (in dark blue) for (pseudo)exon skipping or modified U1 snRNA (in black) to favour exon inclusion in cases where mutations (in red) are found in the donor splice site. Trans-splicing occurs between two independent RNA molecules—The original transcript and the exogenous molecule without the mutation. In all cases, splicing is modulated to obtain a transcript with full or residual function. Post-translational gene silencing can be achieved by degrading the RNA transcript using AONs (dark blue), Cas13 (green) with a guide RNA (dark yellow) or (s)iRNA and hhRz (in green). These approaches can be used for dominant-negative mutations by promoting allele-specific degradation. Mutations are indicated in red. With RNA editing using CRISPR/Cas technology, dead Cas13 (in green) is conjugated with an adenosine deaminase (dark yellow) acting at the RNA level (ADAR, in light red). This molecule is guided to the mutation using a guide RNA binding on top of the mutation (in red) to induce a G-to-A transversion. (**C**) Representative examples of compound therapies. Translational read-through allows the ribosome to continue protein synthesis despite a premature stop codon (in red) in the presence of the translational read-through-inducing drugs (TRIDs). Restoring proteostasis can be accomplished by using chaperones to properly fold proteins. QLT091001 is a pathway-specific therapy that acts in the visual cycle and can be used when for example, *RPE65* or *LRAT* are mutated.

Finally, there is the possibility of topical delivery by the use of eye drops. However, this approach can result in lower bioavailability and increased clearance in comparison to the different types of injections. In addition, ocular barriers decrease the bioavailability of topically applied therapeutic agents to less than 5% [181]. Therefore, the effectiveness of this method is less than those reported with the systems previously described.

3.2. Vectors

Besides the routes of administration, a wide range of viral and non-viral gene delivery approaches has been developed over the last twenty years, in order to allow an efficient transfer of therapeutic molecules to the right target cell. Choosing one over another depends on the cell or tissue type to be targeted, the cloning capacity of each of the vectors and safety concerns [23].

3.2.1. Viral Vectors

Adeno-associated viruses (AAVs): Most commonly but not exclusively, therapeutic genes are delivered to their target cells by viral vectors. AAVs are the most common viral vectors used for gene therapy in IRDs, mainly due to their low immunogenicity and toxicity, and allow for long-term transgene expression [182,183].

Recombinant AAV (rAAV) is the most popular viral vector for delivery in IRDs. Its tropism for different types of retinal cells allows efficient transduction of these cells and relatively fast and stable transgene expression [184]. rAAV is available in two forms, single-stranded AAV (ssAAV) and self-complimentary AAV (scAAV). Once a cell is transduced with ssAAV, the single-stranded DNA of the virus needs to be converted into the double-stranded form; this is a rate-limiting step that can be circumvented with scAAVs [25]. The scAAVs are engineered in a way that upon infection two complementary halves will generate a double-stranded DNA, promoting faster and increased transgene expression [185]. However, the main disadvantage of scAAVs is their reduced cargo capacity (2.4 kb), compared to ssAAV (4.8 kb) which limits its transgene selection. scAAV vectors have been demonstrated to transduce retinal ganglion cells, photoreceptors and RPE cells, and can lead to transgene expression within two days after injection in mice while ssAAV requires several weeks [186]; this rapid and increased transgene expression was independent of the AAV serotype tested (i.e. -1, -2 or -5) [25].

Despite its numerous advantages, AAV presents a limited packaging capacity (4.8 kb) [22,25,45]. To overcome this, various strategies have been developed. For instance, with the use of dual AAV vectors, a cDNA can be split in two separate fragments, after which the two parts recombine inside the cells using HDR, trans-splicing or both [41,187]. With this, the capacity can be increased up to 9 kb [41,43,187]. The dual AAV system has been used in preclinical studies to deliver some genes mutated in IRD such as *ABCA4* [188] and *MYO7A* [189], with promising results. However, dual AAVs may still not be sufficient for several other genes mutated in IRD. The use of triple AAV approaches allows to increase the cargo capacity to 14 kb [43,189,190], enabling the development of gene therapies for IRDs caused by mutations in even larger genes. Maddalena and colleagues demonstrated the potential of this system to restore *CDH23* (cDNA size 11.1 kB, mutated in Usher syndrome type 1D) and *ALMS1* (cDNA size 12.9 kb, mutated in Almstrom syndrome) gene expression. Certainly, the enclosed and small subretinal space may facilitate co-infection of the same cell by three independent AAV vectors [43].

To date, up to 12 AAV serotypes and more than 100 variants have been identified in humans and NHPs [25]. From these, AAV2, AAV5 and AAV8 have been most extensively studied, being used as delivery vector in several clinical and preclinical studies for different genes such as *RPE65, CNGB3, RS1* or *PDE6B* (Table 1) [25]. AAV serotypes 2, 5, 7, 8 and 9 are able to transduce photoreceptors, while virtually every AAV serotype is capable of efficiently infecting RPE cells [23]. So far, AAV2 is the only vector described to transduce retinal ganglion cells upon intravitreal delivery [191,192]. However, alternative serotypes of AAV have also been developed. Some examples are the serotypes AAV7m8 [193] and AAV8BP2 [194]. Both of them were designed to alter AAV capsids aiming to improve uptake into the retina and be able to target photoreceptors following intravitreal injection [193,194]. AAV7m8 serotype was generated by in vivo directed evolution in the mouse retina by Dalkara and collaborators [193,195]. They reported that the intravitreal delivery of AAV7m8 resulted in effective pan-retinal photoreceptor and RPE cell transduction in mice. This serotype was also tested in NHP retinas via intravitreal administration. The results indicated a higher transduction rate of foveal and extrafoveal photoreceptors in comparison with the parental serotype AAV2. However, authors also noted toxicity in an NHP injected with a high titre of AAV7m8 [193]. Therefore, a study of safety and efficiency of transduction using lower doses of this serotype is required if this capsid is planned to be used in primates, including humans. The AAV8BP2 serotype was generated in vivo by Cronin and colleagues, it targets ON-bipolar cells and cone photoreceptors efficiently following both intravitreal and subretinal injections in mouse [194]. This research group performed a comparative study between these two novel serotypes. Both vectors showed promising results in mice but in NHPs, either subretinal or intravitreal delivery did not allow to transduce all target cells within the retina. Specifically, AAV7m8 showed some toxicity effects (as previously reported) as well as severe inflammation when using a high titre [195]. For AAV8BP2, a lower transduction of bipolar cells was observed, even at high doses. Taken together, the results of both serotypes indicate that studies in rodents might not provide sufficient information to understand the cellular transduction and pharmacological properties of these engineered AAVs and further studies in for example NHPs are needed before using them in humans. Carvalho and collaborators characterized an *in silico* designed serotype named Anc80 for retinal gene transfer [196]. Three Anc80 variants were evaluated, Anc80L27, Anc80L65 and Anc80L12, in mice and NHP. All of them were capable of efficiently targeting retinal cells following subretinal delivery, although Anc80L65 showed a higher efficiency for targeting retinal cells as well as higher expression levels compared to AAV8. These data support the use of Anc80L65 for gene delivery to the retina. Taken together, all these studies characterizing novel serotypes have illustrated the impact of minimal changes in capsid composition on aspects relevant to experimental and clinical gene transfer applications. This will prove useful for improving delivery to the retina and thus for their use in developing new treatments for IRDs.

Lentiviral vectors: Lentiviruses (LV) are RNA viruses of the retrovirus family. In IRDs, the retroviral variant of human immunodeficiency virus type 1 (HIV-1) or the equine infectious anaemia virus (EIAV) have been tested. LVs have the ability to pass through the cells' intact nuclear membrane and infect both dividing and non-dividing cells [197]. Moreover, LVs efficiently integrate their genome into that of the host-cell, leading to stable expression. LVs are modified to stop replication, so these vectors are not pathogenic after initial gene delivery. LVs present a transgene capacity cargo of ~8–10 kb and, in terms of IRD, are capable of infecting RPE cells and to a lesser extent of differentiated photoreceptors [23,25]. EIAVs have been used for *ABCA4*, as its cDNA size (6.8 kb) outplaced the cargo capacity of AAV but not that of lentiviruses [198]. To assess this strategy in human subjects, a clinical trial (NCT01367444) has been ongoing for several years (Table 1), whilst no clear efficacy data have been reported.

Adenoviruses and helper-dependent adenoviruses: In comparison to the previously mentioned viral vectors, adenoviruses (AdVs) have a cargo capacity of about 8 kb, while its 'gutted' helper-dependent adenovirus (HDAd) has an extremely large capacity of up to 36 kb. It is demonstrated that adenoviral vectors infect RPE cells efficiently but because the coxsackie-AdV receptor is presumed to be absent on the cell membrane of photoreceptors [199,200], these vectors do not efficiently transduce photoreceptor cells [201]. Overall, AdVs have been only sparsely used in the treatment of IRDs [202,203].

3.2.2. Non-Viral Vectors

Although various viral vectors have demonstrated their potential in the treatment of IRDs, there is a continuing need for refinement delivery vectors for the eye. Therefore, research efforts have also been directed towards the development of non-viral delivery systems, such as nanoparticles (NPs), naked DNA or liposomes [174].

Naked DNA is the most elementary form of non-viral gene therapy [204]. As naked DNA does typically not enter into the cells, it is not considered as a suitable therapy for the eye. Different studies have used electroporation or iontophoresis to obtain a significant uptake and expression in the target cells, however both delivery ways presented significant challenges. The side effects of electroporation make it an unlikely method to be clinically feasible, whilst iontophoresis so far presents conflicting information about the real effectiveness of this method [174,204].

In contrast, NPs are well capable of delivering plasmid DNA containing a functional copy of a gene into the retina [205]. The three determinants of the effectiveness of gene delivery using this kind of vectors are cellular uptake, endosomal escape and transfer of the plasmid DNA into the nucleus. All forms of NPs-(metal, lipid or polymers) have some capability to pass through the cell membrane, avoid endosomal trapping and deliver the plasmid DNA into the nucleus. Lipid-based NPs are biocompatible and stable particles; furthermore, there is no inflammatory response to these NPs when injected into the eye. However, there are also some disadvantages, such as lower gene expression when compared to the same transgenes delivered by viral vectors [174]. A new type of delivery system was recently developed by Trigueros and colleagues using gold nanoparticles (DNA-gold NPs), as these are relatively easy to generate and can be adapted to different shapes and sizes [206]. Gold is well-tolerated inside an organism and presents low rates of toxicity. However, they present a low clearance rate, thereby hampering their uptake in specific cells or tissues [207]. Therefore, Trigueros et al. further optimized this system for IRDs. In this study, they compared this new system with DNA-liposome complexes and demonstrated higher expression of a reporter gene. Their results showed that RPE cells responded differently to pristine-gold NPs and DNA-gold NPs, probably because of changes in the membrane-NP interface. Moreover, both types of NPs used different alternative endocytic ways for internalization, as indicated by their detection in different endosomal compartments. DNA-gold NPs were located in early endosomes that later will not mature into late endosome vesicles, resulting in an earlier expression of the reporter gene compared to pristine-gold NPs. This study was the first step to use non-cytotoxic gold NPs for an in vivo gene therapy to treat IRDs. However, some biological questions are still unclear, such as the internalization routes that are used and the exact nature of intracellular endosome trafficking. Furthermore, before using these particles as a delivery method in the retina, it is necessary to understand the complexity of cell–NP interaction, enhance the cargo delivery by avoiding degradative pathways (such as the lysosomal pathway) and ensure a constant expression of the therapeutic gene [206].

Finally, cationic lipids (liposomes) offer an alternative way to deliver DNA into the eye. In addition to the two most common ways of retinal delivery (see above), other delivery methods such as topical or intravenous administration have already reported positive results in eye diseases [174]. Liposomes however also present some limitations such as retinal toxicity and aggregation following administration [208]. Consequently, researchers developed a new type of liposome-PEGylated with perfluoropropane gas-that appears to be safer and more efficient for transfection but, as happened with other lipid-based vectors, presented a drop in gene expression four days after administration [174].

4. Other IRD Treatments

While gene-based therapies may stop or at least delay, the progression of the disease, other promising approaches that are less dependent of the genetic cause of the disease are also gaining momentum. This is for instance the case for stem cell-derived retinal cell transplantation (cell therapy) or the use of prosthetic implants.

4.1. Cell Therapy

Retinal cells, like other cells within the central nervous system, present a low regeneration potential. Therefore, cell therapies could be applied in those IRDs that present an advanced degeneration stage. The use of this type of therapy aims to result in an integration of exogenously delivered cells and subsequent re-activation of visual function [45]. Patient-derived somatic cells could be used to reprogram induced pluripotent stem cells (iPSCs) that subsequently could be differentiated to retinal precursor cells and introduced into the eye to replace either photoreceptors or supporting cells (e.g., RPE) that provide trophic and metabolic maintenance to prevent further degeneration of the remaining photoreceptors [209]. Genome editing tools (such as those described in Section 2.1.2) can be used to repair patient-specific mutations, to eventually transplant the corrected cells back to the patient [210]. The use of embryonic stem cells (ESCs) would not require this genetic modification and it has been demonstrated that these cells also have a high capacity to differentiate into retinal precursors [45,211]. However, the use of ESC is associated with ethical considerations not present with the use of iPSCs generated from the patients. Moreover, the transplantation of iPSC-derived retinal cells would avoid the risk of immune rejection after surgery [45].

Following up on the promising advances that demonstrated that stem cell-derived photoreceptor transplantation can restore rod- and cone-mediated vision [211–214], recent studies showed that these transplanted cells are not able to integrate well into non-degenerative host retinas. Instead, it seems that post-mitotic donor and host photoreceptors can exchange RNA and proteins, including rhodopsin [215,216]. The visual improvements measured after stem cell-derived photoreceptor transplantation could thus also be the result of endogenous photoreceptors that have taken up donor cell-derived proteins. Recently, it was demonstrated that cell integration as well as cytoplasmic transfer can occur but the relative contributions of each depend on the environment within the host retina [45,216].

Some cell therapies that are already tested in the clinic use hESC or hiPSC-derived RPE, for treating diseases such as AMD or Stardgardt disease [217–220]. For the study employing iPSC-derived RPE transplantation, a one-year follow-up analysis indicated that the transplantation did not generate any adverse effect and no immune response was induced, even in the absence of immunosuppression. One of the studies using hESC-derived RPE also reported an improvement of vision in patients with age-related macular degeneration as well as those with Stargardt disease [218]. Nevertheless, more studies are needed to provide reproducible protocols to generate iPSC-derived photoreceptor precursor cells. In addition, if such cells are transplanted after gene mutation repair, stringent quality controls of the iPSCs before and after genome editing are extremely important [45].

4.2. Retinal Prosthetic Implants

Inner retinal neurons largely retain their capability of signal transmission and are still present in advanced stages of retinal degradation. This fact encouraged the use of a stimulation mechanism (prosthetic implants) that is able to restore vision to some extent. Such a device would bypass the degraded photoreceptor layer and directly interact with the still functioning inner retinal neurons [84]. Retinal prostheses work as an integral system that contain an image acquisition device (which is integrated by thousands of light-sensitive microphotodies), an image processor, a stimulator chip and an electrode array [84,221]. In this system, light emanating from visible objects is converted by the microphotodies into little currents of hundreds of microelectrodes, which are directed onto remaining neurons within the neuronal network, the middle and the inner retina [221]. These systems have demonstrated a partial visual restoration, presenting the first evidence of this strategy in the field of vision [222]. To date, several stimulation modalities have been built [84] and four of them have obtained market approval for use in Europe and/or United States (Argus II, IRIS, IMS and AMS) [222]. These devices are classified according to their anatomical placement.

Epiretinal prostheses (Argus II, IRIS and EPI-IRET3) are implanted on the surface of the neurosensory retina, adjacent to nerve fibre and ganglion cell layers. Its location ensures certain advantages such as easy surgical delivery and safe heat dispersion [84,222]. Functionally, the stimulation is directly applied to the retinal ganglion cells, bypassing the residual intraretinal processing system, thereby inhibiting the capacity to mimic the physiological topographic organization. Besides this, as the epiretinal prostheses are close to passing axonal nerve fibres, ectopic visual perceptions from axonal stimulation can occur, thereby decreasing spatial resolution and confusing the intended stimulation pattern. As a note, the epiretinal prostheses have an external camera positioned outside the eye that provides power induction and a data signal that is transmitted to the intraocular simulator [84,221,222]. From these prostheses, Argus II is the most widely-used and it has been implanted in more than 250 patients to date, reporting encouraging results [223].

Subretinal prostheses (ASR, IMS/AMS, PRIMA and BSI) are placed between the degenerated photoreceptor layer and the RPE, such that the intrinsic signal processing capability of the retinal interneurons can be used optimally, generating vision similar to the one that is physiologically generated in the eye [84,222]. Moreover, the device is placed closer to the retina and is therefore favoured over the natural retinal signal amplification, requiring lower stimulation intensities. Unless the system has intrinsic photosensitivity and amplification capacity, it, like the epiretinal devices, requires a power source and a connection serving the delivery of data. Surgically, some studies have indicated that positioning these devices could be technically complicated because of the RPE adhesion caused by the retinal degeneration. Moreover, this surgical approach is less known and practiced outside routine retinal surgery [222]. To date, there are two methods to subretinal stimulation—one that employs a standard electrode array and another that uses a microphotodiode array (MPDA) that is present in all devices with exception of BSI (Boston retinal implant). This last one itself is able to capture light, allowing to avoid the use of cameras, while the visual scene is perceived by the lens on the array [84].

Suprachoroidal prostheses (STS and BVA) are located in the suprachoroidal space. This space is highly vascular and therefore there is a high risk of haemorrhage and fibrosis post-implantation. In comparison with the other two counterparts mentioned above, suprachoroidal devices are relatively far away from the retina. This implies that the design requires greater stimulation power to elicit visual perception [84,222]. Larger numbers are needed to establish solid conclusions about the efficacy of both suprachoroidal and transscleral implants in their present formats; however, results to date suggest greater limitations to these approaches compared to epiretinal or subretinal implants [84].

5. Concluding Remarks

The approval of Luxturna^{TM} as the first approved gene augmentation therapy for an ocular disease has provided an enormous impulse to the development of retinal therapeutics, both in academic centres as well as in industry. As summarized in this review, current developments range from gene augmentation, splice modulation, genome editing, optogenetics and compound therapies to cell replacement strategies and retinal prostheses. Patients with progressive vision loss are in need of treatment, to improve their quality of life by (partially) restoring vision or at least slow down or halt the progression of their diseases. Which strategy has the highest chance of being safe and efficacious depends on many factors, including the person's genetic defect(s) and the stage of disease accompanied by the appearance of the retina. However, therapeutic development also requires appropriate cellular and/or animal models to test the efficacy of a given approach, as well as clinical endpoints to determine whether an improvement of therapeutic intervention can be measured. Only when fundamental and translational scientists, clinicians, funding agencies, patient organizations, industry and regulatory bodies join forces, we can fight these devastating conditions and provide hope and vision, for thousands of visually impaired individuals worldwide.

Author Contributions: I.V.D., A.G. and R.W.J.C. collected data, wrote the manuscript, and performed careful proofreading. All authors approve the final content of the manuscript.

References

1. Sohocki, M.M.; Daiger, S.P.; Bowne, S.J.; Rodriquez, J.A.; Northrup, H.; Heckenlively, J.R.; Saperstein, D.A. Prevalence of mutations causing retinitis pigmentosa and other inherited retinopathies. *Hum. Mutat.* **2001**, *17*, 42–51. [CrossRef]
2. Khan, M.; Fadaie, Z.; Cornelis, S.S.; Cremers, F.P.; Roosing, S. Identification and Analysis of Genes Associated with Inherited Retinal Diseases. *Methods Mol. Biol.* **2019**, *1834*, 3–27. [PubMed]
3. Kaur, C.; Foulds, W.; Ling, E. Blood–retinal barrier in hypoxic ischaemic conditions: Basic concepts, clinical features and management. *Prog. Retin. Eye Res.* **2008**, *27*, 622–647. [CrossRef] [PubMed]
4. Anand, V.; Duffy, B.; Yang, Z.; Dejneka, N.S.; Maguire, A.M.; Bennett, J. A Deviant Immune Response to Viral Proteins and Transgene Product Is Generated on Subretinal Administration of Adenovirus and Adeno-associated Virus. *Mol. Ther.* **2002**, *5*, 125–132. [CrossRef] [PubMed]
5. Bennett, J. Immune response following intraocular delivery of recombinant viral vectors. *Gene Ther.* **2003**, *10*, 977–982. [CrossRef] [PubMed]
6. Öner, A. Recent Advancements in Gene Therapy for Hereditary Retinal Dystrophies. *Turk. J. Ophthalmol.* **2017**, *47*, 338–343. [CrossRef] [PubMed]
7. Gupta, P.R.; Huckfeldt, R.M. Gene therapy for inherited retinal degenerations: Initial successes and future challenges. *J. Neural Eng.* **2017**, *14*, 051002. [CrossRef]
8. Liang, F.Q.; Anand, V.; Maguire, A.M.; Bennett, J. Intraocular delivery of recombinant virus. *Methods Mol. Med.* **2001**, *47*, 125–139.
9. Ong, T.; Pennesi, M.E.; Birch, D.G.; Lam, B.L.; Tsang, S.H. Adeno-Associated Viral Gene Therapy for Inherited Retinal Disease. *Pharm. Res.* **2019**, *36*, 34. [CrossRef]
10. Sahel, J.-A.; Marazova, K.; Audo, I. Clinical Characteristics and Current Therapies for Inherited Retinal Degenerations. *Cold Spring Harb. Perspect. Med.* **2014**, *5*, a017111. [CrossRef]
11. Robson, A.G. Pattern ERG Correlates of Abnormal Fundus Autofluorescence in Patients with Retinitis Pigmentosa and Normal Visual Acuity. *Investig. Opthalmology Vis. Sci.* **2003**, *44*, 3544–3550. [CrossRef] [PubMed]
12. Koizumi, H.; Spaide, R.F.; Fisher, Y.L.; Freund, K.B.; Klancnik, J.M.; Yannuzzi, L.A. Three-Dimensional Evaluation of Vitreomacular Traction and Epiretinal Membrane Using Spectral-Domain Optical Coherence Tomography. *Am. J. Ophthalmol.* **2008**, *145*, 509–517. [CrossRef] [PubMed]
13. Hagiwara, A.; Yamamoto, S.; Ogata, K.; Sugawara, T.; Hiramatsu, A.; Shibata, M.; Mitamura, Y. Macular abnormalities in patients with retinitis pigmentosa: Prevalence on OCT examination and outcomes of vitreoretinal surgery. *Acta Ophthalmol.* **2011**, *89*, e122–e125. [CrossRef] [PubMed]
14. Lewin, A.S.; Rossmiller, B.; Mao, H. Gene Augmentation for adRP Mutations in RHO. *Cold Spring Harb. Perspect. Med.* **2014**, *4*, a017400. [CrossRef] [PubMed]
15. Salsman, J.; Dellaire, G. Precision genome editing in the CRISPR era. *Biochem. Cell Boil.* **2017**, *95*, 187–201. [CrossRef] [PubMed]
16. Kaczmarek, J.C.; Kowalski, P.S.; Anderson, D.G. Advances in the delivery of RNA therapeutics: From concept to clinical reality. *Genome Med.* **2017**, *9*, 60. [CrossRef] [PubMed]
17. Mead, B.; Berry, M.; Logan, A.; Scott, R.A.; Leadbeater, W.; Scheven, B.A. Stem cell treatment of degenerative eye disease. *Stem Cell Res.* **2015**, *14*, 243–257. [CrossRef] [PubMed]
18. Weiland, J.D.; Humayun, M.S. Retinal prosthesis. *IEEE Trans. Biomed. Eng.* **2014**, *61*, 1412–1424. [CrossRef] [PubMed]
19. Berger, W.; Kloeckener-Gruissem, B.; Neidhardt, J. The molecular basis of human retinal and vitreoretinal diseases. *Prog. Retin. Eye Res.* **2010**, *29*, 335–375. [CrossRef]
20. Smith, J.; Ward, D.; Michaelides, M.; Moore, A.T.; Simpson, S. New and emerging technologies for the treatment of inherited retinal diseases: A horizon scanning review. *Eye* **2015**, *29*, 1131–1140. [CrossRef]
21. Schön, C.; Biel, M.; Michalakis, S. Retinal gene delivery by adeno-associated virus (AAV) vectors: Strategies and applications. *Eur. J. Pharm. Biopharm.* **2015**, *95*, 343–352. [CrossRef] [PubMed]

22. Bennett, J. Taking Stock of Retinal Gene Therapy: Looking Back and Moving Forward. *Mol. Ther.* **2017**, *25*, 1076–1094. [CrossRef] [PubMed]
23. Moore, N.A.; Morral, N.; Ciulla, T.A.; Bracha, P. Gene therapy for inherited retinal and optic nerve degenerations. *Expert Opin. Biol. Ther.* **2018**, *18*, 37–49. [CrossRef] [PubMed]
24. Zuris, J.A.; Thompson, D.B.; Shu, Y.; Guilinger, J.P.; Bessen, J.L.; Hu, J.H.; Liu, D.R. Cationic lipid-mediated delivery of proteins enables efficient protein-based genome editing in vitro and in vivo. *Nat. Biotechnol.* **2015**, *33*, 73–80. [CrossRef] [PubMed]
25. Arbabi, A.; Liu, A.; Ameri, H. Gene Therapy for Inherited Retinal Degeneration. *J. Ocul. Pharmacol. Ther.* **2019**, *35*, 79–97. [CrossRef] [PubMed]
26. Zangi, L.; Lui, K.O.; Von Gise, A.; Ma, Q.; Ebina, W.; Ptaszek, L.M.; Später, D.; Xu, H.; Tabebordbar, M.; Gorbatov, R.; et al. Modified mRNA directs the fate of heart progenitor cells and induces vascular regeneration after myocardial infarction. *Nat. Biotechnol.* **2013**, *31*, 898–907. [CrossRef] [PubMed]
27. Ameri, H. Prospect of retinal gene therapy following commercialization of voretigene neparvovec-rzyl for retinal dystrophy mediated by RPE65 mutation. *J. Curr. Ophthalmol.* **2018**, *30*, 1–2. [CrossRef] [PubMed]
28. Rowe-Rendleman, C.L.; Durazo, S.A.; Kompella, U.B.; Rittenhouse, K.D.; Di Polo, A.; Weiner, A.L.; Grossniklaus, H.E.; Naash, M.I.; Lewin, A.S.; Horsager, A.; et al. Drug and Gene Delivery to the Back of the Eye: From Bench to Bedside. *Investig. Opthalmol. Vis. Sci.* **2014**, *55*, 2714–2730. [CrossRef] [PubMed]
29. Soofiyani, S.R.; Baradaran, B.; Lotfipour, F.; Kazemi, T.; Mohammadnejad, L. Gene Therapy, Early Promises, Subsequent Problems, and Recent Breakthroughs. *Adv. Pharm. Bull.* **2013**, *3*, 249–255.
30. Jacobson, S.G.; Cideciyan, A.V.; Roman, A.J.; Sumaroka, A.; Schwartz, S.B.; Héon, E.; Hauswirth, W.W. Improvement and Decline in Vision with Gene Therapy in Childhood Blindness. *N. Engl. J. Med.* **2015**, *372*, 1920–1926. [CrossRef]
31. Gao, G.; Vandenberghe, L.H.; Wilson, J.M. New recombinant serotypes of AAV vectors. *Curr. Gene Ther.* **2005**, *5*, 285–297. [CrossRef] [PubMed]
32. Vandenberghe, L.H.; Wilson, J.M.; Gao, G. Tailoring the AAV vector capsid for gene therapy. *Gene Ther.* **2009**, *16*, 311–319. [CrossRef] [PubMed]
33. Le Meur, G.; Stieger, K.; Smith, A.J.; Weber, M.; Deschamps, J.Y.; Nivard, D.; Ali, R.R. Restoration of vision in RPE65-deficient Briard dogs using an AAV serotype 4 vector that specifically targets the retinal pigmented epithelium. *Gene Ther.* **2007**, *14*, 292–303. [CrossRef] [PubMed]
34. Fischer, M.D.; McClements, M.E.; De La Camara, C.M.-F.; Bellingrath, J.-S.; Dauletbekov, D.; Ramsden, S.C.; Hickey, D.G.; Barnard, A.R.; MacLaren, R.E. Codon-Optimized RPGR Improves Stability and Efficacy of AAV8 Gene Therapy in Two Mouse Models of X-Linked Retinitis Pigmentosa. *Mol. Ther.* **2017**, *25*, 1854–1865. [CrossRef] [PubMed]
35. Georgiadis, A.; Duran, Y.; Ribeiro, J.; Abelleira-Hervas, L.; Robbie, S.J.; Sünkel-Laing, B.; Fourali, S.; Cordero, A.G.; Cristante, E.; Michaelides, M.; et al. Development of an optimized AAV2/5 gene therapy vector for Leber congenital amaurosis owing to defects in RPE65. *Gene Ther.* **2016**, *23*, 857–862. [CrossRef] [PubMed]
36. McClements, M.E.; MacLaren, R.E. Gene therapy for retinal disease. *Transl. Res.* **2013**, *161*, 241–254. [CrossRef] [PubMed]
37. Wilson, J.H.; Wensel, T.G. The Nature of Dominant Mutations of Rhodopsin and Implications for Gene Therapy. *Mol. Neurobiol.* **2003**, *28*, 149–158. [CrossRef]
38. Farrar, G.J.; Millington-Ward, S.; Chadderton, N.; Humphries, P.; Kenna, P.F. Gene-based therapies for dominantly inherited retinopathies. *Gene Ther.* **2012**, *19*, 137–144. [CrossRef]
39. O'Reilly, M.; Palfi, A.; Chadderton, N.; Millington-Ward, S.; Ader, M.; Cronin, T.; Tuohy, T.; Auricchio, A.; Hildinger, M.; Tivnan, A.; et al. RNA Interference–Mediated Suppression and Replacement of Human Rhodopsin In Vivo. *Am. J. Hum. Genet.* **2007**, *81*, 127–135. [CrossRef]
40. Dyka, F.M.; Boye, S.L.; Chiodo, V.A.; Hauswirth, W.W.; Boye, S.E. Dual adeno-associated virus vectors result in efficient in vitro and in vivo expression of an oversized gene, MYO7A. *Hum. Gene Ther. Methods* **2014**, *25*, 166–177. [CrossRef]
41. Trapani, I.; Colella, P.; Sommella, A.; Iodice, C.; Cesi, G.; de Simone, S.; Farrar, G.J. Effective delivery of large genes to the retina by dual AAV vectors. *EMBO Mol. Med.* **2014**, *6*, 194–211. [CrossRef] [PubMed]

42. Colella, P.; Trapani, I.; Cesi, G.; Sommella, A.; Manfredi, A.; Puppo, A.; Iodice, C.; Rossi, S.; Simonelli, F.; Giunti, M.; et al. Efficient gene delivery to the cone-enriched pig retina by dual AAV vectors. *Gene Ther.* **2014**, *21*, 450–456. [CrossRef] [PubMed]
43. Maddalena, A.; Tornabene, P.; Tiberi, P.; Minopoli, R.; Manfredi, A.; Mutarelli, M.; Auricchio, A. Triple Vectors Expand AAV Transfer Capacity in the Retina. *Mol. Ther.* **2018**, *26*, 524–541. [CrossRef] [PubMed]
44. Baye, L.M.; Patrinostro, X.; Swaminathan, S.; Beck, J.S.; Zhang, Y.; Stone, E.M.; Sheffield, V.C.; Slusarski, D.C. The N-terminal region of centrosomal protein 290 (CEP290) restores vision in a zebrafish model of human blindness. *Hum. Mol. Genet.* **2011**, *20*, 1467–1477. [CrossRef] [PubMed]
45. Sanjurjo-Soriano, C.; Kalatzis, V. Guiding Lights in Genome Editing for Inherited Retinal Disorders: Implications for Gene and Cell Therapy. *Neural Plast.* **2018**, *2018*, 1–15. [CrossRef] [PubMed]
46. Gaj, T.; Gersbach, C.A.; Barbas, C.F., III. ZFN, TALEN and CRISPR/Cas-based methods for genome engineering. *Trends Biotechnol.* **2013**, *31*, 397–405. [CrossRef] [PubMed]
47. Yao, X.; Wang, X.; Hu, X.; Liu, Z.; Liu, J.; Zhou, H.; Shen, X.; Wei, Y.; Huang, Z.; Ying, W.; et al. Homology-mediated end joining-based targeted integration using CRISPR/Cas9. *Cell Res.* **2017**, *27*, 801–814. [CrossRef] [PubMed]
48. Schierling, B.; Dannemann, N.; Gabsalilow, L.; Wende, W.; Cathomen, T.; Pingoud, A. A novel zinc-finger nuclease platform with a sequence-specific cleavage module. *Nucleic Acids Res.* **2012**, *40*, 2623–2638. [CrossRef] [PubMed]
49. Greenwald, D.L.; Cashman, S.M.; Kumar-Singh, R. Engineered Zinc Finger Nuclease–Mediated Homologous Recombination of the Human Rhodopsin Gene. *Investig. Opthalmol. Vis. Sci.* **2010**, *51*, 6374–6380. [CrossRef] [PubMed]
50. Low, B.E.; Krebs, M.P.; Joung, J.K.; Tsai, S.Q.; Nishina, P.M.; Wiles, M.V. Correction of the Crb1rd8 Allele and Retinal Phenotype in C57BL/6N Mice Via TALEN-Mediated Homology-Directed Repair. *Investig. Opthalmol. Vis. Sci.* **2014**, *55*, 387–395. [CrossRef] [PubMed]
51. Nelson, C.E.; Hakim, C.H.; Ousterout, D.G.; Thakore, P.I.; Moreb, E.A.; Rivera RM, C.; Asokan, A. In vivo genome editing improves muscle function in a mouse model of Duchenne muscular dystrophy. *Science* **2016**, *351*, 403–407. [CrossRef] [PubMed]
52. Hung, S.S.C.; Chrysostomou, V.; Li, F.; Lim, J.K.H.; Wang, J.-H.; Powell, J.E.; Tu, L.; Daniszewski, M.; Lo, C.; Wong, R.C.; et al. AAV-Mediated CRISPR/Cas Gene Editing of Retinal Cells In Vivo. *Investig. Opthalmol. Vis. Sci.* **2016**, *57*, 3470. [CrossRef] [PubMed]
53. Tabebordbar, M.; Zhu, K.; Cheng, J.K.; Chew, W.L.; Widrick, J.J.; Yan, W.X.; Cong, L. In vivo gene editing in dystrophic mouse muscle and muscle stem cells. *Science* **2016**, *351*, 407–411. [CrossRef] [PubMed]
54. Long, C.; Amoasii, L.; Mireault, A.A.; McAnally, J.R.; Li, H.; Sanchez-Ortiz, E.; Olson, E.N. Postnatal genome editing partially restores dystrophin expression in a mouse model of muscular dystrophy. *Science* **2016**, *351*, 400–403. [CrossRef] [PubMed]
55. Kim, S.; Kim, D.; Cho, S.W.; Kim, J.; Kim, J.-S. Highly efficient RNA-guided genome editing in human cells via delivery of purified Cas9 ribonucleoproteins. *Genome Res.* **2014**, *24*, 1012–1019. [CrossRef] [PubMed]
56. Hsu, P.D.; Scott, D.A.; Weinstein, J.A.; Ran, F.A.; Konermann, S.; Agarwala, V.; Li, Y.; Fine, E.J.; Wu, X.; Shalem, O.; et al. DNA targeting specificity of RNA-guided Cas9 nucleases. *Nat. Biotechnol.* **2013**, *31*, 827–832. [CrossRef] [PubMed]
57. Cho, S.W.; Kim, S.; Kim, Y.; Kweon, J.; Kim, H.S.; Bae, S.; Kim, J.S. Analysis of off-target effects of CRISPR/Cas-derived RNA-guided endonucleases and nickases. *Genome Res.* **2014**, *24*, 132–141. [CrossRef] [PubMed]
58. Kim, Y.; Kweon, J.; Kim, A.; Chon, J.K.; Yoo, J.Y.; Kim, H.J.; Kim, S.; Lee, C.; Jeong, E.; Chung, E.; et al. A library of TAL effector nucleases spanning the human genome. *Nat. Biotechnol.* **2013**, *31*, 251–258. [CrossRef] [PubMed]
59. Peddle, C.F.; MacLaren, R.E. The Application of CRISPR/Cas9 for the Treatment of Retinal Diseases. *Yale J. Boil. Med.* **2017**, *90*, 533–541.
60. Slaymaker, I.M.; Gao, L.; Zetsche, B.; Scott, D.A.; Yan, W.X.; Zhang, F. Rationally engineered Cas9 nucleases with improved specificity. *Science* **2016**, *351*, 84–88. [CrossRef]
61. Jo, D.H.; Koo, T.; Cho, C.S.; Kim, J.H.; Kim, J.-S.; Kim, J.H. Long-Term Effects of In Vivo Genome Editing in the Mouse Retina Using Campylobacter jejuni Cas9 Expressed via Adeno-Associated Virus. *Mol. Ther.* **2019**, *27*, 130–136. [CrossRef]

62. Li, F.; Hung, S.S.; Khalid, M.K.N.M.; Wang, J.-H.; Chrysostomou, V.; Wong, V.H.; Singh, V.; Wing, K.; Tu, L.; Bender, J.A.; et al. Utility of self-destructing CRISPR/Cas constructs for targeted gene editing in the retina. *Hum. Gene Ther.* **2019**. [CrossRef]
63. Zelinka, C.P.; Sotolongo-Lopez, M.; Fadool, J.M. Targeted disruption of the endogenous zebrafish rhodopsin locus as models of rapid rod photoreceptor degeneration. *Mol. Vis.* **2018**, *24*, 587–602.
64. Xia, C.-H.; Ferguson, I.; Li, M.; Kim, A.; Onishi, A.; Li, L.; Su, B.; Gong, X. Essential function of NHE8 in mouse retina demonstrated by AAV-mediated CRISPR/Cas9 knockdown. *Exp. Eye Res.* **2018**, *176*, 29–39. [CrossRef]
65. Moreno, A.M.; Fu, X.; Zhu, J.; Katrekar, D.; Shih, Y.-R.V.; Marlett, J.; Cabotaje, J.; Tat, J.; Naughton, J.; Lisowski, L.; et al. In Situ Gene Therapy via AAV-CRISPR-Cas9-Mediated Targeted Gene Regulation. *Mol. Ther.* **2018**, *26*, 1818–1827. [CrossRef]
66. Giannelli, S.G.; Luoni, M.; Castoldi, V.; Massimino, L.; Cabassi, T.; Angeloni, D.; Broccoli, V. Cas9/sgRNA selective targeting of the P23H Rhodopsin mutant allele for treating retinitis pigmentosa by intravitreal AAV9.PHP.B-based delivery. *Hum. Mol. Genet.* **2018**, *27*, 761–779. [CrossRef]
67. Burnight, E.R.; Gupta, M.; Wiley, L.A.; Anfinson, K.R.; Tran, A.; Triboulet, R.; Hoffmann, J.M.; Klaahsen, D.L.; Andorf, J.L.; Jiao, C.; et al. Using CRISPR-Cas9 to Generate Gene-Corrected Autologous iPSCs for the Treatment of Inherited Retinal Degeneration. *Mol. Ther.* **2017**, *25*, 1999–2013. [CrossRef]
68. Kim, E.; Koo, T.; Park, S.W.; Kim, D.; Kim, K.; Cho, H.-Y.; Song, D.W.; Lee, K.J.; Jung, M.H.; Kim, S.; et al. In vivo genome editing with a small Cas9 orthologue derived from Campylobacter jejuni. *Nat. Commun.* **2017**, *8*, 14500. [CrossRef]
69. Latella, M.C.; Di Salvo, M.T.; Cocchiarella, F.; Benati, D.; Grisendi, G.; Comitato, A.; Marigo, V.; Recchia, A. In vivo Editing of the Human Mutant Rhodopsin Gene by Electroporation of Plasmid-based CRISPR/Cas9 in the Mouse Retina. *Mol. Ther. Nucleic Acids* **2016**, *5*, e389. [CrossRef]
70. Bassuk, A.G.; Zheng, A.; Li, Y.; Tsang, S.H.; Mahajan, V.B. Precision Medicine: Genetic Repair of Retinitis Pigmentosa in Patient-Derived Stem Cells. *Sci. Rep.* **2016**, *6*, 19969. [CrossRef]
71. Wu, W.-H.; Tsai, Y.-T.; Justus, S.; Lee, T.-T.; Zhang, L.; Lin, C.-S.; Bassuk, A.G.; Mahajan, V.B.; Tsang, S.H. CRISPR Repair Reveals Causative Mutation in a Preclinical Model of Retinitis Pigmentosa. *Mol. Ther.* **2016**, *24*, 1388–1394. [CrossRef]
72. Zhong, H.; Chen, Y.; Li, Y.; Chen, R.; Mardon, G. CRISPR-engineered mosaicism rapidly reveals that loss of Kcnj13 function in mice mimics human disease phenotypes. *Sci. Rep.* **2015**, *5*, 8366. [CrossRef]
73. Swiech, L.; Heidenreich, M.; Banerjee, A.; Habib, N.; Li, Y.; Trombetta, J.; Zhang, F. In vivo interrogation of gene function in the mammalian brain using CRISPR-Cas9. *Nat. Biotechnol.* **2015**, *33*, 102–106. [CrossRef]
74. Wang, D.; Mou, H.; Li, S.; Li, Y.; Hough, S.; Tran, K.; Li, J.; Yin, H.; Anderson, D.G.; Sontheimer, E.J.; et al. Adenovirus-Mediated Somatic Genome Editing of Pten by CRISPR/Cas9 in Mouse Liver in Spite of Cas9-Specific Immune Responses. *Hum. Gene Ther.* **2015**, *26*, 432–442. [CrossRef]
75. Lin, S.; Staahl, B.T.; Alla, R.K.; Doudna, J.A. Enhanced homology-directed human genome engineering by controlled timing of CRISPR/Cas9 delivery. *eLife* **2014**, *3*, 04766. [CrossRef]
76. Kim, K.; Park, S.W.; Kim, J.H.; Lee, S.H.; Kim, D.; Koo, T.; Kim, K.-E.; Kim, J.H.; Kim, J.-S. Genome surgery using Cas9 ribonucleoproteins for the treatment of age-related macular degeneration. *Genome Res.* **2017**, *27*, 419–426. [CrossRef]
77. Suzuki, K.; Tsunekawa, Y.; Hernandez-Benitez, R.; Wu, J.; Zhu, J.; Kim, E.J.; Hatanaka, F.; Yamamoto, M.; Araoka, T.; Li, Z.; et al. In vivo genome editing via CRISPR/Cas9 mediated homology-independent targeted integration. *Nature* **2016**, *540*, 144–149. [CrossRef]
78. Diakatou, M.; Manes, G.; Bocquet, B.; Meunier, I.; Kalatzis, V. Genome Editing as a Treatment for the Most Prevalent Causative Genes of Autosomal Dominant Retinitis Pigmentosa. *Int. J. Mol. Sci.* **2019**, *20*, 2542. [CrossRef]
79. Garanto, A.; Van Beersum, S.E.C.; Peters, T.A.; Roepman, R.; Cremers, F.P.M.; Collin, R.W.J. Unexpected CEP290 mRNA Splicing in a Humanized Knock-In Mouse Model for Leber Congenital Amaurosis. *PLoS ONE* **2013**, *8*, e79369. [CrossRef]
80. Maeder, M.L.; Stefanidakis, M.; Wilson, C.J.; Baral, R.; Barrera, L.A.; Bounoutas, G.S.; Bumcrot, D.; Chao, H.; Ciulla, D.M.; DaSilva, J.A.; et al. Development of a gene-editing approach to restore vision loss in Leber congenital amaurosis type 10. *Nat. Med.* **2019**, *25*, 229–233. [CrossRef]
81. Duebel, J.; Marazova, K.; Sahel, J.A. Optogenetics. *Curr. Opin. Ophthalmol.* **2015**, *26*, 226–232. [CrossRef]

82. Simunovic, M.; Shen, W.; Lin, J.; Protti, D.; Lisowski, L.; Gillies, M. Optogenetic approaches to vision restoration. *Exp. Eye Res.* **2019**, *178*, 15–26. [CrossRef]
83. Deisseroth, K.; Feng, G.; Majewska, A.K.; Miesenböck, G.; Ting, A.; Schnitzer, M.J. Next-Generation Optical Technologies for Illuminating Genetically Targeted Brain Circuits. *J. Neurosci.* **2006**, *26*, 10380–10386. [CrossRef]
84. Yue, L.; Weiland, J.D.; Roska, B.; Humayun, M.S. Retinal stimulation strategies to restore vision: Fundamentals and systems. *Prog. Retin. Eye Res.* **2016**, *53*, 21–47. [CrossRef]
85. Zhang, F.; Vierock, J.; Yizhar, O.; Fenno, L.E.; Tsunoda, S.; Kianianmomeni, A.; Prigge, M.; Berndt, A.; Cushman, J.; Polle, J.; et al. The Microbial Opsin Family of Optogenetic Tools. *Cell* **2011**, *147*, 1446–1457. [CrossRef]
86. Bernstein, J.G.; Boyden, E.S. Optogenetic tools for analyzing the neural circuits of behavior. *Trends Cogn. Sci.* **2011**, *15*, 592–600. [CrossRef]
87. Ahnelt, P.K.; Kolb, H. The mammalian photoreceptor mosaic-adaptive design. *Prog. Retin. Eye Res.* **2000**, *19*, 711–777. [CrossRef]
88. Gaub, B.M.; Berry, M.H.; Holt, A.E.; Isacoff, E.Y.; Flannery, J.G. Optogenetic Vision Restoration Using Rhodopsin for Enhanced Sensitivity. *Mol. Ther.* **2015**, *23*, 1562–1571. [CrossRef]
89. Sengupta, A.; Chaffiol, A.; Macé, E.; Caplette, R.; Desrosiers, M.; Lampič, M.; Forster, V.; Marre, O.; Lin, J.Y.; Sahel, J.; et al. Red-shifted channelrhodopsin stimulation restores light responses in blind mice, macaque retina, and human retina. *EMBO Mol. Med.* **2016**, *8*, 1248–1264. [CrossRef]
90. Liu, M.M.; Zack, D.J. Alternative splicing and retinal degeneration. *Clin. Genet.* **2013**, *84*, 142–149. [CrossRef]
91. Hammond, S.M.; Wood, M.J. Genetic therapies for RNA mis-splicing diseases. *Trends Genet.* **2011**, *27*, 196–205. [CrossRef]
92. Garanto, A.; Collin, R.W.J. Applications of antisense oligonucleotides for the treatment of inherited retinal diseases. *Curr. Opin. Ophthalmol.* **2017**, *28*, 1–266.
93. Bacchi, N.; Casarosa, S.; Denti, M.A. Splicing-Correcting Therapeutic Approaches for Retinal Dystrophies: Where Endogenous Gene Regulation and Specificity Matter. *Investig. Opthalmol. Vis. Sci.* **2014**, *55*, 3285–3294. [CrossRef]
94. Chan, J.H.; Lim, S.; Wong, W.F. Antisense oligonucleotides: from design to therapeutic application. *Clin. Exp. Pharmacol. Physiol.* **2006**, *33*, 533–540. [CrossRef]
95. Goyenvalle, A.; Vulin, A.; Fougerousse, F.; Leturcq, F.; Kaplan, J.-C.; García, L.; Danos, O. Rescue of Dystrophic Muscle Through U7 snRNA-Mediated Exon Skipping. *Science* **2004**, *306*, 1796–1799. [CrossRef]
96. Garanto, A.; Chung, D.C.; Duijkers, L.; Corral-Serrano, J.C.; Messchaert, M.; Xiao, R.; Bennett, J.; Vandenberghe, L.H.; Collin, R.W. In vitro and in vivo rescue of aberrant splicing in CEP290-associated LCA by antisense oligonucleotide delivery. *Hum. Mol. Genet.* **2016**, *25*, 2552–2563.
97. Vitravene Study Group. Safety of intravitreous fomivirsen for treatment of cytomegalovirus retinitis in patients with AIDS. *Am. J. Ophthalmol.* **2002**, *133*, 484–498.
98. Vitravene Study Group. Randomized dose-comparison studies of intravitreous fomivirsen for treatment of cytomegalovirus retinitis that has reactivated or is persistently active despite other therapies in patients with AIDS. *Am. J. Ophthalmol.* **2002**, *133*, 475–483.
99. Den Hollander, A.I.; Koenekoop, R.K.; Yzer, S.; Lopez, I.; Arends, M.L.; Voesenek, K.E.J.; Zonneveld, M.N.; Strom, T.M.; Meitinger, T.; Brunner, H.G.; et al. Mutations in the CEP290 (NPHP6) Gene Are a Frequent Cause of Leber Congenital Amaurosis. *Am. J. Hum. Genet.* **2006**, *79*, 556–561. [CrossRef]
100. Collin, R.W.; Hollander, A.I.D.; Van Der Velde-Visser, S.D.; Bennicelli, J.; Bennett, J.; Cremers, F.P. Antisense Oligonucleotide (AON)-based Therapy for Leber Congenital Amaurosis Caused by a Frequent Mutation in CEP290. *Mol. Ther. Nucleic Acids* **2012**, *1*, e14. [CrossRef]
101. Gerard, X.; Perrault, I.; Hanein, S.; Silva, E.; Bigot, K.; Defoort-Delhemmes, S.; Rio, M.; Munnich, A.; Scherman, D.; Kaplan, J.; et al. AON-mediated Exon Skipping Restores Ciliation in Fibroblasts Harboring the Common Leber Congenital Amaurosis CEP290 Mutation. *Mol. Ther. Nucleic Acids* **2012**, *1*, e29. [CrossRef]
102. Parfitt, D.A.; Lane, A.; Ramsden, C.M.; Carr, A.-J.F.; Munro, P.M.; Jovanovic, K.; Schwarz, N.; Kanuga, N.; Muthiah, M.N.; Hull, S.; et al. Identification and Correction of Mechanisms Underlying Inherited Blindness in Human iPSC-Derived Optic Cups. *Cell Stem Cell* **2016**, *18*, 769–781. [CrossRef]

103. Duijkers, L.; van den Born, L.; Neidhardt, J.; Bax, N.; Pierrache, L.; Klevering, B.; Garanto, A. Antisense Oligonucleotide-Based Splicing Correction in Individuals with Leber Congenital Amaurosis due to Compound Heterozygosity for the c.2991+1655A>G Mutation in CEP290. *Int. J. Mol. Sci.* **2018**, *19*, 753. [CrossRef]
104. Dulla, K.; Aguila, M.; Lane, A.; Jovanovic, K.; Parfitt, D.A.; Schulkens, I.; Collin, R.W. Splice-Modulating Oligonucleotide QR-110 Restores CEP290 mRNA and Function in Human c.2991+1655A>G LCA10 Models. *Mol. Ther. Nucleic Acids* **2018**, *12*, 730–740. [CrossRef]
105. Cideciyan, A.V.; Jacobson, S.G.; Drack, A.V.; Ho, A.C.; Charng, J.; Garafalo, A.V.; Pfeifer, W.L. Effect of an intravitreal antisense oligonucleotide on vision in Leber congenital amaurosis due to a photoreceptor cilium defect. *Nat. Med.* **2019**, *25*, 225–228. [CrossRef]
106. Barny, I.; Perrault, I.; Michel, C.; Goudin, N.; Defoort-Dhellemmes, S.; Ghazi, I.; Kaplan, J.; Rozet, J.-M.; Gerard, X. AON-Mediated Exon Skipping to Bypass Protein Truncation in Retinal Dystrophies Due to the Recurrent CEP290 c.4723A > T Mutation. Fact or Fiction? *Genes* **2019**, *10*, 368. [CrossRef]
107. Bonifert, T.; Menendez, I.G.; Battke, F.; Theurer, Y.; Synofzik, M.; Schöls, L.; Wissinger, B. Antisense Oligonucleotide Mediated Splice Correction of a Deep Intronic Mutation in OPA1. *Mol. Ther. Nucleic Acids* **2016**, *5*, e390. [CrossRef]
108. Garanto, A.; Van Der Velde-Visser, S.D.; Cremers, F.P.M.; Collin, R.W.J. Antisense Oligonucleotide-Based Splice Correction of a Deep-Intronic Mutation in CHM Underlying Choroideremia. In *Results and Problems in Cell Differentiation*; Springer: Cham, Switzerland, 2018; pp. 83–89.
109. Slijkerman, R.W.; Vaché, C.; Dona, M.; García-García, G.; Claustres, M.; Hetterschijt, L.; Peters, T.A.; Hartel, B.P.; Pennings, R.J.; Millan, J.M.; et al. Antisense Oligonucleotide-based Splice Correction for USH2A-associated Retinal Degeneration Caused by a Frequent Deep-intronic Mutation. *Mol. Ther. Nucleic Acids* **2016**, *5*, e381. [CrossRef]
110. Albert, S.; Garanto, A.; Sangermano, R.; Khan, M.; Bax, N.M.; Hoyng, C.B.; Zernant, J.; Lee, W.; Allikmets, R.; Collin, R.W.; et al. Identification and Rescue of Splice Defects Caused by Two Neighboring Deep-Intronic ABCA4 Mutations Underlying Stargardt Disease. *Am. J. Hum. Genet.* **2018**, *102*, 517–527. [CrossRef]
111. Sangermano, R.; Garanto, A.; Khan, M.; Runhart, E.H.; Bauwens, M.; Bax, N.M.; Born, L.I.V.D.; Khan, M.I.; Cornelis, S.S.; Verheij, J.B.G.M.; et al. Deep-intronic ABCA4 variants explain missing heritability in Stargardt disease and allow correction of splice defects by antisense oligonucleotides. *Genet. Med.* **2019**, *21*, 1751–1760. [CrossRef]
112. Bauwens, M.; Garanto, A.; Sangermano, R.; Naessens, S.; Weisschuh, N.; De Zaeytijd, J.; Khan, M.; Sadler, F.; Balikova, I.; Van Cauwenbergh, C.; et al. ABCA4-associated disease as a model for missing heritability in autosomal recessive disorders: Novel noncoding splice, cis-regulatory, structural, and recurrent hypomorphic variants. *Genet. Med.* **2019**, *21*, 1761–1771. [CrossRef] [PubMed]
113. Garanto, A.; Duijkers, L.; Tomkiewicz, T.Z.; Collin, R.W. Antisense Oligonucleotide Screening to Optimize the Rescue of the Splicing Defect Caused by the Recurrent Deep-Intronic ABCA4 Variant c.4539+2001G>A in Stargardt Disease. *Genes* **2019**, *10*, 452. [CrossRef] [PubMed]
114. Tanner, G.; Glaus, E.; Barthelmes, D.; Ader, M.; Fleischhauer, J.; Pagani, F.; Berger, W.; Neidhardt, J. Therapeutic strategy to rescue mutation-induced exon skipping in rhodopsin by adaptation of U1 snRNA. *Hum. Mutat.* **2009**, *30*, 255–263. [CrossRef] [PubMed]
115. Schmid, F.; Glaus, E.; Barthelmes, D.; Fliegauf, M.; Gaspar, H.; Nürnberg, G.; Nürnberg, P.; Omran, H.; Berger, W.; Neidhardt, J. U1 snRNA-mediated gene therapeutic correction of splice defects caused by an exceptionally mild BBS mutation. *Hum. Mutat.* **2011**, *32*, 815–824. [CrossRef] [PubMed]
116. Glaus, E.; Schmid, F.; Da Costa, R.; Berger, W.; Neidhardt, J. Gene Therapeutic Approach Using Mutation-adapted U1 snRNA to Correct a RPGR Splice Defect in Patient-derived Cells. *Mol. Ther.* **2011**, *19*, 936–941. [CrossRef]
117. Schmid, F.; Hiller, T.; Korner, G.; Glaus, E.; Berger, W.; Neidhardt, J. A Gene Therapeutic Approach to Correct Splice Defects with Modified U1 and U6 snRNPs. *Hum. Gene Ther.* **2013**, *24*, 97–104. [CrossRef] [PubMed]
118. Abad, X.; Vera, M.; Jung, S.P.; Oswald, E.; Romero, I.; Amin, V.; Fortes, P.; Gunderson, S.I. Requirements for gene silencing mediated by U1 snRNA binding to a target sequence. *Nucleic Acids Res.* **2008**, *36*, 2338–2352. [CrossRef]

119. Berger, A.; Lorain, S.; Joséphine, C.; Desrosiers, M.; Peccate, C.; Voit, T.; Garcia, L.; Sahel, J.-A.; Bemelmans, A.-P. Repair of Rhodopsin mRNA by Spliceosome-Mediated RNA Trans. -Splicing: A New Approach for Autosomal Dominant Retinitis Pigmentosa. *Mol. Ther.* **2015**, *23*, 918–930. [CrossRef]
120. Lei, Q.; Li, C.; Zuo, Z.; Huang, C.; Cheng, H.; Zhou, R. Evolutionary Insights into RNA trans-Splicing in Vertebrates. *Genome Boil. Evol.* **2016**, *8*, 562–577. [CrossRef]
121. Li, N.; Zheng, J.; Li, H.; Deng, J.; Hu, M.; Wu, H.; Li, W.; Li, F.; Lan, X.; Lu, J.; et al. Identification of chimeric TSNAX–DISC1 resulting from intergenic splicing in endometrial carcinoma through high-throughput RNA sequencing. *Carcinogenesis* **2014**, *35*, 2687–2697. [CrossRef]
122. Guerra, E.; Trerotola, M.; Arciprete, R.D.; Bonasera, V.; Palombo, B.; El-Sewedy, T.; Ciccimarra, T.; Crescenzi, C.; Lorenzini, F.; Rossi, C.; et al. A Bicistronic CYCLIN D1-TROP2 mRNA Chimera Demonstrates a Novel Oncogenic Mechanism in Human Cancer. *Cancer Res.* **2008**, *68*, 8113–8121. [CrossRef] [PubMed]
123. Hirano, M.; Noda, T. Genomic organization of the mouse Msh4 gene producing bicistronic, chimeric and antisense mRNA. *Gene* **2004**, *342*, 165–177. [CrossRef] [PubMed]
124. Dooley, S.J.; McDougald, D.S.; Fisher, K.J.; Bennicelli, J.L.; Mitchell, L.G.; Bennett, J. Spliceosome-Mediated Pre-mRNA trans-Splicing Can Repair CEP290 mRNA. *Mol. Ther. Nucleic Acids* **2018**, *12*, 294–308. [CrossRef] [PubMed]
125. Saurabh, S.; Vidyarthi, A.S.; Prasad, D. RNA interference: Concept to reality in crop improvement. *Planta* **2014**, *239*, 543–564. [CrossRef] [PubMed]
126. Qiu, S.; Adema, C.M.; Lane, T. A computational study of off-target effects of RNA interference. *Nucleic Acids Res.* **2005**, *33*, 1834–1847. [CrossRef] [PubMed]
127. Ryoo, N.-K.; Lee, J.; Lee, H.; Hong, H.K.; Kim, H.; Lee, J.B.; Woo, S.J.; Park, K.H.; Kim, H. Therapeutic effects of a novel siRNA-based anti-VEGF (siVEGF) nanoball for the treatment of choroidal neovascularization. *Nanoscale* **2017**, *9*, 15461–15469. [CrossRef] [PubMed]
128. Yau, E.H.; Butler, M.C.; Sullivan, J.M. A Cellular High-Throughput Screening Approach for Therapeutic trans-Cleaving Ribozymes and RNAi against Arbitrary mRNA Disease Targets. *Exp. Eye Res.* **2016**, *151*, 236–255. [CrossRef] [PubMed]
129. Lagos-Quintana, M.; Rauhut, R.; Meyer, J.; Borkhardt, A.; Tuschl, T. New microRNAs from mouse and human. *RNA* **2003**, *9*, 175–179. [CrossRef]
130. Zuzic, M.; Arias, J.E.R.; Wohl, S.G.; Busskamp, V. Retinal miRNA Functions in Health and Disease. *Genes* **2019**, *10*, 377. [CrossRef]
131. Mangos, M.M.; Min, K.-L.; Viazovkina, E.; Galarneau, A.; Elzagheid, M.I.; Parniak, M.A.; Damha, M.J. Efficient RNase H-Directed Cleavage of RNA Promoted by Antisense DNA or 2′F-ANA Constructs Containing Acyclic Nucleotide Inserts. *J. Am. Chem. Soc.* **2003**, *125*, 654–661. [CrossRef]
132. Honcharenko, D.; Barman, J.; Varghese, O.P. Comparison of the RNase H Cleavage Kinetics and Blood Serum Stability of theNorth-Conformationally Constrained and 2′-Alkoxy Modified Oligonucleotides†. *Biochemistry* **2007**, *46*, 5635–5646. [CrossRef] [PubMed]
133. Murray, S.F.; Jazayeri, A.; Matthes, M.T.; Yasumura, D.; Yang, H.; Peralta, R.; Watt, A.; Freier, S.; Hung, G.; Adamson, P.S.; et al. Allele-Specific Inhibition of Rhodopsin With an Antisense Oligonucleotide Slows Photoreceptor Cell Degeneration. *Investig. Opthalmol. Vis. Sci.* **2015**, *56*, 6362–6375. [CrossRef] [PubMed]
134. Naessens, S.; Ruysschaert, L.; Lefever, S.; Coppieters, F.; De Baere, E. Antisense Oligonucleotide-Based Downregulation of the G56R Pathogenic Variant Causing NR2E3-Associated Autosomal Dominant Retinitis Pigmentosa. *Genes* **2019**, *10*, 363. [CrossRef] [PubMed]
135. Cox, D.B.; Gootenberg, J.S.; Abudayyeh, O.O.; Franklin, B.; Kellner, M.J.; Joung, J.; Zhang, F. RNA editing with CRISPR-Cas13. *Science* **2017**, *358*, 1019–1027. [CrossRef] [PubMed]
136. Shmakov, S.; Smargon, A.; Scott, D.; Cox, D.; Pyzocha, N.; Yan, W.; Abudayyeh, O.O.; Gootenberg, J.S.; Makarova, K.S.; Wolf, Y.I.; et al. Diversity and evolution of class 2 CRISPR–Cas systems. *Nat. Rev. Genet.* **2017**, *15*, 169–182. [CrossRef] [PubMed]
137. Abudayyeh, O.O.; Gootenberg, J.S.; Essletzbichler, P.; Han, S.; Joung, J.; Belanto, J.J.; Lander, E.S. RNA targeting with CRISPR-Cas13. *Nature* **2017**, *550*, 280–284. [CrossRef]
138. Stafforst, T.; Schneider, M.F. An RNA-Deaminase Conjugate Selectively Repairs Point Mutations. *Angew. Chem. Int. Ed.* **2012**, *51*, 11166–11169. [CrossRef] [PubMed]
139. Wettengel, J.; Reautschnig, P.; Geisler, S.; Kahle, P.J.; Stafforst, T. Harnessing human ADAR2 for RNA repair - Recoding a PINK1 mutation rescues mitophagy. *Nucleic Acids Res.* **2017**, *45*, 2797–2808. [CrossRef]

140. Vighi, E.; Trifunović, D.; Veiga-Crespo, P.; Rentsch, A.; Hoffmann, D.; Sahaboglu, A.; Strasser, T.; Kulkarni, M.; Bertolotti, E.; Heuvel, A.V.D.; et al. Combination of cGMP analogue and drug delivery system provides functional protection in hereditary retinal degeneration. *Proc. Natl. Acad. Sci. USA* **2018**, *115*, E2997–E3006. [CrossRef]

141. Nagel-Wolfrum, K.; Möller, F.; Penner, I.; Baasov, T.; Wolfrum, U. Targeting Nonsense Mutations in Diseases with Translational Read-Through-Inducing Drugs (TRIDs). *BioDrugs* **2016**, *30*, 49–74. [CrossRef]

142. Schwarz, N.; Carr, A.J.; Lane, A.; Moeller, F.; Chen, L.L.; Aguila, M.; Nagel-Wolfrum, K. Translational read-through of the RP2 Arg120stop mutation in patient iPSC-derived retinal pigment epithelium cells. *Hum. Mol. Genet.* **2015**, *24*, 972–986. [CrossRef] [PubMed]

143. Guérin, K.; Gregory-Evans, C.; Hodges, M.D.J.; Moosajee, M.; Mackay, D.; Gregory-Evans, K.; Flannery, J.G.; Mackay, D. Systemic aminoglycoside treatment in rodent models of retinitis pigmentosa. *Exp. Eye Res.* **2008**, *87*, 197–207. [CrossRef] [PubMed]

144. Goldmann, T.; Overlack, N.; Möller, F.; Belakhov, V.; Van Wyk, M.; Baasov, T.; Wolfrum, U.; Nagel-Wolfrum, K. A comparative evaluation of NB30, NB54 and PTC124 in translational read-through efficacy for treatment of an USH1C nonsense mutation. *EMBO Mol. Med.* **2012**, *4*, 1186–1199. [CrossRef] [PubMed]

145. Goldmann, T.; Rebibo-Sabbah, A.; Overlack, N.; Nudelman, I.; Belakhov, V.; Baasov, T.; Ben-Yosef, T.; Wolfrum, U.; Nagel-Wolfrum, K. Beneficial Read-Through of a USH1C Nonsense Mutation by Designed Aminoglycoside NB30 in the Retina. *Investig. Opthalmol. Vis. Sci.* **2010**, *51*, 6671–6680. [CrossRef] [PubMed]

146. Nudelman, I.; Glikin, D.; Smolkin, B.; Hainrichson, M.; Belakhov, V.; Baasov, T. Repairing faulty genes by aminoglycosides: Development of new derivatives of geneticin (G418) with enhanced suppression of diseases-causing nonsense mutations. *Bioorganic Med. Chem.* **2010**, *18*, 3735–3746. [CrossRef] [PubMed]

147. Nudelman, I.; Rebibo-Sabbah, A.; Cherniavsky, M.; Belakhov, V.; Hainrichson, M.; Chen, F.; Schacht, J.; Pilch, D.S.; Ben-Yosef, T.; Baasov, T. Development of novel aminoglycoside (NB54) with reduced toxicity and enhanced suppression of disease-causing premature stop mutations. *J. Med. Chem.* **2009**, *52*, 2836–2845. [CrossRef] [PubMed]

148. Nudelman, I.; Rebibo-Sabbah, A.; Shallom-Shezifi, D.; Hainrichson, M.; Stahl, I.; Ben-Yosef, T.; Baasov, T. Redesign of aminoglycosides for treatment of human genetic diseases caused by premature stop mutations. *Bioorganic Med. Chem. Lett.* **2006**, *16*, 6310–6315. [CrossRef]

149. Rebibo-Sabbah, A.; Nudelman, I.; Ahmed, Z.M.; Baasov, T.; Ben-Yosef, T. In vitro and ex vivo suppression by aminoglycosides of PCDH15 nonsense mutations underlying type 1 Usher syndrome. *Qual. Life Res.* **2007**, *122*, 373–381. [CrossRef]

150. Welch, E.M.; Barton, E.R.; Zhuo, J.; Tomizawa, Y.; Friesen, W.J.; Trifillis, P.; Paushkin, S.; Patel, M.; Trotta, C.R.; Hwang, S.; et al. PTC124 targets genetic disorders caused by nonsense mutations. *Nature* **2007**, *447*, 87–91. [CrossRef]

151. Shimizu-Motohashi, Y.; Komaki, H.; Motohashi, N.; Takeda, S.; Yokota, T.; Aoki, Y. Restoring Dystrophin Expression in Duchenne Muscular Dystrophy: Current Status of Therapeutic Approaches. *J. Pers. Med.* **2019**, *9*, 1. [CrossRef]

152. Sermet-Gaudelus, I.; De Boeck, K.; Casimir, G.J.; Vermeulen, F.; Leal, T.; Mogenet, A.; Roussel, D.; Fritsch, J.; Hanssens, L.; Hirawat, S.; et al. Ataluren (PTC124) Induces Cystic Fibrosis Transmembrane Conductance Regulator Protein Expression and Activity in Children with Nonsense Mutation Cystic Fibrosis. *Am. J. Respir. Crit. Care Med.* **2010**, *182*, 1262–1272. [CrossRef] [PubMed]

153. Xue, X.; Mutyam, V.; Tang, L.; Biswas, S.; Du, M.; Jackson, L.A.; Dai, Y.; Belakhov, V.; Shalev, M.; Chen, F.; et al. Synthetic Aminoglycosides Efficiently Suppress Cystic Fibrosis Transmembrane Conductance Regulator Nonsense Mutations and Are Enhanced by Ivacaftor. *Am. J. Respir. Cell Mol. Boil.* **2014**, *50*, 805–816. [CrossRef] [PubMed]

154. Moosajee, M.; Tracey-White, D.; Smart, M.; Weetall, M.; Torriano, S.; Kalatzis, V.; Da Cruz, L.; Coffey, P.; Webster, A.R.; Welch, E. Functional rescue of REP1 following treatment with PTC124 and novel derivative PTC-414 in human choroideremia fibroblasts and the nonsense-mediated zebrafish model. *Hum. Mol. Genet.* **2016**, *25*, 3416–3431. [CrossRef] [PubMed]

155. Torriano, S.; Erkilic, N.; Baux, D.; Cereso, N.; De Luca, V.; Meunier, I.; Moosajee, M.; Roux, A.-F.; Hamel, C.P.; Kalatzis, V. The effect of PTC124 on choroideremia fibroblasts and iPSC-derived RPE raises considerations for therapy. *Sci. Rep.* **2018**, *8*, 8234. [CrossRef] [PubMed]

156. Sarkar, H.; Mitsios, A.; Smart, M.; Skinner, J.; Welch, A.A.; Kalatzis, V.; Coffey, P.J.; Dubis, A.M.; Webster, A.R.; Moosajee, M. Nonsense-mediated mRNA decay efficiency varies in choroideremia providing a target to boost small molecule therapeutics. *Hum. Mol. Genet.* **2019**, *28*, 1865–1871. [CrossRef] [PubMed]
157. Madni, A.; Sarfraz, M.; Rehman, M.; Ahmad, M.; Akhtar, N.; Ahmad, S.; Tahir, N.; Ijaz, S.; Al-Kassas, R.; Löbenberg, R.; et al. Liposomal Drug Delivery: A Versatile Platform for Challenging Clinical Applications. *J. Pharm. Pharm. Sci.* **2014**, *17*, 401–426. [CrossRef] [PubMed]
158. Parfitt, D.A.; Cheetham, M.E. Targeting the Proteostasis Network in Rhodopsin Retinitis Pigmentosa. *Adv. Exp. Med. Biol.* **2016**, *854*, 479–484. [PubMed]
159. Faber, S.; Roepman, R. Balancing the Photoreceptor Proteome: Proteostasis Network Therapeutics for Inherited Retinal Disease. *Genes* **2019**, *10*, 557. [CrossRef] [PubMed]
160. Parfitt, D.A.; Aguila, M.; McCulley, C.H.; Bevilacqua, D.; Mendes, H.F.; Athanasiou, D.; Novoselov, S.S.; Kanuga, N.; Munro, P.M.; Coffey, P.J.; et al. The heat-shock response co-inducer arimoclomol protects against retinal degeneration in rhodopsin retinitis pigmentosa. *Cell Death Dis.* **2014**, *5*, e1236. [CrossRef]
161. Athanasiou, D.; Aguila, M.; Bellingham, J.; Li, W.; McCulley, C.; Reeves, P.J.; Cheetham, M.E. The molecular and cellular basis of rhodopsin retinitis pigmentosa reveals potential strategies for therapy. *Prog. Retin Eye Res.* **2018**, *62*, 1–23. [CrossRef]
162. Mendes, H.F.; Cheetham, M.E. Pharmacological manipulation of gain-of-function and dominant-negative mechanisms in rhodopsin retinitis pigmentosa. *Hum. Mol. Genet.* **2008**, *17*, 3043–3054. [CrossRef] [PubMed]
163. Bogéa, T.H.; Wen, R.H.; Moritz, O.L. Light Induces Ultrastructural Changes in Rod Outer and Inner Segments, Including Autophagy, in a Transgenic Xenopus laevis P23H Rhodopsin Model of Retinitis Pigmentosa. *Investig. Opthalmol. Vis. Sci.* **2015**, *56*, 7947–7955. [CrossRef] [PubMed]
164. Sakami, S.; Maeda, T.; Bereta, G.; Okano, K.; Golczak, M.; Sumaroka, A.; Roman, A.J.; Cideciyan, A.V.; Jacobson, S.G.; Palczewski, K. Probing Mechanisms of Photoreceptor Degeneration in a New Mouse Model of the Common Form of Autosomal Dominant Retinitis Pigmentosa due to P23H Opsin Mutations. *J. Boil. Chem.* **2011**, *286*, 10551–10567. [CrossRef] [PubMed]
165. Lax, P.; Pinilla, I.; Cuenca, N.; Fernández-Sánchez, L.; Martín-Nieto, J. Tauroursodeoxycholic Acid Prevents Retinal Degeneration in Transgenic P23H Rats. *Investig. Opthalmol. Vis. Sci.* **2011**, *52*, 4998–5008.
166. Tao, Y.; Dong, X.; Lu, X.; Qu, Y.; Wang, C.; Peng, G.; Zhang, J. Subcutaneous delivery of tauroursodeoxycholic acid rescues the cone photoreceptors in degenerative retina: A promising therapeutic molecule for retinopathy. *Biomed. Pharmacother.* **2019**, *117*, 109021. [CrossRef] [PubMed]
167. Lobysheva, E.; Taylor, C.; Marshall, G.; Kisselev, O. Tauroursodeoxycholic acid binds to the G-protein site on light activated rhodopsin. *Exp. Eye Res.* **2018**, *170*, 51–57. [CrossRef] [PubMed]
168. Remondelli, P.; Renna, M. The Endoplasmic Reticulum Unfolded Protein Response in Neurodegenerative Disorders and Its Potential Therapeutic Significance. *Front. Mol. Neurosci.* **2017**, *10*, 187. [CrossRef]
169. Tolone, A.; Belhadj, S.; Rentsch, A.; Schwede, F.; Paquet-Durand, F. The cGMP Pathway and Inherited Photoreceptor Degeneration: Targets, Compounds, and Biomarkers. *Genes* **2019**, *10*, 453. [CrossRef] [PubMed]
170. Palczewski, K. Retinoids for Treatment of Retinal Diseases. *Trends Pharmacol. Sci.* **2010**, *31*, 284–295. [CrossRef]
171. Scholl, H.P.N.; Moore, A.T.; Koenekoop, R.K.; Wen, Y.; Fishman, G.A.; Born, L.I.V.D.; Bittner, A.; Bowles, K.; Fletcher, E.C.; Collison, F.T.; et al. Safety and Proof-of-Concept Study of Oral QLT091001 in Retinitis Pigmentosa Due to Inherited Deficiencies of Retinal Pigment Epithelial 65 Protein (RPE65) or Lecithin:Retinol Acyltransferase (LRAT). *PLoS ONE* **2015**, *10*, e0143846. [CrossRef]
172. Patel, A.; Cholkar, K.; Agrahari, V.; Mitra, A.K. Ocular drug delivery systems: An overview. *World J. Gastrointest. Pharmacol. Ther.* **2013**, *2*, 47–64. [CrossRef] [PubMed]
173. Bordet, T.; Behar-Cohen, F. Ocular gene therapies in clinical practice: Viral vectors and nonviral alternatives. *Drug Discov. Today* **2019**, *24*, 1685–1693. [CrossRef]
174. Conley, S.M.; Cai, X.; Naash, M.I. Non-Viral Ocular Gene Therapy: Assessment and Future Directions. *Curr. Opin. Mol. Ther.* **2008**, *10*, 456–463. [PubMed]
175. Chiang, B.; Jung, J.H.; Prausnitz, M.R. The suprachoroidal space as a route of administration to the posterior segment of the eye. *Adv. Drug Deliv. Rev.* **2018**, *126*, 58–66. [CrossRef] [PubMed]
176. Rodrigues, G.A.; Shalaev, E.; Karami, T.K.; Cunningham, J.; Slater, N.K.H.; Rivers, H.M. Pharmaceutical Development of AAV-Based Gene Therapy Products for the Eye. *Pharm. Res.* **2018**, *36*, 29. [CrossRef] [PubMed]

177. Olsen, T.W.; Feng, X.; Wabner, K.; Conston, S.R.; Sierra, D.H.; Folden, D.V.; Smith, M.E.; Cameron, J.D. Cannulation of the Suprachoroidal Space: A Novel Drug Delivery Methodology to the Posterior Segment. *Am. J. Ophthalmol.* **2006**, *142*, 777–787.e2. [CrossRef] [PubMed]
178. Einmahl, S.; Savoldelli, M.; D'Hermies, F.; Tabatabay, C.; Gurny, R.; Behar-Cohen, F. Evaluation of a novel biomaterial in the suprachoroidal space of the rabbit eye. *Investig. Ophthalmol. Vis. Sci.* **2002**, *43*, 1533–1539.
179. Mandelcorn, E.D.; Kitchens, J.W.; Fijalkowski, N.; Moshfeghi, D.M. Active Aspiration of Suprachoroidal Hemorrhage Using a Guarded Needle. *Ophthalmic Surg. Lasers Imaging Retin.* **2014**, *45*, 150–152. [CrossRef] [PubMed]
180. Goldstein, D.A.; Do, D.; Noronha, G.; Kissner, J.M.; Srivastava, S.K.; Nguyen, Q.D. Suprachoroidal Corticosteroid Administration: A Novel Route for Local Treatment of Noninfectious Uveitis. *Transl. Vis. Sci. Technol.* **2016**, *5*, 14. [CrossRef] [PubMed]
181. Gote, V.; Sikder, S.; Sicotte, J.; Pal, D. Ocular Drug Delivery: Present Innovations and Future Challenges. *J. Pharmacol. Exp. Ther.* **2019**, *370*, 602–624. [CrossRef] [PubMed]
182. Bennett, J.; Ashtari, M.; Wellman, J.; Marshall, K.A.; Cyckowski, L.L.; Chung, D.C.; McCague, S.; Pierce, E.A.; Chen, Y.; Bennicelli, J.L.; et al. AAV2 Gene Therapy Readministration in Three Adults with Congenital Blindness. *Sci. Transl. Med.* **2012**, *4*, 120ra15. [CrossRef] [PubMed]
183. Trapani, I.; Puppo, A.; Auricchio, A. Vector platforms for gene therapy of inherited retinopathies. *Prog. Retin. Eye Res.* **2014**, *43*, 108–128. [CrossRef] [PubMed]
184. Stieger, K.; Lhériteau, E.; Moullier, P.; Rolling, F. AAV-Mediated Gene Therapy for Retinal Disorders in Large Animal Models. *ILAR J.* **2009**, *50*, 206–224. [CrossRef] [PubMed]
185. Petrs-Silva, H.; Dinculescu, A.; Li, Q.; Deng, W.T.; Pang, J.J.; Min, S.H.; Agbandje-McKenna, M. Novel properties of tyrosine-mutant AAV2 vectors in the mouse retina. *Mol. Ther.* **2011**, *19*, 293–301. [CrossRef] [PubMed]
186. Kong, F.; Li, W.; Li, X.; Zheng, Q.; Dai, X.; Zhou, X.; Boye, S.L.; Hauswirth, W.W.; Qu, J.; Pang, J.-J. Self-complementary AAV5 Vector Facilitates Quicker Transgene Expression in Photoreceptor and Retinal Pigment Epithelial Cells of Normal Mouse. *Exp. Eye Res.* **2010**, *90*, 546–554. [CrossRef] [PubMed]
187. Ghosh, A.; Yue, Y.; Duan, D. Efficient transgene reconstitution with hybrid dual AAV vectors carrying the minimized bridging sequences. *Hum. Gene Ther.* **2011**, *22*, 77–83. [CrossRef] [PubMed]
188. Trapani, I. Dual AAV Vectors for Stargardt Disease. *Methods Mol. Biol.* **2018**, *1715*, 153–175. [PubMed]
189. Trapani, I. Adeno-Associated Viral Vectors as a Tool for Large Gene Delivery to the Retina. *Genes* **2019**, *10*, 287. [CrossRef]
190. Patel, A.; Zhao, J.; Duan, D.; Lai, Y. Design of AAV Vectors for Delivery of Large or Multiple Transgenes. *Adv. Struct. Saf. Stud.* **2019**, *1950*, 19–33.
191. Auricchio, A.; Kobinger, G.; Anand, V.; Hildinger, M.; O'Connor, E.; Maguire, A.M.; Wilson, J.M.; Bennett, J. Exchange of surface proteins impacts on viral vector cellular specificity and transduction characteristics: The retina as a model. *Hum. Mol. Genet.* **2001**, *10*, 3075–3081. [CrossRef]
192. Martin, K.R.; Klein, R.L.; Quigley, H.A. Gene delivery to the eye using adeno-associated viral vectors. *Methods* **2002**, *28*, 267–275. [CrossRef]
193. Dalkara, D.; Byrne, L.C.; Klimczak, R.R.; Visel, M.; Yin, L.; Merigan, W.H.; Flannery, J.G.; Schaffer, D.V. In Vivo-Directed Evolution of a New Adeno-Associated Virus for Therapeutic Outer Retinal Gene Delivery from the Vitreous. *Sci. Transl. Med.* **2013**, *5*, 189ra76. [CrossRef] [PubMed]
194. Cronin, T.; Vandenberghe, L.H.; Hantz, P.; Juttner, J.; Reimann, A.; Kacsó, Á.E.; Huckfeldt, R.M.; Busskamp, V.; Kohler, H.; Lagali, P.S.; et al. Efficient transduction and optogenetic stimulation of retinal bipolar cells by a synthetic adeno-associated virus capsid and promoter. *EMBO Mol. Med.* **2014**, *6*, 1175–1190. [CrossRef] [PubMed]
195. Ramachandran, P.S.; Lee, V.; Wei, Z.; Song, J.Y.; Casal, G.; Cronin, T.; Willett, K.; Huckfeldt, R.; Morgan, J.I.; Aleman, T.S.; et al. Evaluation of Dose and Safety of AAV7m8 and AAV8BP2 in the Non-Human Primate Retina. *Hum. Gene Ther.* **2017**, *28*, 154–167. [CrossRef] [PubMed]
196. Carvalho, L.S.; Xiao, R.; Wassmer, S.J.; Langsdorf, A.; Zinn, E.; Pacouret, S.; Shah, S.; Comander, J.I.; Kim, L.A.; Lim, L.; et al. Synthetic Adeno-Associated Viral Vector Efficiently Targets Mouse and Nonhuman Primate Retina In Vivo. *Hum. Gene Ther.* **2018**, *29*, 771–784. [CrossRef] [PubMed]
197. Greenberg, K.P.; Lee, E.S.; Schaffer, D.V.; Flannery, J.G. Gene delivery to the retina using lentiviral vectors. *Adv. Exp. Med. Biol.* **2006**, *572*, 255–266.

198. Han, Z.; Conley, S.M.; Naash, M.I. Gene Therapy for Stargardt Disease Associated with ABCA4 Gene. *Adv. Exp. Med. Biol.* **2014**, *801*, 719–724.
199. Bergelson, J.M.; Modlin, J.F.; Wieland-Alter, W.; Cunningham, J.A.; Crowell, R.L.; Finberg, R.W. Clinical Coxsackievirus B Isolates Differ from Laboratory Strains in Their Interaction with Two Cell Surface Receptors. *J. Infect. Dis.* **1997**, *175*, 697–700. [CrossRef]
200. Cashman, S.M.; Sadowski, S.L.; Morris, D.J.; Frederick, J.; Kumar-Singh, R. Intercellular Trafficking of Adenovirus-Delivered HSV VP22 from the Retinal Pigment Epithelium to the Photoreceptors—Implications for Gene Therapy. *Mol. Ther.* **2002**, *6*, 813–823. [CrossRef]
201. Mallam, J.N.; Hurwitz, M.Y.; Mahoney, T.; Che´vez-Barrios, P.; Hurwitz, R.L. Efficient gene transfer into retinal cells using adenoviral vectors: Dependence on receptor expression. *Investig. Opthalmol. Vis. Sci.* **2004**, *45*, 1680–1687. [CrossRef]
202. Kumar-Singh, R.; Farber, D.B. Encapsidated adenovirus mini-chromosome-mediated delivery of genes to the retina: Application to the rescue of photoreceptor degeneration. *Hum. Mol. Genet.* **1998**, *7*, 1893–1900. [CrossRef] [PubMed]
203. Bergelson, J.M.; Cunningham, J.A.; Droguett, G.; Kurt-Jones, E.A.; Krithivas, A.; Hong, J.S.; Horwitz, M.S.; Crowell, R.L.; Finberg, R.W. Isolation of a Common Receptor for Coxsackie B Viruses and Adenoviruses 2 and 5. *Science* **1997**, *275*, 1320–1323. [CrossRef] [PubMed]
204. Andrieu-Soler, C.; Bejjani, R.-A.; De Bizemont, T.; Normand, N.; Benezra, D.; Behar-Cohen, F. Ocular gene therapy: A review of nonviral strategies. *Mol. Vis.* **2006**, *12*, 1334–1347. [PubMed]
205. Foroozandeh, P.; Aziz, A.A. Insight into Cellular Uptake and Intracellular Trafficking of Nanoparticles. *Nanoscale Res. Lett.* **2018**, *13*, 339. [CrossRef] [PubMed]
206. Trigueros, S.; Domènech, E.B.; Toulis, V.; Marfany, G. In Vitro Gene Delivery in Retinal Pigment Epithelium Cells by Plasmid DNA-Wrapped Gold Nanoparticles. *Genes* **2019**, *10*, 289. [CrossRef] [PubMed]
207. Zhang, X. Gold Nanoparticles: Recent Advances in the Biomedical Applications. *Cell Biophys.* **2015**, *72*, 771–775. [CrossRef]
208. Peeters, L.; Sanders, N.N.; Braeckmans, K.; Boussery, K.; Van De Voorde, J.; De Smedt, S.C.; Demeester, J. Vitreous: A barrier to nonviral ocular gene therapy. *Investig. Opthalmol. Vis. Sci.* **2005**, *46*, 3553–3561. [CrossRef] [PubMed]
209. Chen, F.; McLenachan, S.; Edel, M.; Da Cruz, L.; Coffey, P.; Mackey, D. iPS Cells for Modelling and Treatment of Retinal Diseases. *J. Clin. Med.* **2014**, *3*, 1511–1541. [CrossRef]
210. Takahashi, K.; Tanabe, K.; Ohnuki, M.; Narita, M.; Ichisaka, T.; Tomoda, K.; Yamanaka, S. Induction of Pluripotent Stem Cells from Adult Human Fibroblasts by Defined Factors. *Cell* **2007**, *131*, 861–872. [CrossRef] [PubMed]
211. Lamba, D.A.; Gust, J.; Reh, T.A. Transplantation of human embryonic stem cells derived photoreceptors restores some visual function in Crx deficient mice. *Cell Stem Cell* **2009**, *4*, 73–79. [CrossRef] [PubMed]
212. Pearson, R.A.; Barber, A.C.; Rizzi, M.; Hippert, C.; Xue, T.; West, E.L.; Duran, Y.; Smith, A.J.; Chuang, J.Z.; Azam, S.A.; et al. Restoration of vision after transplantation of photoreceptors. *Nature* **2012**, *485*, 99–103. [CrossRef] [PubMed]
213. West, E.L.; Gonzalez-Cordero, A.; Hippert, C.; Osakada, F.; Martinez-Barbera, J.P.; Pearson, R.A.; Ali, R.R. Defining the integration capacity of embryonic stem cell-derived photoreceptor precursors. *Stem Cells* **2012**, *30*, 1424–1435. [CrossRef] [PubMed]
214. Barber, A.C.; Hippert, C.; Duran, Y.; West, E.L.; Bainbridge, J.W.; Warre-Cornish, K.; Pearson, R.A. Repair of the degenerate retina by photoreceptor transplantation. *Proc. Natl. Acad Sci. USA* **2013**, *110*, 354–359. [CrossRef] [PubMed]
215. Pearson, R.A.; Cordero, A.G.; West, E.L.; Ribeiro, J.R.; Aghaizu, N.; Goh, D.; Sampson, R.D.; Georgiadis, A.; Waldron, P.V.; Duran, Y.; et al. Donor and host photoreceptors engage in material transfer following transplantation of post-mitotic photoreceptor precursors. *Nat. Commun.* **2016**, *7*, 13029. [CrossRef] [PubMed]
216. Santos-Ferreira, T.; Llonch, S.; Börsch, O.; Postel, K.; Haas, J.; Ader, M. Retinal transplantation of photoreceptors results in donor–host cytoplasmic exchange. *Nat. Commun.* **2016**, *7*, 13028. [CrossRef] [PubMed]
217. Liu, Y.; Xu, H.W.; Wang, L.; Li, S.Y.; Zhao, C.J.; Hao, J.; Li, Q.Y.; Zhao, T.T.; Wu, W.; Wang, Y.; et al. Human embryonic stem cell-derived retinal pigment epithelium transplants as a potential treatment for wet age-related macular degeneration. *Cell Discov.* **2018**, *4*, 50. [CrossRef] [PubMed]

218. Schwartz, S.D.; Regillo, C.D.; Lam, B.L.; Eliott, D.; Rosenfeld, P.J.; Gregori, N.Z.; Hubschman, J.-P.; Davis, J.L.; Heilwell, G.; Spirn, M.; et al. Human embryonic stem cell-derived retinal pigment epithelium in patients with age-related macular degeneration and Stargardt's macular dystrophy: Follow-up of two open-label phase 1/2 studies. *Lancet* **2015**, *385*, 509–516. [CrossRef]
219. Song, W.K.; Park, K.-M.; Kim, H.-J.; Lee, J.H.; Choi, J.; Chong, S.Y.; Shim, S.H.; Del Priore, L.V.; Lanza, R. Treatment of Macular Degeneration Using Embryonic Stem Cell-Derived Retinal Pigment Epithelium: Preliminary Results in Asian Patients. *Stem Cell Rep.* **2015**, *4*, 860–872. [CrossRef] [PubMed]
220. Mandai, M.; Watanabe, A.; Kurimoto, Y.; Hirami, Y.; Morinaga, C.; Daimon, T.; Fujihara, M.; Akimaru, H.; Sakai, N.; Shibata, Y.; et al. Autologous Induced Stem-Cell–Derived Retinal Cells for Macular Degeneration. *N. Engl. J. Med.* **2017**, *376*, 1038–1046. [CrossRef] [PubMed]
221. Zrenner, E. Will Retinal Implants Restore Vision? *Science* **2002**, *295*, 1022–1025. [CrossRef] [PubMed]
222. Bloch, E.; Luo, Y.; Da Cruz, L. Advances in retinal prosthesis systems. *Ther. Adv. Ophthalmol.* **2019**, *11*, 2515841418817501. [CrossRef] [PubMed]
223. da Cruz, L.; Dorn, J.D.; Humayun, M.S.; Dagnelie, G.; Handa, J.; Barale, P.O.; Salzmann, J. Five-Year Safety and Performance Results from the Argus II Retinal Prosthesis System Clinical Trial. *Ophthalmology* **2016**, *123*, 2248–2254. [CrossRef] [PubMed]

12

Noble Metals and Soft Bio-Inspired Nanoparticles in Retinal Diseases Treatment

Valeria De Matteis [1,*] and Loris Rizzello [2,3,4]

1. Department of Mathematics and Physics "Ennio De Giorgi", University of Salento, Via Arnesano, 73100 Lecce, Italy
2. Department of Chemistry, University College London, 20 Gordon Street, London WC1H 0AJ, UK; lrizzello@ibecbarcelona.eu
3. Institute for Bioengineering of Catalonia (IBEC), The Barcelona Institute of Science and Technology, Baldiri Reixac 10-12, 08028 Barcelona, Spain
4. Department of Pharmaceutical Sciences, University of Milan, via Mangiagalli 25, 20133 Milano, Italy

* Correspondence: valeria.dematteis@unisalento.it

Abstract: We are witnessing an exponential increase in the use of different nanomaterials in a plethora of biomedical fields. We are all aware of how nanoparticles (NPs) have influenced and revolutionized the way we supply drugs or how to use them as therapeutic agents thanks to their tunable physico-chemical properties. However, there is still a niche of applications where NP have not yet been widely explored. This is the field of ocular delivery and NP-based therapy, which characterizes the topic of the current review. In particular, many efforts are being made to develop nanosystems capable of reaching deeper sections of the eye such as the retina. Particular attention will be given here to noble metal (gold and silver), and to polymeric nanoparticles, systems consisting of lipid bilayers such as liposomes or vesicles based on nonionic surfactant. We will report here the most relevant literature on the use of different types of NPs for an efficient delivery of drugs and bio-macromolecules to the eyes or as active therapeutic tools.

Keywords: retinal diseases; noble metals NPs; bio-inspired NPs; drug delivery

---

1. Introduction

The human eye is a unique and fragile structure prone to different types of pathologies. It is characterized by an anterior and the posterior segment [1]. Pupil, cornea, iris, ciliary body, aqueous humor and lens make up the anterior segment, whereas vitreous humor, macula, retina, choroid, and optic nerve are parts of the posterior segment [1]. The macula is a small area of the retina that contains photoreceptor, special light-sensitive cells, connected to a neuronal network [2]. Retina contains five types of neurons: photoreceptor, bipolar, ganglion, horizontal, and amacrine cells (Figure 1) [3,4]. The retina is the nerve layer that receives visual information, creating impulses that are transmitted through the optic nerve to the visual cortex in the brain [5]. Two types of photoreceptor cells exist: the rods and the cones. It is estimated that there are approximately 120 million rods and about six million cones in the human eye. The unique properties of photoreceptor cells expose them to a variety of genetic and environmental threats. Any dysfunction or deterioration of vital ocular tissue has a dramatic impact on a patient's quality of life. Therefore, the retina is susceptible to several diseases that result in visual loss and blindness. As countries become wealthier and the per capita income increases, prevalence of blindness decreases, and causes of blindness change. In a poor African country, the major of blinding conditions are likely to be cataract and corneal scar. In the middle-income countries such as Latin America, the leading causes of blindness are glaucoma and diabetic retinopathy. Because cataract surgery is more readily available, fewer people become blind from cataract [6]. In wealthy countries, glaucoma and cataract continue to be very common and important conditions, but most of the blindness is due to retinal degenerative diseases (RDDs) [7], an heterogeneous group of phatologies characterized by progressive death of photoreceptors. RDDs can be caused by defects in proteins involved in photo transduction, synaptic transmission, retinal pigment epithelial (RPE) integrity function, intracellular trafficking and cilia function. It can be also related to toxic accumulation of retinoids. Each of these RDDs can lead to visual loss or complete blindness [8].

The most common RDDs include age-related macular degeneration (AMD), diabetic retinopathy (DR), and retinitis pigmentosa (RP). Cytomegalovirus (CMV) retinitis, proliferative vitreoretinopathy, Stargardt disease, and retinoblastoma can also occur and are usually associated with toxic retinoid biogenesis and accumulation [9]. Retinal diseases are already the most common cause of childhood blindness [10] with an incidence of 1.5 million people suffering worldwide. RP is characterized by a progressive loss of photoreceptors and its specific mechanisms are not fully understood. Following the loss of photoreceptor functionality, a retinal remodeling phenomenon is triggered as the final step, which then culminates with cell death and topological restructuring of the retina. The progression of retinal remodeling is similar to negative plasticity that occurs in some pathologies like trauma and epilepsy constituting substantial impediments to rescue strategies of all types [11]. Another process that involve the retina segment is neovascularization, a pathological phenomenon that provokes vision loss causing blindness due to its correlation with diabetic retinopathy and AMD [12]. In the neovascularization phenomenon, endothelial growth factor (VEGF) pathway has a key role [13,14].

Ocular diseases, and retinal diseases in particular, are still approached using rather invasive treatments, which are also not completely effective. The development of efficacious therapeutics is thus a primary research goal. So far, many delivery strategies have been explored, and the progress in the field of molecular genetics has led to the identification of genes involved in retinal disruption. For this reason, gene delivery systems represent one of the most promising approaches [15,16]. Delivery approaches can be broadly classified in two groups, whether they are based on a viral or non-viral method of delivery. Each system comes with advantages and disadvantages. For instance, although Adeno-Associated Virus (AAV) based vectors have high gene transduction efficiency, they face a major obstacle in terms of biosafety for clinical applications. The development of effective non-viral approaches for ocular disease is thus crucial. However, how to adequately deliver therapeutic agents to the back of eye (i.e., retina) remains a challenge. With the development of nanotechnology and bioengineering science, a wide range of innovations in this area have been achieved. This holds the promise for developing more effective ocular drug delivery systems.

In this review, we carefully report the last studies in which noble metal and soft (bioinspired) NPs were applied as new delivery agents for treatment of ocular disease in vitro and in vivo. We also provide perspective on opportunities and challenges for future nanotechnology in retinal drug delivery and therapies.

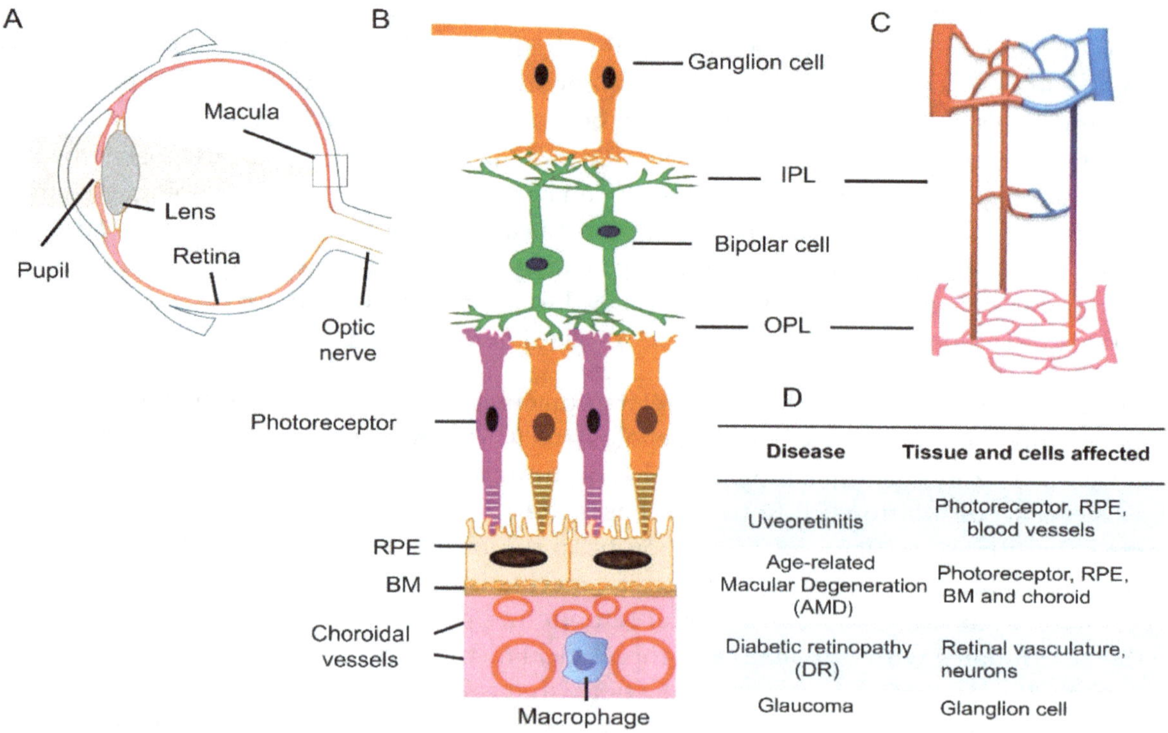

Disease	Tissue and cells affected
Uveoretinitis	Photoreceptor, RPE, blood vessels
Age-related Macular Degeneration (AMD)	Photoreceptor, RPE, BM and choroid
Diabetic retinopathy (DR)	Retinal vasculature, neurons
Glaucoma	Glanglion cell

Figure 1. Retinal neuronal and vascular structure and retinal disease. (**A**) Diagram of a human eye. Light passes through the pupil and is focused by lens onto macula of the retinal layer at the back of the eye. (**B**) Retina consists of three layers of neurons, photoreceptor, bipolar, and ganglion cells. The retinal pigment epithelial (RPE) monolayer together with Bruch's membrane (BM) form outer blood retinal barrier that separates the neuroretina from the choroid. Choroidal circulation provides oxygen and nutrients to outer retina. (**C**) The retina has an interconnected network of three vascular layers located in the ganglion cell/nerve fiber layer, inner plexiform layer (IPL), and outer plexiform layer (OPL). (**D**) retinal tissue and cells that are affected under different disease conditions. Adapted from reference [17].

2. Drug Ocular Administrations

The delivery of drugs in the eyes presents many difficulties. As in the case of the brain, it presents multiple physical boundaries: corneal and conjunctival epithelium, blood-aqueous barriers (BAB), and blood-retinal barriers (BRB). These barriers finely control the transit of molecules and fluids across eye and, in most cases, the drug is unable to enrich the deeper layers. The BRB consists of two different barriers: (i) the outer BRB characterized by endothelial cells lining the choroidal vasculature (fenestrated blood vessels) and by tight-junction-coupled RPE cells, and (ii) inner BRB. The latter is made by endothelial cells in conjunction with pericytes, astrocytes, and Müller glial cells. The inner BRB shows a lot of similarities with blood–brain barrier (BBB) with the exception of Müller glia [18]. In general, the most common drug administration is through eye drops and suspensions' that target only the anterior segment of eye, mainly due to the patient compliance. With such a method, less than 5% of topically applied dose is delivered to deeper ocular tissues, such as in vitreous cavity [19]. The chemical nature of bioactive molecules also influences the uptake. For example, BRB is selectively permeable to lipophilic molecules in the presence of specific eye drugs transporters. In this way, the formulation of new therapies should take in consideration this limitation [20]. Ocular transporters are divided in two groups: the solute carrier (SLC) family and the ATP-binding cassette (ABC) family. The electrochemical gradient was used by SLC transporters to induce the uptake of molecules through cell membrane, whereas ABC transporters employ ATP [21]. However, physiological eye phenomena, such as tear turnover, reflex blinking, ocular static, or lacrimal drainage reduce the action of the drug and consequently the eye drop administration fails to treat retina disease [22]. As a matter of fact, in unstimulated conditions, total aqueous tear volume is 7 μL and the normal tear turn-over is about 1.2 μL/min [23]. Thus, the precorneal drug half-life is about 3 minutes [24]. Therefore, treatment of posterior segment injuries still remains a challenge. For all the reasons explained above, medical research seeks alternative routes such as intravitreal injections. This method consists of direct administration into vitreus via *pars plana* using a needle. In this way, a high concentration of drug is guaranteed at the retina level, but the molecule half-life depends on its molecular weight. In fact, proteins and peptides characterized by high molecular weight (ranging from 40 kDa to 70 kDa) and steric hindrance showed longer retention [25,26]. However, a lot of complications (hemorrhages, retinal detachment, cataracts) can manifest after injection [27]. An alternative method is periocular route (Figure 2) that was demonstrated to be an effective route to direct drugs to the posterior eye segment consisting of subconjunctival, sub-tenon, retrobulbar, peribulbar, and posterior juxtascleral [28]. Administration of drug by sub-tenon injection was found to be more suitable as demonstrated by Ghate et al. [29], where sodium fluorescein was used in rabbits' eyes by subocular administration. The study concluded that injection of drug via sub-tenon resulted in highest vitreous concentration of sodium fluorescein (two sodium fluorescein (NaF) concentrations, 2.5 mg in 0.1 mL (c1) and 2.5 mg in 0.5 mL (c2)) compared to the other routes. However, also in this case, a lot of adverse effects have been observed, such as strabismus, hyphema, and intraocular pressure [30].

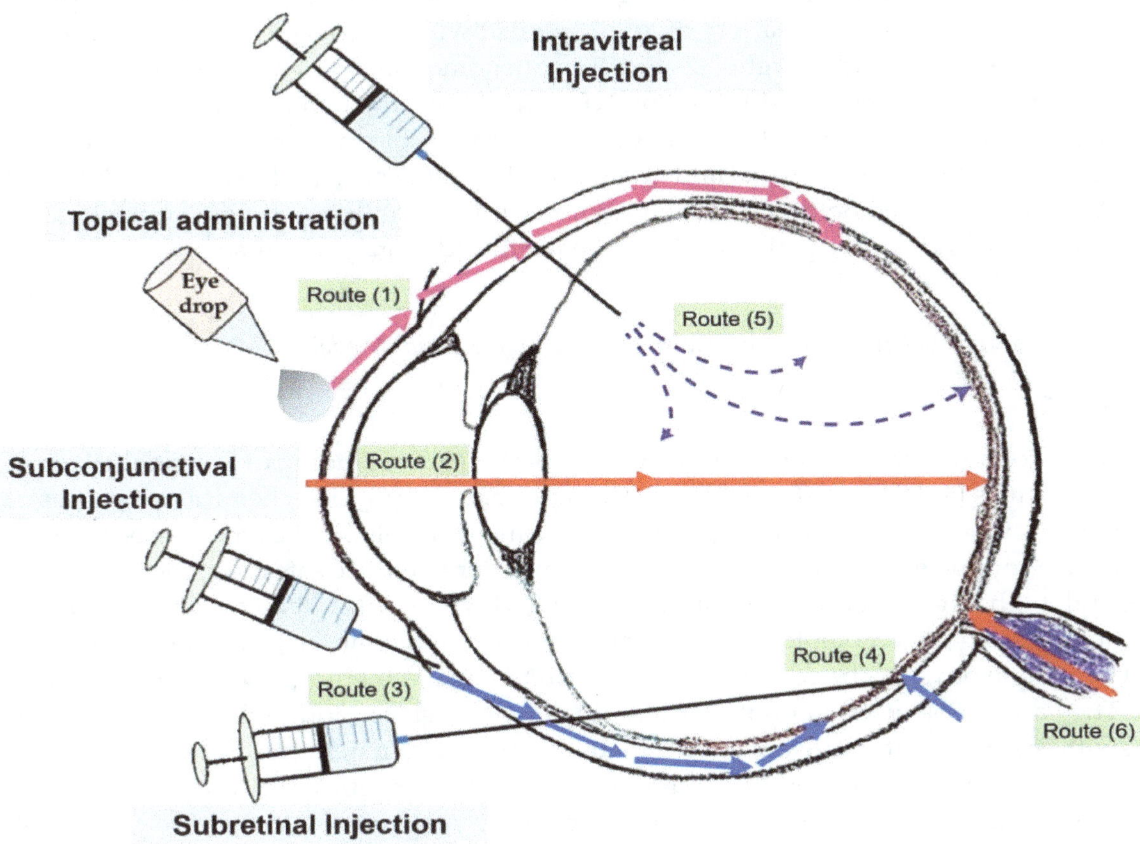

Figure 2. Common drug administration routes through the eye. Topical administration (**1**,**2**), subconjunctival injection (periocular route) (**3**), subretinal injection (**4**), and intravitreal injection (**5**). Adapted from reference [31].

3. Physico-Chemical Properties of Nanomaterials

A "Nanomaterial" is defined as a "material with any external dimension in the nanoscale or having internal structure or surface structure in the nanoscale" (ISO, 2010) [32]. Similarly, a definition of "nanoparticle" is a "nano-object with all three external dimensions in the nanoscale" where nanoscale was defined as size ranging from 1 nm to 100 nm (ISO, 2008) [33]. NPs can be obtained by many synthetic routes, starting from chemical elements such as carbon, metals, metal oxide, biological molecules, and polymers [34]. The biological effects are strongly affected by physico-chemical properties of NPs such as surface charge, size, shape, and solubility. In addition, they exhibit greater surface area per unit mass compared to bulk materials [35]. Because of the above mentioned properties and of the material they are made, NPs are ideal tools to treat retinal disease as active components of the therapy without the help of drugs [36,37]. In addition, NPs with a smaller size (<20 nm) are demonstrated to have the ability to cross eye barriers including cornea, conjunctiva, and BRB [38,39]. NPs for ocular therapy include inorganic NPs (metal oxide and noble metal NPs), as well as soft-biopolymer-based NPs. Metal NPs are more suitable as active therapy tools (for their intrinsic properties), and soft-NPs are more efficient in encapsulating drugs and macromolecules due to their ability to form aqueous-suspended vesicles having a hollow lumen. All these nanomaterials are different in charge, shape, and size, but they are able to be internalized by cells to treat retinal disease [40]. Finally, recent applications of soft nanorobot (with size range in the molecular scale) have been studied. These structures have the capability to deliver active biomolecules in ocular sections due to their ability to make changes in a controlled and predictable manner to the environment following external stimuli [41].

3.1. *Noble Metal NPs: The Case of Gold (Au) and Silver (Ag)*

Noble metals, especially AuNPs and AgNPs, are characterized by unique optical properties. For this reason they are used for a variety of applications owing to collective oscillations of conduction electrons coupled with incident light [42–45]. This phenomenon, known as Localized Surface Plasmon Resonance (LSPR) is strongly influenced by NPs' shape and the metal they are formed. The surface plasmon resonance bands of metal NPs can be tuned from visible to Near Infrared Region (NIR), which is a typical wavelength to penetrate and analyze biological tissues [46]. Even if AuNPs are the most studied in nanomedicine field due to their good chemical stability and well-controlled size/surface functionalization and biocompatibility, AgNPs have the advantage of possessing an antibacterial and antiangiogenesis effect [47,48].

3.2. *Au and AgNPs: Safety Studies in In Vitro and In Vivo Retinal Models*

3.2.1. AuNPs

The use of novel nanomaterials necessitates a better understanding of potential adverse effects on biological entities [49]. These effects are strictly dependent on physico-chemical properties of NPs and evaluation of cytotoxicity is critical, especially from a medical field application perspective [50]. A lot of studies were conducted to assess biocompatibility in order to ensure safe drug release with low toxicity. In general, high degree of biocompatibility is verified when NPs interact with the living organisms without triggering unacceptable toxic, thrombogenic, carcinogenic, and immunogenic responses [51].

The unique physico-chemical properties of AuNPs make them a powerful tool in the biomedical field. They are widely used in photothermal treatment of cancer and in drug and gene delivery. For their synthesis, auric salts such as $HAuCl_4$ are used as starting materials to obtain stable AuNPs with a size ranging from 1–100 nm (Brust or Turkevish [52,53]). In recent years, green syntheses of AuNPs has also been developed to reduce solvents and reduce/cap agents' toxicity so that AuNPs can be synthetized from plant extracts or biomass [54,55]. AuNPs are easy to functionalize with a wide range of ligands ranging to polymer, DNA, peptides, RNA, and fluorescent molecules particularly suitable for bio-imaging applications [56]. Furthermore, various cytotoxicity studies demonstrated their low toxicity due to the inert nature of Au [57,58].

Regarding the biodistribution, a recent work demonstrated a rapid elimination of colloidal AuNPs from blood circulation in a rats model, and liver and spleen accumulation without inducing adverse effects or inflammation [59]. Au comprised in passion fruit-like nanoarchitectures (NAs) were studied in murine models demonstrating the excretion by renal and biliary pathways without nephrotoxicity up to 150 mg kg^{-1} [60]. Some studies reported pro-inflammatory cytokines expressions induced by

AuNPs in different organs of rats [61] and mice [62]. However, the cytotoxic effects were temporary and normalized in a short time. The biocompatibility of Au is strictly correlated to their size, shape, concentration, as well as surface area as demonstrated by Biswas's group [63]. They investigated the effects of Au spheres (5, 10, 20, 30, 50, and 100 nm), cubes (50 nm), and rods (10 × 90 nm) in cells in adult retinal pigment epithelial cell line 19 (ARPE-19). The cubes with an average diameter of 50 nm and spheres (50–100 nm) resulted in being biocompatible up to 750 μg of concentration. NPs with a smaller size (<30 nm) and nanorods (10 nm) showed higher toxicity, but they are more able to be uptaked by cells. Kim et al. [64] used C57BL/6 mice to demonstrate the ability of AuNPs (20 nm) to cross BRB and enriched retinal layers after intravenous administration. NPs greatly accumulated in neurons (75 ± 5%), followed by endothelial cells (17 ± 6%) and peri-endothelial glial cells (8 ± 3%) without affecting both viability of endothelial cells, astrocytes, retinoblastoma cells, and expression of functional biomolecules. After five weeks of post administration, the thickness of retinal layers was undisturbed without any damage. Bakri et al. [65] used Dutch-belted rabbits to test biocompatibility of AuNPs. They used two groups of rabbits receiving a 67 μmol/0.1 mL and 670 μmol/0.1 mL of AuNPs into one eye respectively by intravitreal injection. After one month, evident inflammation or adverse effects were not detected also at a high dosage. Soderstjerna et al. [66] used AuNPs and AgNPs with 19 and 89 nm citrate capped to test biocompatibility in in vitro cultured retinas using 800 NPs/cell. The retina tissue model offered a sustained long-term retinal organization and controlled serum-free conditions. This study demonstrated that low concentrations of Au and AgNPs have adverse effects on retina and can induce apoptosis and oxidative stress. A strong connection between NPs hydrodynamic diameter, surface functionalization/concentration and the biological effects is evident. In particular, the authors showed that NPs size should be large enough to avoid their fast flow into circulation, but small enough to be administrated and easy cross the BRB [67].

Starting from this assumption, the application of AuNPs is influenced by these parameters that should be taken in consideration to customize nanotools for a specific biomedical application.

3.2.2. AgNPs

Numerous in vitro and in vivo studies demonstrated the toxicity of AgNPs that perturbs several cellular pathways [4]. The most accepted mechanism through which they induce side effects, despite still under investigation, seems to be related to Ag ions released from NPs surface [68–70]. In terms of production process, AgNPs can be synthetized by different chemical routes such as chemical-based reduction [71], sol-gel, or green synthesis [72,73].

Jun et al. [74] used zebrafish embryos as model organism to test their delivery at an ocular level. They investigated the toxicity of AgNPs at concentration of 0.4 mg/L and observed down- expressions of different lens crystalline genes by unknown mechanisms that either induced apoptosis or blocked nuclear DNA or RNA export.

Sriram et al. [75] demonstrated the cytotoxicity and Reactive Oxygen Species (ROS)-induced apoptosis after exposure of AgNPs with two different size (22.4 and 42.5 nm) in bovine retinal endothelial cells (BRECs) finding size-dependent toxicity. As a matter of fact, smaller NPs induced adverse effects on cells. Kim and colleagues [76] exposed New Zealand white rabbits (according to OECD test guidelines) to AgNPs in order to understand the possible eye irritation effect. Oedema and conjunctival redness have been observed after 1 h of AgNPs incubation, but the cornea, iris, or conjunctiva resulted unaffected after 24, 48, and 72 h of NPs exposure. In similar experiments, the instillation of AgNPs (5000 ppm) were tested on another in vivo model, the guinea pigs, observing a transient conjunctivae irritation during 24 h of early observation [77].

4. Noble-Metal NPs as Therapy and Diagnostic for Retinal Disease

AuNPs scatter or absorb light at specific wavelengths as a function of their physico-chemical properties. This characteristic is particularly suitable for bioimaging and to treat some diseases like cancer by NIR-triggered photothermal therapy (PTT), in which light is converted to heat in the tumor site where NPs accumulate [78]. In the NIR (650–900 nm), the absorption coefficients of haemoglobin and water are very low, and for this reason, the penetration of NIR wavelength in tissues is very high, allowing NPs stimulation without causing damage [79]. Song et al. [80] reported application of gold nanodisks (GNDs) on human retinal microvascular endothelial cells (HRMEC) and mouse oxygen-induced retinopathy model. The GNDs were optically suitable for nanomedicine applications due to their ability to produce detectable signals regardless of polarization or direction of light source and to scatter in NIR region (830 nm). In addition, GNDs were internalized less efficiently in cells with respect to AuNPs or Au rods (AuNRs), thus minimizing the ROS production and other several adverse effects. The authors used differently charged anisotropic NPs (nanorods or nanodisks) and compared them with AuNPs. After simulating the role of different sizes to select the best diameter (160 nm), they showed that GNDs were able to bind vascular endothelial growth factor (VEGF) inhibiting in vitro angiogenesis with high performance and abolished the VEGF-induced migration of endothelial cells. When these nanostructures were applied to mice eyes, a strong signal in optical coherence tomography (OCT) was detected with a consequent reduction of retinal degeneration (Figure 3). The OCT system involves the use of light energy that, once absorbed by tissues, causes a thermos-elastic expansion generating ultrasonic waves detected by a transducer.

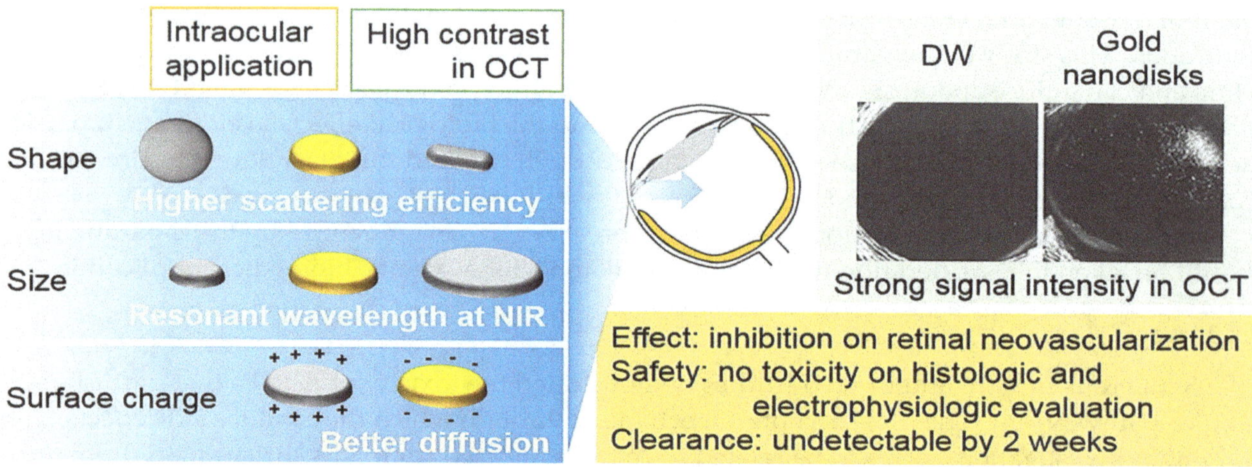

Figure 3. Schematic representation of gold nanodisks (GNDs) effects in retinal degeneration and Optical Coherence Tomography (OCT) imaging. The GNDs were particularly suitable for their optical properties connected to the shape: GNDs absorbed in the Near Infrared Region (NIR). The size and surface charge also influenced the eye diffusion. In OCT images, GNDs exhibited a strong signal compared to the dual window (DW) processing method, which is used to detect modulation of OCT signals due to scattering or absorption.

Recent therapies to treat some diseases strictly connected to retinal degeneration consider the transplantation of photoreceptor precursors (PRPs) as efficient support improving visual acuity [81]. The analysis of cell survivor in the host retina is a key factor in this kind of treatment. Chemla et al. [82] used AuNPs in order to improve the tracking of transplanted PRPs. Cells were labelled with photothermic AuNPs and transplanted in the vitreous and sub-retinal space of Long-Evans pigmented rats (4–8 weeks old) by gauge needle.

By using coherence tomography, computed tomography and fluorescence fundus imaging, NPs have been tracked for 1 month without recording adverse effects. Real-time tracking is essential for evaluating the efficiency of retinal cell replacement therapies. These studies confirmed the possibility to use AuNPs to improve retinal cell therapy in humans. AuNPs-based photothermal therapy has been also used to treat eye tumors in vitro and in vivo. Some eye cancers provoke retinal detachment leading to a decreased visual eye activity.

In this framework, Kim et al. [83] tested anticancer properties of Doxorubicin (Dox)-conjugated Fucoidan (Fu)-encapsulated AuNPs (Dox-Fu@AuNPs) for the treatment of VX2 squamous carcinoma cells and xenograft tumors in New Zealand White rabbits. After intra-tumoral injection of Dox-Fu@AuNPs in the eye, a complete suppression of the tumor has been observed by dual-chemotherapy and PTT treatment. No damage to retina has been also detected. These composite nanostructures enabled the improvement of the OCT imaging technique (thanks to the selective light absorption of AuNPs) [84].

The quality of photoacoustic-based imaging was also improved thanks to selective light absorption of AuNPs. In this way, a double effect in terms of therapy and diagnostic was achieved.

As reported above, OCT is largely used for imaging in ocular clinical research due to the possibility to take structural information based on the reflectivity of tissue. In this respect, Gordon and colleagues [85] confirmed that Au nanorods (with a peak absorption of 750 nm and diameter of 10–35 nm) injected in the retina of Wild-type C57BL/6 mice are able to enhance the contrast, thus significantly improving the quality of a scanned lesion. Additionally, intravitreal injection of Au nanorods functionalized by anti-VEGF antibody triggered a reduction in the extent of anatomic laser damage and lesion-associated photothermal signal density in mice treated in laser induced choroidal neovascularization (LCNV) model and injected with ICAM2-targeted GNR. AuNPs (3–5 nm) were also used as inhibitor of VEGF on choroid-retina endothelial cells (RF/6A) [86]. A similar effect was showed using AgNPs, which have been found to reduce the VEGF activation and induced cell proliferation and migration in bovine retinal endothelial cells [87]. In addition, AgNPs were shown to inhibit the angiogenesis, typical of metastasising cells and of retinal neovascularization development. Ag is widely used because it has the great advantage of being a cost-effective material. For this reason, it is a good candidate for the replacement of the current therapies used for the treatment of various retinal angiogenic disorders. In this respect, Sheikpranbabu and co-workers [88] investigated the effect of green AgNPs, obtained from *Bacillus licheniformis*, on VEGF-and Interleukin 1 β (IL-1β) expression—that induced retinal endothelial cell permeability. AgNPs were able to stop VEGF-and IL-1β-induced permeability in retinal endothelial cells from porcine retina.

5. Bio-Inspired NPs for Ocular Drug Delivery

The use of bio-inspired materials mimicking natural components for applications in living organisms has widely spread recently [89]. In fact, inorganic NPs have the serious drawback of not being degradable and are also difficult to get excreted from the body [90]. Bio-inspired nanomaterials, including liposomes, niosomes, and chitosan/alginate NPs have been then explored as valid alternatives to metal NPs for treatment of several diseases [91]. In addition, these 'soft' NPs have been applied for drug delivery in the posterior segment of eye, including retinal photoreceptors.

5.1. Liposomes as Drug Delivery Carrier

Liposomes consist of a lipid bilayer, resembling a cellular membrane, that surrounds an aqueous core. These structures are widely used in pre-clinical studies to improve drug delivery, for example through Blood Brain Barrier (BBB) [92]. The BBB and BRB have the same functional properties [93,94]: so liposomes improve drug delivery to the retina and its photoreceptors due to their high half-life, permitting the long term drug absorption [95]. Liposomes also offer the ability to significantly improve pharmacokinetics and pharmacodynamics of any loaded drug compared to its free-circulating counterpart. They are also considered as highly biocompatible and biodegradable as well up to some extent both in vitro and in vivo. For this reason, several anticancer drugs such as doxorubicin, daunorubicin, and epirubicin were encapsulated in liposomes core with results demonstrating a significant decrease of many severe adverse effects (nausea, weakness, vomiting) with respect to the same concentration of free (non-encapsulated) drug. In this context, Zhang et al. [96] subcutaneously injected tacrolimus-encapsulated liposomes in Lewis rats with autoimmune uveoretinitis (EAU) by subcutaneous injection. Confocal analysis over rhodamine-conjugated liposomes (containing also the tacrolimus) revealed that such vesicles remained in ocular fluids even after 14 days. They found a reduced intraocular inflammation and decrease of EAU development without observing significant adverse effects.

Liposomes encapsulated with the anti-inflammatory and anti-angiogenic drugs berberine hydrochloride and chrysophanol were applied in myoblasts and in ischemic animal models. These drugs have the ability to contrast oxidative stress by enhancing the activities of antioxidant enzymes such as superoxide dismutase (SOD) and glutathione peroxidase (GSH-Px) [97,98]. Berberine hydrochloride and chrysophanol have been used in ocular liposome-mediated delivery to overcome their low stability. In this respect, a recent study [99] showed a liposome system that can entrap the two drugs at same times using the third polyamidoamine dendrimer (PAMAM G3.0) as a delivery carrier for age-related macular degeneration (AMD) therapy in the ocular posterior chamber.

PAMAM G3.0-coated compound liposomes were used to evaluated HCECs (Human Corneal Epithelial Cells) internalization, trans-corneal permeability in New Zealand white rabbits (weighing 2.0–2.5 kg) and male Sprague–Dawley rats (weighing 210–250 g). Pharmacokinetics were evaluated together with in vitro assessments of anti-reactive oxygen species (ROS) efficacy. The PAMAM G3.0-coated compound liposomes enhanced bio-adhesion on rabbit corneal epithelium after topical administration and exhibited great permeability in HCECs cells. The possibility to deliver a protective agent against photo-oxidative retinal damage in a light-damaged animal model was also investigated through the use of dendrimers (Figure 4A). Results showed that dendrimers encapsulated with chrysophanol–berberine hydrochloride induced the greatest protection of retinal function in light-exposed rats compared to unloaded dendrimers and free drug. In addition, no inflammation and damage of cornea, iris, and conjunctiva was observed after drug-loaded dendrimers instillation for 14 days. Upon exploring the fundus of the eye (interior surface of eye opposite the lens including the retina, optic disc, macula, fovea, and posterior pole) [100], modifications in the vessel structure and distribution have not been observed after different treatments. (Figure 4B).

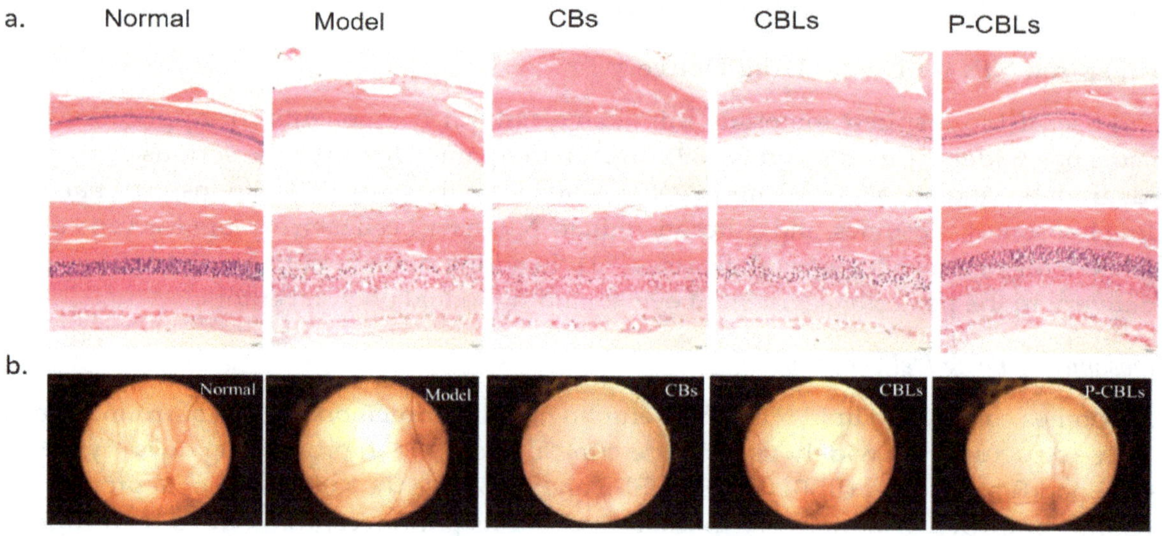

Figure 4. (**A**) Protection evaluation against photo-oxidative retinal damage in a light-damaged animal model by the use of different formulation: chrysophanol–berberine hydrochloride suspension (CBs), compound liposomes (CBLs), and PAMAM coated compound liposomes (P-CBLs). Retina was stained with hematoxilyn/eosin (scale bare = 20 μm). (**B**) Fundus retinography after incubation with the different formulations. Adapted from [99] under the terms of the Creative Commons Attribution 4.0 International License.

Liposomes offer also the great ability of an easy surface functionalization with a plethora of active macromolecules and targeting moieties that bind in a selective manner some specific receptors constitutive of different cell lines [101,102].

The surface modification of liposomes has also been widely studied to improve their specificity of targeting and to deliver them in different eye compartments. It has been reported [103] that the cationic PEGylated liposomes having an average zeta potentials below +20 mV were able to efficiently penetrate the murine retina. In contrast, liposome having surface zeta potential values above +20 mV were retained on vitreous section. This did not change whether PEGylated or non-PEGylated liposomes were used. Another critical factor for a liposome-based therapy is the phospholipids composition characterizing them. For example, edaravone-loaded egg L-phosphatidylcholine liposomes prevent retinal ganglion cells (RGCs) from undesired apoptotic processes [104]. This drug is a free radical scavenger used for acute brain infarction and amyotrophic lateral sclerosis treatment [105]. Surprisingly, minor RGC protection was observed with edaravone-loaded distearoyl phosphatidylcholine (DSPC) liposomes. This evidence suggest a link between the viscoelastic properties of the lipid bilayer and the final biological effect. In this specific case, the higher fluidity was a key factor to improve the ocular therapy. Another study [106] also tested the use of liposomes for the treatment of different kinds of hereditary degeneration of the retina. The degeneration of retina affects rod photoreceptors important for capturing light under low illumination conditions. Because of the pathology development, the patients affected by retina degeneration become aware of defects only when lesions are in an advanced stage. A key factor for this disease seems to be rods-specific Pde6b gene mutation in the transduction pathway that triggers an excessive accumulation of cGMP (that have two effectors: cyclic nucleotide gated ion channels (CNGCs) and cGMP-dependent protein kinase (PKG) [107]. Consequently, rod cell death was induced and in some cases the secondary loss of cones was observed [108]. The authors identified a liposomal cGMP analogue that was able to overcome the blood–retinal barrier (BRB) while strongly preserving retinal function and reducing rod photoreceptor loss in three different in vivo models for retina degeneration [106,109]. The vesicle structure of liposomes was suitable to confine proteins and peptides into aqueous core overcoming potential agglomeration and protein misfolding events. However, the surface functionalization with peptides is the most common method used for retina therapy. For example, liposomes functionalized with tanticoagulant annexin A5 have been demonstrated to have enhanced uptake levels through corneal epithelial barriers [110].

This vector has been injected topically to deliver 127 ng/g of bevacizumab to posterior segment of both rats and rabbit eye. Annexin A5-functionalized liposomes loaded with bevacizumab were also rapidly delivered to retina of the two animal models. Annexin A5 unilamellar liposomes made by different polymers (2-dipalmitoyl-sn-glycero-3-phosphocholine,1,2-dioleoyl-sn-glycero-3-phospho-L-serine and cholesterol) have been also used to target transforming growth factor (TGF)-ß1 into the vitreous of rabbits [111]. It has been found that a higher concentration of molecule with respect to the experimental group treated with the unloaded drug only. The choice for human recombinant TGF-β1 relied on the drug's ability to prevent retinal damage elicited by Aβ oligomers.

5.2. *Niosomes for Drug and Gene Delivery*

Gene therapies is an approach where diseases are cured by modifying the expression of specific genes regulating pathology. This happens through the administration of nucleic acids aiming to replace abnormal gene sequence [112]. Liposomes and lipoplexes have been taken into consideration as suitable non-viral vectors platform for gene editing. Non-viral gene delivery approaches were widely applied in clinical trials since 2004 to attempt replacing the use of viral vectors that possess high risk of inducing oncogenesis, immunogenicity, mutagenicity phenomena [113].

Among non-viral vectors, niosomes have been recently tested as a potential candidate for gene delivery. Niosomes are vesicular systems comprising of bilayer made up of nonionic surfactants and they can internalize several types of bio-macromolecules such as nucleic acids and drugs. The most commonly used surfactant are Sorbitan fatty acid esters, Spans (Span 20, 40, 60, 65, 80, and 85), Tweens (20, 40, 60, and 80) [114] and brij (30, 35, 52, 58, 72, and 76) [115].

In a recent study [116], niosomes made by cationic lipid 1,2-di-octadecenyl-3-trimethylammonium propane, Squalene, and Tween 20 have been combined with GFP-encoding genetic materials consisting on minicircle (MC-GFP, 2.3 kb), its parental plasmid (pGFP, 3.5 kb), and a larger plasmid (pEGFP, 5.5 kb). Their efficacy in retinal disease treatment has been investigated. These noisome-DNA complexes, named as nioplexes, demonstrated good transfection ability in human ARPE19 retinal pigment epithelium cells (in vitro) and in embrionary rat retinal primary cells (in vivo). Fluorescence showed GFP positive signal emission after transfection with the nioplexes carrying plasmidic DNA. In addition, such transfected cells showed physiological glial cell morphology confirming good cell viability in all tested cases. (Figure 5). The successive injections of nioplexes in rat retinas confirmed the higher capacity of cationic niosomes vectoring minicircle DNA to deliver genetic material into retina cells. Therefore, nioplexes based on cationic niosomes vectoring minicircle DNA are demonstrated as powerful agents in retinal diseases therapies. Cationic formulations made by a combination of Tween-60:DOTMA:lycopene have been used to transfect ARPE-19 cells with pCMS-EGFP plasmid with a transfection efficiency close to 35% [117]. Also in case, in vivo experiments in rat eye showed the efficiency of nioplexes to transfect outer segments of the retina, Niosomes constituted by Span 40 or Span 60 and cholesterol were produced to encapsulate and topically deliver in vivo acetazolamide. The intraocular pressure (IOP) after drug delivery system application was reduced in rabbits. In particular, multilamellar acetazolamide niosomes developed with Span 60 and cholesterol (7:4 molar ratio) were more efficient in reducing IOP, and at same time, no irritation and retinal damage were observed [118]. Gugleva et al. [119] prepared niosomes by different surfactants to deliver doxycycline hyclate in rats eye. Doxycycline hyclate is an antibiotic used for the treatment of eye infections. It was demonstrated to inhibit effect on matrix metalloprotease 9 (MMP-9) activity and mitogen activated protein kinase in experimental murine dry eye [120]. Niosomes were synthesized using several surfactants (Span 20, Span 60, Span 80, Tween 60) and cholesterol in different molar ratios and tested on male albino rabbits. The experiments clearly showed that the prepared niosomal formulations were high tolerated and did not induce any irritations.

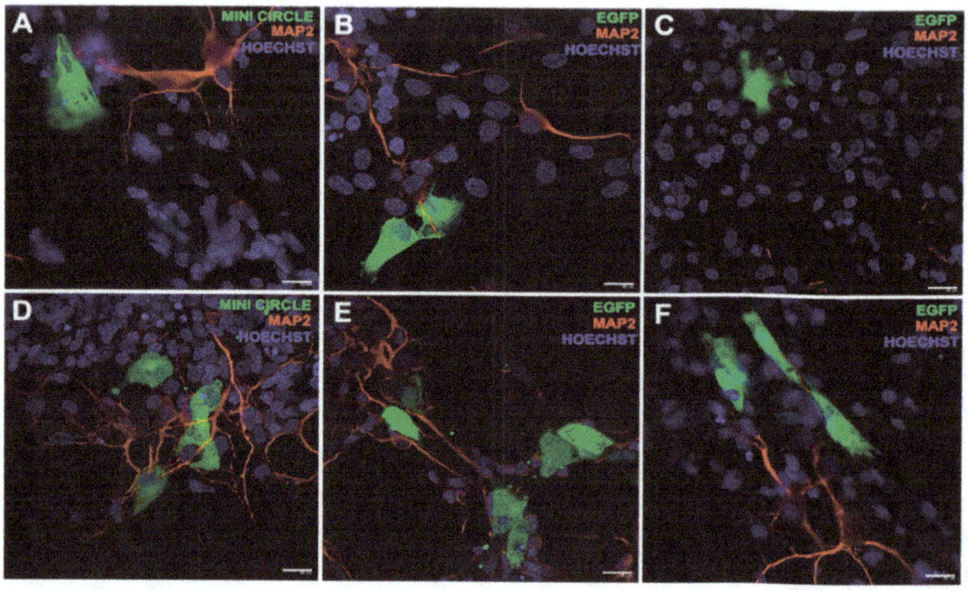

Figure 5. Fluorescence immonostaining by GFP expression in embrionary rat retinal primary cells. The green signal was referred to the transfection event of DST20 nioplexes with MC-GFP, (**B**) pGFP 3.5 kb, or (**C**) pEGFP 5.5 kb. (**D–F**) Positive controls incubated with Lipofectamine™ 2000. Nuclei were stained with Hoechst 33,342 (blue) and neuronal dendrites with MAP2 (red). Scale bars: 20 μm.

5.3. *Hydrogels-Based Nanocarriers*

Hydrogels are three-dimensional, cross-linked networks of natural or synthetic water-soluble polymers that are suitable for applications like tissue engineering and controlled/sustained drugs delivery [121,122]. The aqueous environment is particularly advantageous to confine soluble active molecules, oligonucleotides, and proteins. For this reason, they are powerful tools in retinal treatment disease [123]. In addition, smart or environment-responsive hydrogels were synthetized to improve drug delivery efficacy [124].

5.3.1. Natural Hydrogels: Chitosan NPs (CHNPs)

Chitosan is a natural hydrogel cationic polysaccharide of co-polymers glucosamine and N-acetyl glucosamine [125] obtained by alkaline deacetylation of chitin that is constitutive of crustacean shells of shrimps, lobster, and crab. It presents a positive charge that can be exploited to form polyelectrolyte vesicular complexes able to act as delivery systems. The positive charged chitosan is also ideal to bind a negatively charged corneal surface, to improve precorneal retention time and to decreases clearance [126]. In addition to chitosan, also the biocompatible alginate is extensively employed in biomedical applications. Alginate can also be a useful biopolymers for designing responsive hydrogels [127]. Because of its characteristics, alginate is also used for ophthalmic applications often in combination with chitosan [128]. For example, chitosan coated sodium alginate NPs [129] loaded with Fluorouracil (5-FU) have been successfully tested for eye delivery demonstrating a high 5-FU release in aqueous humor compared to free drug in rabbit eye. In another approach, chitosan NPs were encapsulated with levofloxacin for the treatment of ocular infection [130]. The formulation of NPs were optimized to enhance corneal retention without inducing eye irritation. These nanovectors demonstrated strong antibacterial agents against *Pseudomonas aeruginosa* and *Stafiloccocus aureus*.

Andrei and co-workers [131] designed biocompatible chitosan and alginate-based micro/NPs with a specific morphology aiming to deliver cefuroxim, a second-generation cephalosporin antibiotic. The authors performed an in vivo assessment to evaluate the biodistribution following an intravitreal administration of fluorescein-chitosan NPs on wistar rats. They observed an efficient NPs distribution in lens and retina. Similarly, chitosan-dextran NPs have been employed to deliver the antibiotic moxifloxacin that has been retained for a long time in vivo thanks to the mucoadhesive properties of NPs [132].

In recent work, humanin, a neuronal peptide that mediated inflammatory responses, was used in the treatment of age-related macular degeneration (AMD) [133]. This peptide was a suppressor of the IL-6 cytokine receptors and protects neuronal cells from necrosis [134]. The authors studied the effect on the inflammatory response reduction using chitosan NPs as vector vesicle (with a size of 346 ± 52 nm) in which humanin (a micropeptide encoded in the mitochondrial genome) derivative AGA-(CR8) HNG17 (AGA-HNG) were encapsulated. The effects of NPs were assessed in retinal pigment epithelial cells. The percentage release profile of free protein after five days was 60%, after which it enriched a plateau whereas the nanostructured exhibited a slow and substantial release with 80% of protein released after fifteen days. Cheng et al. [135] developed a thermosensitive hydrogel containing latanoprost and curcumin-loaded NPs (CUR-NPs). Curcumin was selected because of its antioxidative and antiinflammatory properties that made it suitable also for treatment of eye pathologies such as chronic anterior uveitis and light-induced retinal degeneration [136]. Latanoprost was chosen because it acted on IOP restore due to uveoscleral outflow increase [137]. In glaucoma disease, IOP is generated by loss of aqueous humor drainage through the uveoscleral or trabecular outflow pathway that can be damaged by oxidative stress at trabecular meshwork level [138]. In this condition, Latanoprost and CUR-NPs were demonstrated to decrease the oxidative stress in trabecular meshwork (TM) cells that resulted in decreased levels of apoptosis, inflammation-related gene expression, and mitochondrial damage [135]. In another work [139], neuroprotective and neuro regenerative agent Erythropoietin (EPO) was encapsulated in chitosan/hyaluronic acid (HA) nanoparticulate (size ≤300 nm). Different formulations have been tested and delivered to porcine corneas, scleras, and conjunctivas by ex vivo permeation, finding out a good combination between targeting efficiency and biocompatibility.

Pandit et al. [140] encapsulated high levels of bevacizumab (an anti-angiogenesis drug) within chitosan-coated PLGA NPs (size 222.28 ± 7.45) and demonstrated its efficient deliver to the retina followed by efficient release. As matter of fact, CS-coated NPs showed better permeability of the bevacizumab across sclera as compared to the free drug solution. Another category of carrier is made by glycol chitosan (GCS) NPs [141]. These biocompatible NPs, demonstrated to load high amount of plasmid DNA, have been successfully delivered to retinal pigment epithelium of adult wild-type albino mice. More importantly, the encapsulated pDNA was intact and maintained a proper conformation.

5.3.2. Synthetic Hydrogel Based Nanocarriers

The synthetic hydrogels are easy to customize and indeed are a close model of biological matrices. Hydrogels exhibit high hydrophilicity and high hydration [142]. The most commonly used are poly(hydroxyethyl methacrylate) (PHEMA), poly(ethylene oxide) (PEO, also called poly(ethyleneglycol) (PEG)), polyvinylpyrrolidone (PVP), poly(acrylic acid)(PAA), polyacrylamide (PAM), and poly(vinyl alcohol) (PVA) [143]. These polymers are all used in several ophthalmic applications with good results [144–147].

Anti-VEGF antibodies (anibizumab or aflibercept) were loaded within poly(lactic-co-glycolic acid) microspheres, and successively suspended within poly(N-isopropylacrylamide)-based hydrogel and injected into a laser-induced rat model of choroidal neovascularization (CNV). Upon ocular administration, the rats showed smaller CNV lesions (less than 60%) with respect to non-treated animals [148].

Agrahari et al. [149] obtained novel pentablock (PB) copolymer (PB-1: PCL–PLA–PEG–PLA–PCL) based nanoformulations suspended in a thermosensitive gelling copolymer (PB-2: mPEG–PCL–PLA–PCL–PEGm) with a size of 150 nm. This composite nanoformulation was used to deliver macromolecules to slowly release drugs without toxic effects on the posterior segment of the eye. In vitro tests performed on ocular and mouse macrophage (RAW 264.7) demonstrated their biocompatibility and potential to be clinically translated.

Yang et al. [150] reported the production of non-toxic polyamidoamine (PAMAM) dendrimer hydrogel/poly(lactic-co-glycolic acid) (PLGA) NP platform (HDNP) to treat glaucoma. The dendrimers were loaded with brimonidine and timolol maleat, which underwent an enhanced uptake together with a slow release in vitro up to 28–35 days. The topical administration of the same drug-loaded denndrimers in normotensive adult Dutch-belted male rabbits strongly reduced the introcular pressure (IOP) of about 18% maintaining a glaucoma reduction for four days. Conversely, Individual Dendrimer Hydrogel Formulations (DH) and NP Formulations (NP) decreased the disease symptoms only for 48 h (Figure 6).

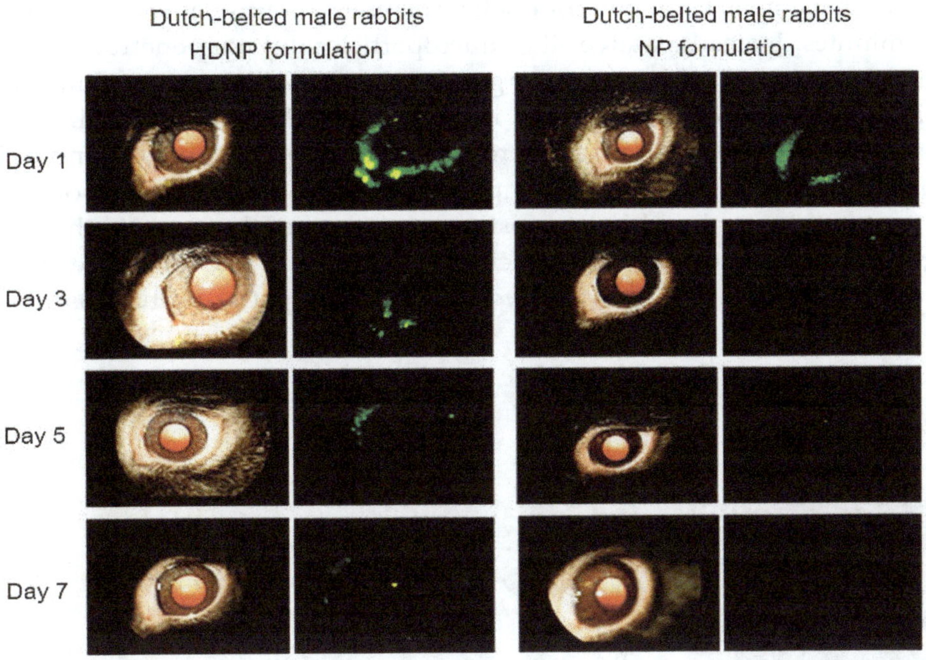

Figure 6. Fundus camera acquisitions of rabbits' eyes after hybrid polyamidoamine (PAMAM) dendrimer hydrogel/poly(lacticco-glycolic acid) (PLGA) nanoparticle platform (HDNP) and NP Formulations (NP) topical administration FluoSpheres were confined in nanosistems to follow the distribution and retention in the eye. The analysis was performed at the end of 1, 3, 5, and 7 days of formulations instillation. Left: regular fundus camera images of the eyes; right: fluorescent fundus camera images.

5.4. *Active and Self-Propelling Nanoparticles: New Generation of Nanobots in Retinal Disease*

The customization of NPs formulation at a molecular level has interesting outcomes for reproduction of fundamental phenomena such as macro- and microorganisms' survival mechanisms [151]. For example, bacteria, uni- or multicellular organisms, and sperm cells are able to sense and actively respond to external stimuli by the generation of movement. In particular, they convert an external energy sources (temperature, magnetic fields, adhesion forces, chemical gradients) into mechanical work that induce migration. This is typical in processes such as thermotaxis, magnetotaxis, haptotaxis, chemotaxis [152]. By taking inspiration from nature, we have also now a panel of NPs able to self-propel towards a gradient of nutrients and to mimic biological taxis [153]. However, the development of such NPs still has many challenges because at nanoscale level, the physical principles of propulsion are different due to the presence of the Brownian effect that can interfere with nanomptors by collisions with solvent molecules. One of these challenges is the generation of particles having asymmetrical geometries at the nanoscale, as this provides guidance for the movement directionality. Bacteria like *Escherichia coli*, in fact, achieve propulsion by non-time-reversible motion of long flagella, and this asymmetric shape of the body is critical for motion generation in a specific direction [154].

It is clear that self-propelling NPs represent a new powerful tool in drug delivery, which is usually dominated by NPs passive diffusion. It should not come as a surprise that such strategies have been employed also for delivery in ocular medicine. For example, Wu et al. [155] designed micro-vehicles that can actively propel through the vitreous humor to enrich retina. The movement can be activated by helical magnetic micropropellers (~120 nm in diameter and ~400 nm in length) with liquid layer coating to reduce the adhesion of biopolymeric network. These nanovectors propelled in nanoporous hyaluronan solution, a fluid mimicking the vitreous. The inspiration for nanotool development is due to the liquid layer that characterizes carnivorous *Nepenthes* pitcher plant, which presents a slippery surface on the peristome to catch insects [156,157]. Porcine eyes were used as a model of human eyes:

applying the external magnetic field, micropropellers exhibited controllable propulsion from eyeball to retina within 30 minutes. Instead, passive silica microparticles did not penetrate the vitreous (Figure 7). Nanorobots were also used to perform microsurgery on the retina and surrounding membranes thanks to the possibility of injecting them elsewhere in the body and bringing the drug to the target eye region [158]. Some intravitreal implants have recently developed to perform more clinical-inspired experiments. These nanotools, constituted by polymeric containers (silicon, poly(vinyl alcohol), or ethylene vinyl acetate), were placed in the posterior segment of the eye and they are permeable to lipophilic drugs. They did not display any toxicity and had a long retention time. These nanosystems have been extremely useful to treat proliferative diabetic retinopathy, retinal vascular occlusion, and uveitis [159].

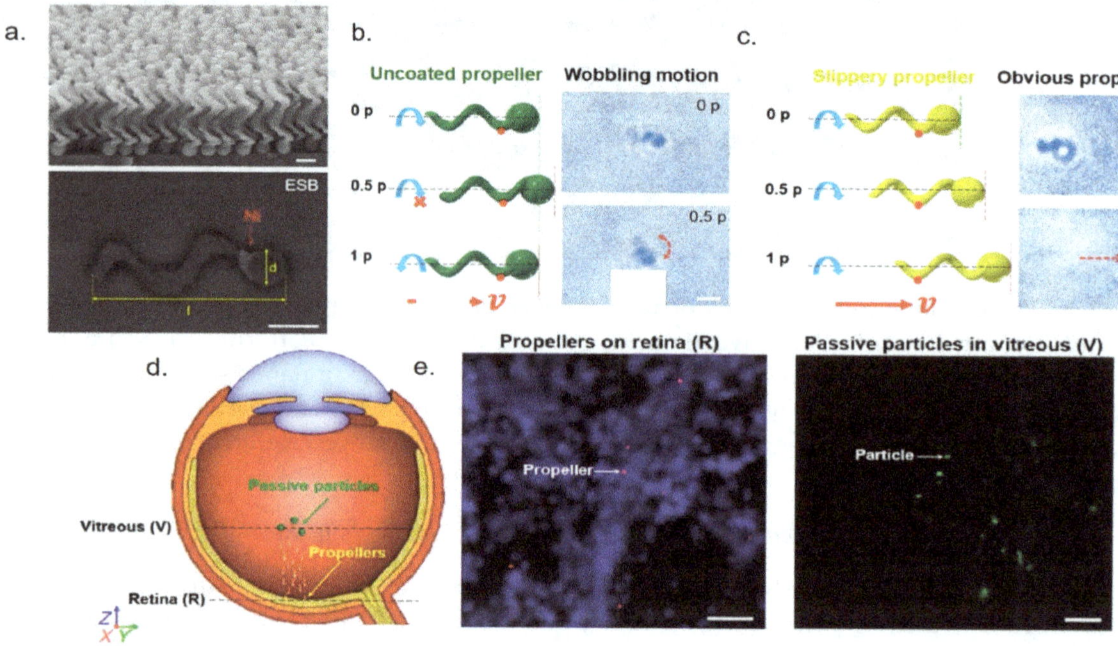

Figure 7. (**a**) SEM and ESB-SEM images of the micropropellers. (**b**,**c**) incomplete rotation of an uncoated micropropeller for one period (p) in the vitreous was showed in schematic and time-lapse microscopy, whereas the coated propeller exhibited propulsion under magnetic stimuli in vitreous for 1.5 s (nine periods). Red arrows showed the propulsion direction of propeller. The original position of nanotools and after the rotating magnetic field application were showed with green and red dashed lines. Scale bars, 1 μm. (**d**) Schematic illustration of micropropeller movement in the vitreous. (**e**) Left: fluorescent acquisitions showed the micropropellers labelled red on retina. Right: passive fluorescent particles were accumulated near center of vitreous. Nuclei of cells were stained with DAPI. Scale bar, 20 μm. Adapted from reference [155] under the terms of the Creative Commons Attribution-Non Commercial license.

6. Conclusions and Perspectives

It is established that eye damage is a leading cause of irreversible vision loss resulting from ocular diseases. The current standard treatments helped in both preventing and curing several pathological conditions, especially when related to the deep sections of the eye. However, many of these methods are rather invasive in terms of procedures, with a consequent possibility of promoting infection, inflammation, or even retinal detachment with potential risk of vision loss. These limitations impose considerable costs on patient quality of life and have an enormous economic impact on the health care system. The progress in the nano-engineering field can help boosting the discovery of a new approach for ocular diagnosis and therapy. Noble metals NPs and bio-inspired NPs represent a powerful tool to overcome all the limitations coming with standard treatments due to their physico-chemical properties. NPs can in fact penetrate deeper inside the ocular segments and also locally deliver high dosages of drugs, enriching local drug concentration when applied topically. In addition, the plasmonic properties of Au and Ag can have an added value to contrast eye diseases. However, numerous challenges still remain to be addressed as there are still limited numbers of in vivo studies. In addition, a deeper toxicology assessment is required for the development of new systems for ocular treatments.

Author Contributions: Conceptualization, V.D.M.; writing—original draft preparation, V.D.M.; review and editing, L.R. All authors have read and agreed to the published version of the manuscript.

Acknowledgments: VDM kindly acknowledges Programma Operativo Nazionale (PON) Ricerca e Innovazione 2014-2020 Asse I "Capitale Umano", Azione I.2, Avviso "A.I.M: Attraction and International Mobility" CUP F88D18000070001.

References

1. Davson, H. *The Physiology of The Eye*; Elsevier: Amsterdam, The Netherlands, 2012.
2. Stephen, R.; Wilkinson, C.; Schachat, A.; Hinton, D.; Wilkinson, C. *Retina*; Elsevier: Amsterdam, The Netherlands, 2012.
3. Günhan, E.; van der List, D.; Chalupa, L.M. Ectopic Photoreceptors and Cone Bipolar Cells in the Developing and Mature Retina. *J. Neurosci.* **2003**, *15*, 1383–1389. [CrossRef]
4. Reichenbach, A.; Schnitzer, J.; Friedrich, A.; Brückner, G.; Schober, W. Development of the rabbit retina. *Anat. Embryol.* **1991**, *183*, 287–297. [CrossRef] [PubMed]
5. Dilnawaz, F.S.S.K. Nanotechnology-Based Ophthalmic Drug Delivery System. In *Focal Controlled Drug Delivery*; Domb, A., Khan, W., Eds.; Advances in Delivery Science and Technology; Springer: Boston, MA, USA, 2014.
6. Rakhi Dandonaa, L.D. Socioeconomic status and blindness. *Br. J. Ophthalmol.* **2001**, *85*, 1484–1488. [CrossRef] [PubMed]
7. Yorston, D. The Retina Retinal Diseases and VISION 2020. *Comm Eye Health* **2003**, *16*, 19–20.
8. Veleri, S.; Lazar, C.H.; Chang, B.; Sieving, P.A.; Banin, E.; Swaroop, A. Biology and therapy of inherited retinal degenerative disease: insights from mouse models. *Dis. Models Mech.* **2015**, *8*, 109–129. [CrossRef] [PubMed]
9. Jiang, S.; Franco, Y.L.; Zhou, Y.; Chen, J. Nanotechnology in retinal drug delivery. *Int. J. Ophthalmol.* **2018**, *11*. [CrossRef]
10. Gilbert, C.; Foster, A. Childhood blindness in the context of VISION 2020—The Right to Sight. *Bull. World Health Organ.* **2001**, *79*, 227–232.
11. Jones, B.W.; Marc, R.E.; Pfeiffer, R.L. Retinal Degeneration, Remodeling and Plasticity. In *Webvision: The Organization of the Retina and Visual System*; Salt Lake City (UT): University of Utah Health Sciences Center, UT, USA, 2016.
12. Rajappa, M.; Saxena, P.K.J. Ocular angiogenesis: Mechanisms and recent advances in therapy. *Adv. Clin. Chem.* **2010**, *50*, 103–121.
13. Aiello, L.P.; Avery, R.L.; Arrigg, P.G.; Keyt, B.A.; Jampel, H.D.; Shah, S.T.; Pasquale, L.R.; Thieme, H.; Iwamoto, M.A.; Park, J.E.; et al. Vascular endothelial growth factor in ocular fluid of patients with diabetic retinopa-thy and other retinal disorders. *N. Engl. J. Med.* **1994**, *331*, 480–1487. [CrossRef]
14. Weis, S.M.; Cheresh, D.A. Pathophysiological consequences of VEGF-induced vascular permeability. *Nature* **2005**, *437*, 497–504. [CrossRef]
15. Kim, S.J. Novel Approaches for Retinal Drug and Gene Delivery. *Transl. Vis. Sci. Technol.* **2014**, *3*, 7. [CrossRef] [PubMed]
16. Bennett, J.; Chung, D.C.; Maguire, A. Gene delivery to the retina: From mouse to man. *Methods Enzym.* **2012**, *507*, 255–257.
17. Xu, H.; Chen, M. Targeting the complement system for the management of retinal in fl ammatory and degenerative diseases. *Eur. J. Pharmacol.* **2016**, *787*, 94–104. [CrossRef] [PubMed]
18. Díaz-Coránguez, M.; Ramos, C.; Antonetti, D.A. The inner Blood-Retinal Barrier: Cellular Basis and Development. *Vis. Res.* **2017**, *139*, 123–137. [CrossRef]

19. Gaudana, R.; Jwala, J.; Boddu, S.H.S.; Mitra, A.K. Recent Perspectives in Ocular Drug Delivery. *Pharm. Res.* **2009**, *26*, 1197–1216. [CrossRef]
20. Kati-Sisko, V.; Hellinen, L. Expression, activity and pharmacokinetic impact of ocular transporters. *Adv. Drug Deliv. Rev.* **2018**, *126*, 3–22.
21. Souto, E.B.; Dias-ferreira, J.; Ana, L.; Ettcheto, M.; Elena, S. Advanced Formulation Approaches for Ocular Drug Delivery: State-Of-The-Art and Recent Patents. *Pharmaceutics* **2019**, *11*, 460. [CrossRef]
22. Le Bourlais, C.; Acar, L.; Zia, H.; Sado, P.A.; Needham, T.; Leverge, R. Ophthalmic drug delivery systems—Recent advances. *Prog. Retin. Eye Res.* **1998**, *17*, 33–58. [CrossRef]
23. Sugrue, M.F. The pharmacology of antiglaucoma drugs. *Pharmacol. Ther.* **1989**, *43*, 91–1989. [CrossRef]
24. Himawan, E.; Ekström, P.; Buzgo, M.; Gaillard, P.; Stefánsson, E.; Marigo, V.; Loftsson, T.; Paquet-Durand, F. Drug delivery to retinal photoreceptors. *Drug Discov. Today* **2019**, *24*, 1637–1643. [CrossRef]
25. Marmor, M.F.; Akira Negi, D.M.M. Kinetics of macromolecules injected into the subretinal space. *Exp. Eye Res.* **1985**, *40*, 687–696. [CrossRef]
26. Meyer, C.H.; Krohne, T.U.; Issa, P.C.; Liu, Z. Routes for Drug Delivery to the Eye and Retina: Intravitreal Injections. *Retin. Pharmacother. Dev. Ophthalmol.* **2016**, *55*, 63–70.
27. Falavarjani, K.G.; Nguyen, Q.D. Adverse events and complications associated with intravitreal injection of anti-VEGF agents: A review of literature. *Eye* **2013**, *27*, 787–794. [CrossRef] [PubMed]
28. Raghava, S.; Hammond, M.K.U. Periocular routes for retinal drug delivery. *Expert Opin. Drug Deliv.* **2004**, *1*, 99–144. [CrossRef]
29. Ghate, D.; Brooks, W.; McCarey, B.E.; Edelhauser, H.F. Pharmacokinetics of Intraocular Drug Delivery by Periocular Injections Using Ocular Fluorophotometry. *Invest. Ophthalmol Vis. Sci.* **2007**, *48*, 2230–2237. [CrossRef] [PubMed]
30. Castellarinand, A.; Pieramici, D.J. Anterior segment complications following periocular and intraocular injections. *Ophthalmol. Clin. N. Am.* **2004**, *17*, 583–590. [CrossRef]
31. Tsai, H.-H.; Wang, P.-Y.; Lin, I.-C.; Huang, H.; Liu, G.; Tseng, C.-L. Ocular Drug Delivery: Role of Degradable Polymeric Nanocarriers for Ophthalmic Application. *Int. J. Mol. Sci.* **2018**, *19*, 2830. [CrossRef]
32. ISO, Int. Organ Stand Nanotechnologies Vocab Part 1 Core Terms ISO/TS 80004-12010. 2010. Available online: https://www.iso.org/standard/51240.html (accessed on 1 March 2020).
33. ISO International Organization for Standardization. *Technical Specification: Nanotechnologies Terminology and Definitions for Nanoobjects Nanoparticle, Nanofibre and Nanoplate*. ISO/TS 80004-2:2008. 2008. Available online: https://www.iso.org/standard/44278.html (accessed on 1 March 2020).
34. De Matteis, V.; Rinaldi, R. Toxicity Assessment in the Nanoparticle Era. In *Cellular and Molecular Toxicology of Nanoparticles*; Springer: Cham, Switzerland, 2018; pp. 1–19.
35. Mu, Q.; Jiang, G.; Chen, L.; Zhou, H.; Fourches, D.; Tropsha, A.; Yan, B. Chemical Basis of Interactions Between Engineered Nanoparticles and Biological Systems. *Chem. Rev.* **2016**, 7740–7781. [CrossRef]
36. Bhatia, S. Nanoparticles Types, Classification, Characterization, Fabrication Methods and Drug Delivery Applications. In *Natural Polymer Drug Delivery Systems*; Springer: Cham, Switzerland, 2016.
37. Ruth Duncan, R.G. Nanomedicine(s) under the Microscope. *Mol. Pharm.* **2011**, *8*, 2101–2214. [CrossRef]
38. Diebold, Y.; Calonge, M. Applications of nanoparticles in ophthalmology. *Prog. Retin. Eye Res.* **2010**, *29*, 596–609. [CrossRef]
39. Farjo, K.M.; Ma, J. The potential of nanomedicine therapies to treat neovascular disease in the retina. *J. Angiogenes Res.* **2010**, *2*, 21. [CrossRef] [PubMed]
40. JeffreyAdijanto, M.I.N. Nanoparticle-based technologies for retinal gene therapy. *Eur. J. Pharm. Biopharm.* **2015**, *95*, 353–367.
41. Soto, F.; Chrostowski, R.; Soto, F. Frontiers of Medical Micro/Nanorobotics: In vivo Applications and Commercialization Perspectives Toward Clinical Uses. *Front. Bioeng. Biotechnol.* **2018**, *6*, 1–12. [CrossRef]
42. Khlebtsovab, N.G.; Dykman, L.A. Optical properties and biomedical applications of plasmonic nanoparticles. *J. Quant. Spectrosc. Radiat. Transf.* **2010**, *111*, 1–35. [CrossRef]
43. Anker, J.N.; Hall, W.P.; Lyandres, O.; Shah, N.C.; Zhao, J.V. Biosensing with plasmonic nanosensors. *Nat. Mater.* **2008**, *7*, 442–453. [CrossRef] [PubMed]
44. Daniel, M.; Astruc, D. Gold Nanoparticles: Assembly, Supramolecular Chemistry, Quantum-Size-Related Properties, and Applications toward Biology, Catalysis, and Nanotechnology. *Chem. Rev.* **2004**, *104*, 293–346. [CrossRef]

45. Asahi, T.; Uwada, T.; Masuhara, H. Single particle spectroscopic study on surface plasmon resonance probing local environmental conditions. *Handai Nanophotonics* **2006**, *2*, 219–228.
46. Boken, J.; Khurana, P.; Thatai, S. Plasmonic nanoparticles and their analytical applications: A review. *Appl. Spectrosc. Rev.* **2017**, *52*, 774–820. [CrossRef]
47. Loiseau, A.; Asila, V.; Boitel-aullen, G.; Lam, M. Silver-Based Plasmonic Nanoparticles for and Their Use in Biosensing. *Biosens* **2019**, *2019*, 9. [CrossRef]
48. Rizzello, L.; Pompa, P.P. Nanosilver-based antibacterial drugs and devices: Mechanisms, methodological drawbacks, and guidelines. *Chem. Soc. Rev.* **2014**, *43*, 1501–1518. [CrossRef]
49. Draslera, B.; Sayreb, P.; Günter, K.; Steinhäuserc, A.-R. In vitro approaches to assess the hazard of nanomaterials. *NanoImpact* **2018**, *9*, 51. [CrossRef]
50. De Matteis, V. Exposure to Inorganic Nanoparticles: Routes of Entry, Immune Response, Biodistribution and In Vitro/In Vivo Toxicity Evaluation. *Toxics* **2017**, *5*, 29. [CrossRef] [PubMed]
51. Naahidi, S.; Jafari, M.; Edalat, F.; Raymond, K.; Khademhosseini, A.C.P. Biocompatibility of engineered nanoparticles for drug delivery. *J. Control. Release* **2013**, *10*, 182–194. [CrossRef] [PubMed]
52. Turkevich, J.; Stevenson, P.C.; Hillier, J. A study of the nucleation and growth processes in the synthesis of colloidal gold. *Faraday Soc.* **1951**, *11*, 55–75. [CrossRef]
53. Brust, M.; Walker, M.; Bethell, D.; Schiffrin, D.J. Synthesis of thiol-derivatised gold nanoparticles in a two-phaseliquid–liquid system. *J. Chem. Soc. Chem. Commun.* **1994**, *7*, 801–802. [CrossRef]
54. Kumar, P.V.; Kala, S.M.J.; Prakash, K.S. Green synthesis of gold nanoparticles using Croton Caudatus Geisel leaf extract and their biological studies. *Mater. Lett.* **2019**, *236*, 19–22. [CrossRef]
55. Molnár, Z.; Bódai, V.; Szakacs, G.; Erdélyi, B.; Fogarassy, Z. Green synthesis of gold nanoparticles by thermophilic filamentous fungi. *Sci. Rep.* **2018**, *8*, 1–12. [CrossRef]
56. Giljohann, D.A.; Seferos, D.S.; Daniel, W.L.; Massich, M.D.; Patel, P.C. Gold Nanoparticles for Biology and Medicine. *Angew. Chem. Int. Ed. Engl.* **2010**, *26*, 3280–3294. [CrossRef]
57. Orlando, A.; Colombo, M.; Prosperi, D.; Corsi, F.; Panariti, A.; Rivolta, I.; Masserini, M.; Cazzinga, E. Evaluation of gold nanoparticles biocompatibility: A multiparametric study on cultured endothelial cells and macrophages. *J. Nanopart. Res.* **2018**, *18*, 58. [CrossRef]
58. Aghaie, T.; Jazayeri, M.H.; Manian, M.; Khani, l.; Erfani, M.; Rezayi, M.; Ferns, G.A.; Avan, A. Gold nanoparticle and polyethylene glycol in neural regeneration in the treatment of neurodegenerative diseases. *J. Cell. Biochem.* **2019**, *120*, 2749–2755. [CrossRef]
59. Bailly, A.-L.; Correard, F.; Popov, A.; Gleb Tselikov, F.; Appay, R.; Al-Kattan, A.; Andrei, V.; Kabashin, D.B.; Esteve, M.-A. In vivo evaluation of safety, biodistribution and pharmacokinetics of lasersynthesized gold nanoparticles. *Sci. Rep.* **2019**, *9*, 12890. [CrossRef] [PubMed]
60. Cassano, D.; Summa, M.; Pocoví-Martínez, S.; Mapanao, A.-K.; Catelani, T.; Bertorelli, R.; Voliani, V. Biodegradable Ultrasmall-in-Nano Gold Architectures: Mid-Period In Vivo Distribution and Excretion Assessment. *Part. Part. Syst. Charact.* **2019**, *36*, 1800464. [CrossRef]
61. Khan, H.A.; Abdelhalim, M.A.K.; Alhomida, A.S.; Al-Ayed, M.S. Effects of Naked Gold Nanoparticles on Proinflammatory Cytokines mRNA Expression in Rat Liver and Kidney. *Biomed. Res. Int.* **2013**, *2013*, 590730. [CrossRef] [PubMed]
62. Khan, H.A.; Alamery, S.; Ibrahim, K.E.; El-Nagar, D.M.; Al-Harbi, N.; Rusop, M.; Alrokayan, S.H. Size and time-dependent induction of proinflammatory cytokines expression in brains of mice treated with gold nanoparticle. *Saudi J. Biol. Sci.* **2019**, *26*. [CrossRef]
63. Karakoçak, B.B.; Raliya, R.; Davis, J.T.; Chavalmane, S.; Wang, W.N.; Ravi, N. Biocompatibility of gold nanoparticles in retinal pigment epithelial cell line. *Toxicol. Vitr.* **2016**, *37*, 61–69. [CrossRef]
64. Kim, J.H.; Kim, J.H.; Kim, K.-W.; Kim, M.H. Intravenously administered gold nanoparticles pass through the blood–retinal barrier depending on the particle size, and induce no retinal toxicity. *Nanotechnology* **2009**, *20*, 505101. [CrossRef]
65. Bakri, S.J.; Pulido, J.S.; Mukherjee, P.; Marler, R.J. Absence of histologic retinal toxicity of intravitreal nanogold in a rabbit model. *Retin* **2008**, *2008*, 147–149. [CrossRef]
66. Söderstjerna, E.; Bauer, P.; Cedervall, T.; Abdshill, H.; Johansson, F.; Johansson, U.E. Silver and Gold Nanoparticles Exposure to In Vitro Cultured Retina—Studies on Nanoparticle Internalization, Apoptosis, Oxidative Stress, Glial- and Microglial Activity. *PLoS ONE* **2014**, *9*, e0105359. [CrossRef]
67. Nakhlband, A. Impacts of nanomedicines in ocular pharmacotherapy. *Bioimpacts* **2011**, *1*, 7–22.

68. Kittler, S.; Greulich Diendorf, M.; Köller, M.E. Toxicity of Silver Nanoparticles Increases during Storage Because of Slow Dissolution under Release of Silver Ions. *Chem. Mater.* **2010**, *22*, 4548–4554. [CrossRef]
69. Yang, X.; Gondikas, A.P.; Marinakos, S.M.; Auffan, M.; Li, J.; Hsu-Kim, H. Mechanism of Silver Nanoparticle Toxicity Is Dependent on Dissolved Silver and Surface Coating in Caenorhabditis elegans. *Environ. Sci. Technol.* **2012**, *46*, 1119–1127. [CrossRef] [PubMed]
70. De Matteis, V.; Malvindi, M.A.; Galeone, A.; Brunetti, V.; De Luca, E.; Kote, S.; Kshirsagar, P.; Sabella, S.; Bardi, G.; Pompa, P.P. Negligible particle-specific toxicity mechanism of silver nanoparticles: The role of Ag + ion release in the cytosol. Nanomedicine Nanotechnology. *Biol. Med.* **2015**, *11*, 731–739. [CrossRef] [PubMed]
71. Abbasi, E.; Milani, M.; Fekri Aval, S.; Kouhi, M.; Akbarzadeh, A.; Tayefi Nasrabadi, H.; Nikasa, P.; Joo, S.W.; Hanifehpour, Y.; Nejati-Koshki, K.; et al. Silver nanoparticles: Synthesis methods, bio- applications and properties. *Crit. Rev. Microbiol.* **2016**, *42*, 173–180. [CrossRef]
72. Zhang, T.; Song, Y.J.; Zhang, X.Y.; Wu, J.Y. Synthesis of silver nanostructures by multistep methods. *Sensors (Switzerland)* **2014**, *14*, 5860–5889. [CrossRef] [PubMed]
73. Singh, C.; Kumar, J.; Kumar, P.; Singh Chauhan, B.; Tiwari, K.N.; Mishra, S.K.; Srikrishna, S.; Saini, R.; Nath, G.; Singth, J. Green synthesis of silver nanoparticles using aqueous leaf extract of *Premna integrifolia* (L.) rich in polyphenols and evaluation of their antioxidant, antibacterial and cytotoxic activity. *Biotechnol. Biotechnol. Equip.* **2019**, 359–371. [CrossRef]
74. Jun, Y.; Zi, Z.; Wanga, Y.; Zhaoa, G.; Liu, J.-X. Silver nanoparticles affect lens rather than retina development in zebrafish embryos. *Ecotoxicol. Environ. Saf.* **2018**, *163*, 279–288.
75. Sriram, M.I.; Kalishwaralal, K.; Barathmanikanth, S. Size-based cytotoxicity of silver nanoparticles in bovine retinal endothelial cells. *Nanosci. Methods* **2012**, *1*, 56–77. [CrossRef]
76. Kim, J.S.; Song, K.S.; Sung, J.H.; Ryu, H.R.; Choi, B.G.; Cho, H.S.; Lee, J.K. Genotoxicity, acute oral and dermal toxicity, eye and dermal irritation and corrosion and skin sensitisation evaluation of silver nanoparticles. *Nanotoxicology* **2013**, *7*, 953. [CrossRef]
77. Maneewattanapinyo, P.; Banlunara, W.; Thammacharoen, C.; Ekgasit, S.; Kaewamatawong, T. An evaluation of acute toxicity of colloidal silver nanoparticles. *J. Vet. Med. Sci.* **2011**, *73*, 1417–1423. [CrossRef]
78. De Matteis, V.; Cascione, M.; Cristina, C.; Rinaldi, R. Engineered Gold Nanoshells Killing Tumor Cells: New Perspectives. *Curr. Pharm. Des.* **2019**, *25*, 1477–1489. [CrossRef]
79. Weissleder, R. A clearer vision for in vivo imaging. *Nat. Biotechnol.* **2001**, *19*, 316–317. [CrossRef] [PubMed]
80. Song, H.B.; Wi, J.S.; Jo, D.H.; Kim, J.H.; Lee, S.W. Intraocular application of gold nanodisks optically tuned for optical coherence tomography: inhibitory effect on retinal neovascularization without unbearable toxicity. *Nanomedicine* **2017**, *13*, 1901–1911. [CrossRef] [PubMed]
81. Gasparini, S.J.; Llonch, S.; Borsch, O. Transplantation of photoreceptors into the degenerative retina: Current state and future perspectives. *Prog. Retin. Eye Res.* **2019**, *69*, 1–37. [CrossRef]
82. Chemla, Y.; Betzer, O.; Markus, A.; Farah, N.; Motiei, M. Gold nanoparticles for multimodal high-resolution imaging of transplanted cells for retinal replacement therapy. *Nanomedicine* **2019**, *14*, 1857–1871. [CrossRef]
83. Kim, H.; Nguyen, V.; Manivasagan, P.; Kim, S.W.; Oh, J. Doxorubicin-fucoidan-gold nanoparticles composite for dualchemo-photothermal treatment on eye tumors. *Oncotarget* **2017**, *8*, 113719–113733. [CrossRef] [PubMed]
84. Valluru, K.S.; Chinni, B.K.; Rao, N.A.; Bhatt, S.; Dogra, V.S. Basics and Clinical Applications of Photoacoustic Imaging. *Ultrasound Clin.* **2009**, *4*, 403–429. [CrossRef]
85. Gordon, A.Y.; Lapierre-Landry, M.; Skala, M.C.; Penn, J.S. Photothermal Optical Coherence Tomography of AntiAngiogenic Treatment in the Mouse Retina Using Gold Nanorods as Contrast Agents. *Transl. Vis. Sci. Technol.* **2019**, *8*, 18. [CrossRef] [PubMed]
86. Chan, C.-M.; Hsiao, C.-Y.; Li, H.-J.; Fang, J.-Y.; Chang, D.-C.; Hung, C.-F. The Inhibitory Effects of Gold Nanoparticles on VEGF-A-Induced Cell Migration in Choroid-Retina Endothelial Cells. *Int. J. Mol. Sci.* **2020**, *21*, 109. [CrossRef]
87. Gurunathanab, S.; Leeb, K.; Kalishwaralala, K.; Sheikpranbabua, S.; Vaidyanathana, R.; Eom, S.H. Antiangiogenic properties of silver nanoparticles. *Biomaterials* **2009**, *30*, 6341–6350. [CrossRef]
88. Sheikpranbabu, S.; Kalishwaralal, K.; Venkataraman, D.; Eom, S.H.; Park, J.; Gurunathan, S. Silver nanoparticles inhibit VEGF-and IL-1β-induced vascular permeability via Src dependent pathway in porcine retinal endothelial cells. *Nanobiotechnol.* **2009**, *7*, 8. [CrossRef]

89. Ngandeu Neubi, G.M.; Opoku-Damoah, Y.; Gu, X.; Han, Y.; Zhou, J.; Ding, Y. Bio-inspired drug delivery systems: an emerging platform for targeted cancer therapy. *Biomater. Sci.* **2018**, *6*, 958–973. [CrossRef] [PubMed]
90. Yang, L.; Kuang, H.; Zhang, W.; Aguilar, Z.P.; Wei, H.; Xu, H. Comparisons of the biodistribution and toxicological examinations after repeated intravenous administration of silver and gold nanoparticles in mice. *Sci. Rep.* **2017**, *7*, 3303. [CrossRef] [PubMed]
91. Madamsetty, V.S.; Mukherjee, A.; Mukherjee, S. Recent Trends of the Bio-Inspired Nanoparticles in Cancer Theranostics. *Front. Pharmacol.* **2019**, *10*, 1264. [CrossRef] [PubMed]
92. Birngruber, T.; Raml, R.; Gladdines, W.; Gatschelhofer, C.; Gander, E.; Ghosh, A.; Kroath, T.; Gaillard, P.J.; Pieber, T.R. Enhanced Doxorubicin Delivery to the Brain Administered Through Glutathione PEGylated Liposomal Doxorubicin (2B3-101) as Compared with Generic Caelyx,®/Doxil®—A Cerebral Open Flow Microperfusion Pilot Study. *J. Pharm. Sci.* **2014**, *203*, 1945–1948. [CrossRef]
93. Trost, A.; Lange, S.; Schroedl, F.; Bruckner, D.; Motloch, K.A.; Bogner, B.; Kaser-Eichberger, A.; Strohmaier, C.; Runge, C.; Aigner, L.; et al. Brain and Retinal Pericytes: Origin, Function and Role. *Front. Cell Neurosci.* **2016**, *4*, 20. [CrossRef] [PubMed]
94. Haque, S.; Shadab, M.D.; Alam, I.; Sahni, J.K.; Ali, J. Nanostructure-based drug delivery systems for brain targeting. *Drug Dev. Ind. Pharm.* **2012**, *38*, 387–411. [CrossRef] [PubMed]
95. Diebold, Y.; Jarrín, M.; Sáez, V.; Carvalho, E.L.; Orea, M.; Calonge, M.; Seijo, B. Ocular drug delivery by liposome-chitosan nanoparticle complexes (LCS-NP). *Biomaterials* **2007**, *28*, 1553–1564. [CrossRef] [PubMed]
96. Zhang, R.; He, R.; Qian, J.; Guo, J.; Xue, K.; Yuan, Y. Immunology and Microbiology Treatment of Experimental Autoimmune Uveoretinitis with Intravitreal Injection of Tacrolimus (FK506) Encapsulated in Liposomes. *Investig. Ophthalmol. Vis. Sci.* **2010**, *51*, 3575–3582. [CrossRef] [PubMed]
97. Yan, J.; Zheng, M. Chrysophanol liposome preconditioning protects against cerebral ischemia–reperfusion injury by inhibiting oxidative stress and apoptosis in mice. *Int. J. Pharmacol.* **2014**, *10*, 55–68. [CrossRef]
98. Choi, Y.H. Berberine hydrochloride protects C_2C_{12} myoblast cells against oxidative stress-induced damage via induction of Nrf-2-mediated HO-1 expression. *Drug Dev. Res.* **2016**, *77*, 8. [CrossRef]
99. Lai, S.; Wei, Y.; Wu, Q.; Zhou, K.; Liu, T.; Zhang, Y.; Jiang, N.; Xiao, W.; Chen, J.; Liu, Q.; et al. Liposomes for efFective drug delivery to the ocular posterior chamber. *J. Nanobiotechnol.* **2019**, *17*, 64. [CrossRef] [PubMed]
100. Wolin, L.R.; Massopust, L.C. Characteristics of the ocular fundus in primates. *J. Anat.* **1967**, *101*, 693–699. [PubMed]
101. Wang, J.-L.; Liu, Y.-L.; Li, Y.; Dai, W.-B.; Guo, Z.-M.; Wang, Z.-H.; Zhang, Q. EphA2 targeted doxorubicin stealth liposomes as a therapy system for choroidal neovascularization in rats. *Ophthalmol. Vis. Sci.* **2012**, *53*, 7348. [CrossRef] [PubMed]
102. Ravar, F.; Saadat, E.; Gholami, M.; Dehghankelishadi, P.; Mahdavi, M.; Azami, S. Hyaluronic acid-coated liposomes for targeted delivery of paclitaxel, in-vitro characterization and in-vivo evaluation. *J. Control. Release* **2016**, *10*, 10–22. [CrossRef]
103. Lee, J.; Goh, U.; Lee, H.J.; Kim, J.; Jeong, M. Effective retinal penetration of lipophilic and lipid-conjugated hydrophilic agents delivered by engineered liposomes. *Mol. Pharm.* **2017**, *14*, 423–430. [CrossRef]
104. Hironaka, K.; Inokuchi, Y.; Fujisawa, T.; Shimazaki, H.; Akane, M.; Tozuka, Y.; Tsuruma, K.; Shimazawa, M.; Hara, H. Edaravone-loaded liposomes for retinal protection against oxidative stress-induced retinal damage. *Eur. J. Pharm. Biopharm.* **2011**, *79*, 119–125. [CrossRef]
105. Yamamoto, Y.; Kuwahara, T.; Watanabe, K. Antioxidant activity of 3-methyl-1-phenyl-2-pyrazolin-5-one. *Redox Rep.* **1996**, *2*, 333–338. [CrossRef]
106. Vighi, E.; Trifunović, D.; Veiga-Crespo, P.; Rentsch, A.; Hoffmann, D.; Sahaboglu, A.; Strasser, T.; Kulkarni, M.; Bertolotti, E.; van den Heuvel, A.; et al. Combination of cGMP analogue and drug delivery system provides functional protection in hereditary retinal degeneration. *Proc. Natl. Acad. Sci. USA* **2018**, *27*, E2997–E3006. [CrossRef]
107. Lucas, K.A.; Pitari, G.M.; Kazerounian, S.; Ruiz-Stewart, I.; Park, J.; Schulz, S.; Chepenik, K.P.; Waldman, S.A. Guanylyl cyclases and signaling by cyclic GMP. *Pharmacol. Rev.* **2000**, *52*, 375–414.
108. Farber, D.B.; Lolley, R.N. Cyclic guanosine monophosphate: Elevation in degenerating photoreceptor cells of the C3H mouse retina. *Science* **1974**, *186*, 449–451. [CrossRef]

109. Campbell, M.; Humphries, M.M.; Kiang, A.-S.; Nguyen, A.T.H.; Gobbo, O.L.; Tam, L.C.S.; Suzuki, M.; Hanrahan, F.; Ozaki, E.; Farrar, G.-J.; et al. Systemic low-molecular weight drug delivery to pre-selected neuronal regions. *EMBO Mol. Med.* **2011**, *3*, 235–245. [CrossRef]
110. Davis, B.M.; Normando, E.M.; Guo, L.; Turner, L.A.; Nizari, S. Topical Delivery of Avastin to the Posterior Segment of the Eye In Vivo Using Annexin A5-associated Liposomes. *Small* **2014**, *24*, 1575–1584. [CrossRef] [PubMed]
111. Platania, C.B.M.; Fisichella, V.; Fidilio, A.; Geraci, F.; Lazzara, F.; Leggio, G.M.; Salomone, S.; Drago, F.; Pignatello, R.; Caraci, F.; et al. Topical Ocular Delivery of TGF- β 1 to the Back of the Eye: Implications in Age-Related Neurodegenerative Diseases. *Int. J. Mol. Sci.* **2017**, *18*, 2076. [CrossRef] [PubMed]
112. Boulyjenkov, V.; Berg, K. *Gene Therapy: Promises, Problems and Prospects*; Genes Resist. to Dis.; Springer: Berlin/Heidelberg, Germany, 2000.
113. Ramamoorth, M.; Narvekar, A. Non viral vectors in gene therapy—An overview. *J. Clin. Diagn. Res.* **2015**, *9*, GE01. [CrossRef]
114. Das, K.G.; Ram, A.R. Niosome ad a novel drug delivery system: A review. *Appl. Pharm.* **2013**, *5*, 1–7.
115. Seleci, D.A.; Seleci, M.; Walter, J.G. Niosomes as Nanoparticular Drug Carriers: Fundamentals and Recent Applications. *J. Nanomat.* **2016**, *2016*, 13. [CrossRef]
116. Gallego, I.; Villate-Beitia, I.; Martínez-Navarrete, G.; Menéndez, M.; López-Méndez, T.; Soto-Sánchez, C.; Zárate, J.; Puras, G.; Fernández, E.; Pedraz, J.L. Non-viral vectors based on cationic niosomes and minicircle DNA technology enhance gene delivery efficiency for biomedical applications in retinal disorders. *Nanomedicine.* **2019**, *17*, 308–318. [CrossRef] [PubMed]
117. Mashal, M.; Attia, N.; Puras, G.; Martinez-Navarrete, G.; Fernandez, E.P. Retinal gene delivery enhancement by lycopene incorporation into cationic niosomes based on DOTMA and polysorbate 60. *J. Control. Release* **2017**, *254*, 55–64. [CrossRef]
118. Guinedi, A.S.; Mortada, N.D.; Mansour, S. Preparation and evaluation of reverse-phase evaporation and multilamellar niosomes as ophthalmic carriers of acetazolamide. *Int. J. Pharm.* **2005**, *306*, 71–82. [CrossRef]
119. Guglevaa, V.; Titevaa, S.; Rangelovb, S.; Momekova, D. Design and in vitro evaluation of doxycycline hyclate niosomes as a potential ocular delivery system. *Int. J. Pharm.* **2019**, *5*, 567. [CrossRef]
120. Cintia, S.; De Paivaa Rosa, M.; Corralesa Arturo, L.; Villarreala William, J.; De-Quan, F.; Lia Michael, E.; Sternb Stephen, C. Corticosteroid and doxycycline suppress MMP-9 and inflammatory cytokine expression, MAPK activation in the corneal epithelium in experimental dry eye. *Exp. Eye Res.* **2006**, *83*, 526–535.
121. Sapino, S.; Chirio, D.; Peira, E.; Abellán Rubio, E.; Brunella, V.; Jadhav, S.A.; Chindamo, G.; Gallarate, M. Ocular Drug Delivery: A Special Focus on the Thermosensitive Approach. *Nanomaterials (Basel)* **2019**, *9*, 884. [CrossRef] [PubMed]
122. Hoare, T.R.; Kohane, D.S. Hydrogels in drug delivery: Progress and challenges. *Polymer (Guildf)* **2008**, *49*, 1993–2007. [CrossRef]
123. Wang, K.; Han, Z. Injectable hydrogels for ophthalmic applications. *J. Control. Release* **2017**, *268*, 212–224. [CrossRef]
124. Ferreira, N.N.; Ferreira, L.M.B.; Cardoso, V.M.O.; Boni, F.I.; Souza, A.L.R.; Gremião, M.P.D. Recent advances in smart hydrogels for biomedical applications: From self-assembly to functional approaches. *Eur. Polym. J.* **2018**, *99*, 117–133. [CrossRef]
125. Elieh-Ali-Komi, D.; Hamblin, M.R. Chitin and Chitosan: Production and Application of Versatile Biomedical Nanomaterials. *Int. J. Adv. Res. (Indore)* **2016**, *4*, 411–427.
126. ValérieDodane, V.D. Pharmaceutical applications of chitosan. *Pharm. Sci. Technol. Today* **1998**, *1*, 246–253.
127. Lee, K.Y.; Mooney, D.J. Alginate: Properties and biomedical applications. *Prog. Polym. Sci.* **2012**, *37*, 106–126. [CrossRef]
128. Paliwal, R.; Paliwal, S.R.; Sulakhiya, K.; Kurmi, B.D.; Kenwat, R.; Mamgain, A. *Chitosan-Based Nanocarriers for Ophthalmic Applications*; Elsevier: Amsterdam, The Netherlands, 2019.
129. Nagarwal, R.C.; Kumar, R. Chitosan coated sodium alginate-chitosan nanoparticles loaded with 5-FU for ocular delivery: in vitro characterization and in vivo study in rabbit eye. *Eur. J. Pharm. Sci.* **2012**, *20*, 678–685. [CrossRef]
130. Ameeduzzafar Imam, S.S.; Abbas Bukhari, S.N.; Ahmad, J. Formulation and optimization of levofloxacin loaded chitosan nanoparticle for ocular delivery: In-vitro characterization, ocular tolerance and antibacterial activity. *Int. J. Biol. Macromol.* **2018**, *108*, 650–659. [CrossRef]

131. Andrei, G.; Peptu, C.A.; Popa, M.; Desbrieres, J.; Peptu, C.; Gardikiotis, F.; Costuleanu, M.; Costin, D.; Dupin, J.C.; Uhart, A. Formulation and evaluation of cefuroxim loaded submicron particles for ophthalmic delivery. *Int. J. Pharm.* **2015**, *30*, 16–29. [CrossRef]
132. Kaskoos, R. Investigation of moxifloxacin loaded chitosan-dextran nanoparticles for topical instillation into eye: In-vitro and ex-vivo evaluation. *Int. J. Pharm. Investig.* **2014**, *4*, 164–173. [CrossRef] [PubMed]
133. Solanki, A.; Smalling, R.; Parola, A.H.; Nathan, I.; Kasher, R.; Pathak, Y.; Sutariya, V. Humanin Nanoparticles for Reducing Pathological Factors Characteristic of Age-related Macular Degeneration. *Curr. Drug Deliv.* **2019**, *16*, 226–232. [CrossRef]
134. Cohen, A.; Lerner-Yardeni, J.; Meridor, D.; Kasher, R.; Nathan, I.; Parola, A. Humanin derivatives inhibit necrotic cell death in neurons. *Mol. Med.* **2015**, *21*, 505. [CrossRef] [PubMed]
135. Cheng, Y.; Ko, Y.; Chang, Y.; Huang, S. Thermosensitive chitosan-gelatin-based hydrogel containing curcumin-loaded nanoparticles and latanoprost as a dual-drug delivery system for glaucoma treatment. *Exp. Eye Res.* **2019**, *179*, 179–187. [CrossRef] [PubMed]
136. Radomska-leśniewska, D.M.; Osiecka-iwan, A.; Hyc, A.; Góźdź, A.; Dąbrowska, A.M.; Skopiński, P. Therapeutic potential of curcumin in eye diseases. *Cent. Eur. J. Immunol.* **2019**, *44*, 2–4. [CrossRef] [PubMed]
137. Nathan Gooch, S.A.M.; Condie, R.; Michael, B.R.; Bonnie Archer, B.K.A.; Ocular, B. Drug Delivery for Glaucoma Management. *Pharmaceutics* **2012**, *4*, 197–211. [CrossRef]
138. Michael, P.; Fautsch, D.H.J. Aqueous Humor Outflow: What Do We Know? Where Will It Lead Us? *Investig. Ophthalmol. Vis. Sci.* **2006**, *47*, 4181–4187.
139. Silva, B.; Marto, J.; Braz, B.S.; Delgado, E.; Almeida, A.J.; Gonçalves, L. New nanoparticles for topical ocular delivery of erythropoietin. *Int. J. Pharm.* **2020**, 119020. [CrossRef]
140. Pandit, J.; Sultana, Y.; Aqil, M. Chitosan-coated PLGA nanoparticles of bevacizumab as novel drug delivery to target retina: optimization, characterization, and in vitro toxicity evaluation. *Artif. Cells Nanomed. Biotechnol.* **2016**, *45*, 1397–1407. [CrossRef]
141. Mitra, R.N.; Han, Z.; Merwin, M.; Taai, M.; Al Conley, S.M. Synthesis and Characterization of Glycol Chitosan DNA Nanoparticles for Retinal Gene Delivery. *ChemMedChem* **2014**, *9*, 189–196. [CrossRef]
142. Lee, J.-H.; Kim, H.-W. Emerging properties of hydrogels in tissue engineering. *J. Tissue Eng.* **2018**, *9*, 2041731418768285. [CrossRef] [PubMed]
143. Chang, D.; Kinam Park, A. Hydrogels for sustained delivery ofbiologics to the back of the eye. *Drug Discov. Today* **2019**, *24*, 1470–1482. [CrossRef] [PubMed]
144. Van Hovea, A.H.; Beltejar, M.G.; Benoit, D.S.W. Development and in vitro assessment of enzymatically-responsive poly(ethylene glycol) hydrogels for the delivery of therapeutic peptides. *Biomaterials* **2014**, *35*, 9719–9730. [CrossRef] [PubMed]
145. Drapala, P.W.; Jiang, B.; Chiu, Y.-C.; Mieler, W.F.; Brey, E.M. The Effect of Glutathione as Chain Transfer Agent in PNIPAAm-Based Thermo-responsive Hydrogels for Controlled Release of Proteins. *Pharm. Res.* **2014**, *31*, 742–753. [CrossRef] [PubMed]
146. Schultz, C.; Breaux, J.; Pharmd, J.S.; Douglas Morck, D.V.M. Drug delivery to the posterior segment of the eye through hydrogel contact lenses. *Clin. Exp. Optom.* **2011**, *94*, 212–218. [CrossRef]
147. Kabiri, M.; Kamal, S.H.; Pawar, S.V.; Roy, P.R.; Derakhshandeh, M.; Kumar, U.; Hatzikiriakos, S.G.; Hossain, S.; Yadav, V.G. A stimulus-responsive, in situ-forming, nanoparticle-laden hydrogel for ocular drug delivery. *Drug Deliv. Transl. Res.* **2018**, *8*, 484–495. [CrossRef]
148. Osswald, C.R.; Kang-Mieler, J.J. Controlled and Extended In Vitro Release of Bioactive Anti-Vascular Endothelial Growth Factors from a Microsphere-Hydrogel Drug Delivery System. *Curr. Eye Res.* **2016**, *41*, 1216–1222. [CrossRef]
149. Agrahari, V.; Agrahari, V.; Hung, W.-T.; Christenson, L.K. Composite Nanoformulation Therapeutics for Long-Term Ocular Delivery of Macromolecules. *Mol. Pharm.* **2016**, *13*, 2912–2922. [CrossRef]
150. Yang, H.; Tyagi, P.; Kadam, R.S.; Holden, C.A. Hybrid dendrimer hydrogel/PLGA nanoparticle platform sustains drug delivery for one week and antiglaucoma effects for four days following one-time topical administration. *ACS Nano* **2012**, *25*, 7595–7606. [CrossRef]
151. Wadhams, G.H.; Armitage, J.P. Making sense of it all: Bacterial chemotaxis. *Nat. Rev. Mol. Cell. Biol.* **2004**, *5*, 1024–1037. [CrossRef] [PubMed]
152. Micali, G.; Endres, R.G. Bacterial chemotaxis: information processing, thermodynamics, and behavior. *Curr. Opin. Microbiol.* **2016**, *30*, 8–15. [CrossRef] [PubMed]

153. Mei, Y.; Alexander, A. Solovev SS and OGS. Rolled-up nanotech on polymers: from basic perception to self-propelled catalytic microengines. *Chem. Soc. Rev.* **2011**, *40*, 2109–2119. [CrossRef] [PubMed]
154. Kumar, M.S.; Philominathan, P. The physics of flagellar motion of E. coli during chemotaxis. *Biophys. Rev.* **2010**, *2*, 13–20. [CrossRef] [PubMed]
155. Wu, Z.; Troll, J.; Jeong, H.-H.; Wei, Q.; Stang, M.; Ziemssen, F.; Wang, Z.; Dong, M.; Schnichels, S.; Qui, T.; et al. A swarm of slippery micropropellers penetrates the vitreous body of the eye. *Sci. Adv.* **2018**, *4*, eaat4388. [CrossRef] [PubMed]
156. Bohn, H.F.; Federle, W. Insect aquaplaning: Nepenthes pitcher plants capture prey with the peristome, a fully wettable water-lubricated anisotropic surface. *Proc. Natl. Acad. Sci. USA* **2004**, *101*, 14138–14143. [CrossRef]
157. Wong, T.-S.; Kang, S.H.; Tang, S.K.Y.; Smythe, E.J.; Hatton, B.D.; Grinthal, A. Bioinspired self-repairing slippery surfaces with pressure-stable omniphobicity. *Nature* **2011**, *477*, 443–447. [CrossRef]
158. Nistor, M.T.; Rusu, A.G. *Nanorobots with Applications in Medicine*; Elsevier: Amsterdam, The Netherlands, 2019.
159. Alhalafi, A.M. Applications of polymers in intraocular drug delivery systems. *Oman J. Ophtalmol.* **2017**, *10*, 3–8. [CrossRef]

Permissions

All chapters in this book were first published by MDPI; hereby published with permission under the Creative Commons Attribution License or equivalent. Every chapter published in this book has been scrutinized by our experts. Their significance has been extensively debated. The topics covered herein carry significant findings which will fuel the growth of the discipline. They may even be implemented as practical applications or may be referred to as a beginning point for another development.

The contributors of this book come from diverse backgrounds, making this book a truly international effort. This book will bring forth new frontiers with its revolutionizing research information and detailed analysis of the nascent developments around the world.

We would like to thank all the contributing authors for lending their expertise to make the book truly unique. They have played a crucial role in the development of this book. Without their invaluable contributions this book wouldn't have been possible. They have made vital efforts to compile up to date information on the varied aspects of this subject to make this book a valuable addition to the collection of many professionals and students.

This book was conceptualized with the vision of imparting up-to-date information and advanced data in this field. To ensure the same, a matchless editorial board was set up. Every individual on the board went through rigorous rounds of assessment to prove their worth. After which they invested a large part of their time researching and compiling the most relevant data for our readers.

The editorial board has been involved in producing this book since its inception. They have spent rigorous hours researching and exploring the diverse topics which have resulted in the successful publishing of this book. They have passed on their knowledge of decades through this book. To expedite this challenging task, the publisher supported the team at every step. A small team of assistant editors was also appointed to further simplify the editing procedure and attain best results for the readers.

Apart from the editorial board, the designing team has also invested a significant amount of their time in understanding the subject and creating the most relevant covers. They scrutinized every image to scout for the most suitable representation of the subject and create an appropriate cover for the book.

The publishing team has been an ardent support to the editorial, designing and production team. Their endless efforts to recruit the best for this project, has resulted in the accomplishment of this book. They are a veteran in the field of academics and their pool of knowledge is as vast as their experience in printing. Their expertise and guidance has proved useful at every step. Their uncompromising quality standards have made this book an exceptional effort. Their encouragement from time to time has been an inspiration for everyone.

The publisher and the editorial board hope that this book will prove to be a valuable piece of knowledge for researchers, students, practitioners and scholars across the globe.

List of Contributors

Yue Ruan, Subao Jiang and Adrian Gericke
Department of Ophthalmology, University Medical Center, Johannes Gutenberg University Mainz, Langenbeckstr. 1, 55131 Mainz, Germany

Tobias Böhmer
Department of Ophthalmology, University Medical Center, Johannes Gutenberg University Mainz, Langenbeckstr. 1, 55131 Mainz, Germany
St. Josef's Hospital Rheingau, Eibinger Str. 9, 65385 Rüdesheim am Rhein, Germany

Suet Lee Shirley Ding
Department of Biomedical Science, Faculty of Medicine and Health Sciences, University Putra Malaysia, 43400 UPM Serdang, Selangor, Malaysia

Suresh Kumar
Department of Medical Microbiology and Parasitology, Faculty of Medicine and Health Sciences, Universiti Putra Malaysia, 43400 UPM Serdang, Selangor, Malaysia
Genetics and Regenerative Medicine Research Centre, Universiti Putra Malaysia, 43400 UPM Serdang, Selangor, Malaysia

Pooi Ling Mok
Department of Biomedical Science, Faculty of Medicine and Health Sciences, University Putra Malaysia, 43400 UPM Serdang, Selangor, Malaysia
Genetics and Regenerative Medicine Research Centre, Universiti Putra Malaysia, 43400 UPM Serdang, Selangor, Malaysia

Emmanuelle Clérin and Thierry Léveillard
Department of Genetics, Sorbonne Université, INSERM, CNRS, Institut de la Vision, 17 rue Moreau, F-75012 Paris, France

Myriam Marussig
Sparing Vision, 55 rue de Lyon, 75012 Paris, France

José-Alain Sahel
Department of Genetics, Sorbonne Université, INSERM, CNRS, Institut de la Vision, 17 rue Moreau, F-75012 Paris, France
CHNO des Quinze-Vingts, DHU Sight Restore, INSERM-DGOS CIC 1423, 28 rue de Charenton, F-75012 Paris, France

Laura R. Bohrer, Luke A. Wiley, Erin R. Burnight, Jessica A. Cooke, Joseph C. Giacalone, Kristin R. Anfinson, Jeaneen L. Andorf, Robert F. Mullins, Edwin M. Stone and Budd A. Tucker
Institute for Vision Research, Department of Ophthalmology and Visual Sciences, University of Iowa, Iowa City, IA 52241, USA

Theodore G. Wensel
Verna and Marrs McLean Department of Biochemistry and Molecular Biology, Baylor College of Medicine, Houston, TX 77030, USA

Marta Zuzic, Jesus Eduardo Rojo Arias and Volker Busskamp
Center for Regenerative Therapies Dresden (CRTD), Technische Universitat Dresden, 01307 Dresden, Germany

Stefanie Gabriele Wohl
Department of Biological and Vision Sciences, The State University of New York, College of Optometry, New York, NY 10036, USA

Marci L. DeRamus, Stephanie J. Davis, Cyril Nyankerh, Delores Stacks, Timothy W. Kraft and Steven J. Pittler
Department of Optometry and Vision Science, Vision Science Research Center, University of Alabama at Birmingham, Birmingham, AL 35294, USA

Sriganesh Ramachandra Rao and Steven J. Fliesler
Departments of Ophthalmology and Biochemistry, State University of New York-University at Buffalo, Buffalo, NY 14209, USA

Siebren Faber and Ronald Roepman
Department of Human Genetics and Radboud Institute for Molecular Life Sciences, Radboud University Medical Center, Geert Grooteplein Zuid 10, 6525 GA Nijmegen, The Netherlands

Xiaoping Qi, Sayak K. Mitter, Maria B. Grant and Michael E. Boulton
Department of Ophthalmology and Visual Sciences, University of Alabama at Birmingham, AL 35294, USA

Yuanqing Yan
Department of Neurosurgery, The University of Texas Health Science Center, Houston, TX 77030, USA

Julia V. Busik
Department of Physiology, Michigan State University, East Lansing, MI 48824, USA

Dilara Hatipoglu, Alecia Cutler, Mariya Ali, Jian Hua Qi, Rupesh Singh, Julia Batoki and Laura Karle
Cole Eye Institute & Lerner Research Institute, Cleveland Clinic Foundation, Cleveland, OH 44195, USA

Alyson Wolk
Cole Eye Institute & Lerner Research Institute, Cleveland Clinic Foundation, Cleveland, OH 44195, USA
Cleveland Clinic Lerner College of Medicine, Department of Molecular Medicine, Case Western Reserve University, Cleveland, OH 44195, USA

Lestella Bell
Cole Eye Institute & Lerner Research Institute, Cleveland Clinic Foundation, Cleveland, OH 44195, USA
Cleveland Clinic Lerner College of Medicine at Case Western Reserve University, Department of Ophthalmology, Cleveland, OH 44195, USA

Vera L. Bonilha and Bela Anand-Apte
Cole Eye Institute & Lerner Research Institute, Cleveland Clinic Foundation, Cleveland, OH 44195, USA
Cleveland Clinic Lerner College of Medicine, Department of Molecular Medicine, Case Western Reserve University, Cleveland, OH 44195, USA
Cleveland Clinic Lerner College of Medicine at Case Western Reserve University, Department of Ophthalmology, Cleveland, OH 44195, USA

Oliver Wessely
Cleveland Clinic Lerner College of Medicine, Department of Molecular Medicine, Case Western Reserve University, Cleveland, OH 44195, USA
Department of Cardiovascular and Metabolic Sciences, Lerner Research Institute, Cleveland Clinic Foundation, Cleveland, OH 44195, USA

Heidi Stoehr
Institute of Human Genetics, University of Regensburg, 93053 Regensburg, Germany

Vincent Hascall
Department of Biomedical Engineering, Lerner Research Institute, Cleveland Clinic Foundation, Cleveland, OH 44195, USA

Irene Vázquez-Domínguez, Alejandro Garanto and Rob W. J. Collin
Department of Human Genetics and Donders Institute for Brain, Cognition and Behaviour, Radboud University Medical Center, 6525GA Nijmegen, The Netherlands

Valeria De Matteis
Department of Mathematics and Physics "Ennio De Giorgi", University of Salento, Via Arnesano, 73100 Lecce, Italy

Loris Rizzello
Department of Chemistry, University College London, 20 Gordon Street, London WC1H 0AJ, UK
Institute for Bioengineering of Catalonia (IBEC), The Barcelona Institute of Science and Technology, Baldiri Reixac 10-12, 08028 Barcelona, Spain
Department of Pharmaceutical Sciences, University of Milan, via Mangiagalli 25, 20133 Milano, Italy

Index

www.ingramcontent.com/pod-product-compliance
Lightning Source LLC
LaVergne TN
LVHW060532210926
848485LV00005B/1185